QUICK & EASY

MEDICAL
TERMINOLOGY

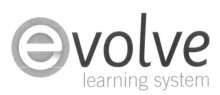
learning system

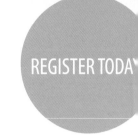
REGISTER TODAY

To Access your Evolve Free Resources visit:

http://evolve.elsevier.com/Leonard/quick

Register today and gain access to:

Student and Instructor

- Study Tips
- Electronic Flashcards
- Games
- Spanish Term Puzzles/Activities
- Audio Glossary
- Body Spectrum Coloring Book
- Glossary (English/Spanish)
- Weblinks

Instructor Only

- Image Collection
- Instructors Resource Material
- Examview Test Bank
- Power Point Lecture Slides with commentary
- TEACH Lesson Plan Manual
- Question Bank for each chapter
- Downloads section

ELSEVIER

QUICK & EASY
MEDICAL
TERMINOLOGY

Sixth Edition

Peggy C. Leonard, MT, MEd

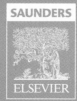

SAUNDERS

ELSEVIER

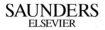

SAUNDERS
ELSEVIER

3251 Riverport Lane
Maryland Heights, MO 63043

Quick & Easy Medical Terminology   ISBN: 978-1-4377-0838-7
Copyright © 2011, 2007, 2003, 2000, 1995, 1990 by Saunders, an imprint of Elsevier Inc.

Notice

Neither the Publisher nor the Author assumes any responsibility for any loss or injury and/or damage to persons or property arising out of or related to any use of the material contained in this book. It is the responsibility of the treating practitioner, relying on independent expertise and knowledge of the patient, to determine the best treatment and method of application for the patient.

The Publisher

Library of Congress Publication Data
Leonard, Peggy C.
  Quick & easy medical terminology / Peggy C. Leonard.—6th ed.
    p. ; cm.
  Includes bibliographical references and index.
  ISBN 978-1-4377-0838-7 (pbk. : alk. paper)   1. Medicine—Terminology.   I. Title.   II. Title:
Quick and easy medical terminology.   III. Title: Medical terminology.
  [DNLM: 1. Terminology as Topic—Programmed Instruction.   W 18.2 L581q 2011]
  R123.L47 2011
  610.1′4—dc22

                                                                      2009045303

Publisher: Jeanne Olson
Associate Developmental Editor: Amy Whittier
Developmental Specialist: Carolyn Kruse
Publishing Services Manager: Patricia Tannian
Senior Project Manager: Sarah Wunderly
Senior Book Designer: Paula Catalano
Artist: Jeanne Robertson

Working together to grow
libraries in developing countries

www.elsevier.com | www.bookaid.org | www.sabre.org

ELSEVIER   BOOK AID International   Sabre Foundation

Printed in China

Last digit is the print number: 9 8 7 6 5 4 3 2

Reviewers

Jessica Alexander, RN, MSN
Assistant Professor
Mississippi University for Women
Columbus, Mississippi

Joseph Cipriani, EdD, OTR/L
Professor
Department of Occupational Therapy
Misericordia University
Dallas, Pennsylvania

Tammy S. Clossen, RDH, PhD
Assistant Professor
Dental Hygiene-Health Sciences
Pennsylvania College of Technology
Williamsport, Pennsylvania

Mary M. Fabick, MSN, MEd, RN-BC, CEN
Associate Professor of Nursing
Milligan College
Milligan College, Tennessee

Barbie Hoover, RN, BSN, MSN
Clinical Instructor
Nursing-School of Health Sciences
Pennsylvania College of Technology
Williamsport, Pennsylvania

Carolyn M. Kruse, BS, DC
Medical Editor
Kruisin Editorial Services
O'Fallon, Missouri

Tricia D. Leggett, MSEd, RT (R) (QM)
Program Director and Assistant Professor
Zane State College
Zanesville, Ohio

Jennifer A. Mai, PT, DPT, MHS, NCS
Assistant Professor of Physical Therapy
Clarke College
Dubuque, Iowa

Linda McCullough
Instructor
Vocational Education and Micro Computer
Occupations
Pittsburg Adult Education
Pittsburg, California

Teresa Pirone, LMT, CNA
Danbury, Connecticut

Melissa Ann Redding, MEd
Teacher
Washington Community High School
Washington, Illinois

Craig Richard, PhD
Associate Professor
Biopharmaceutical Sciences
Bernard J. Dunn School of Pharmacy
Shenandoah University
Winchester, Virginia

Patti Ward, PhD, RT(R)
Professor
Radiologic Technology
Mesa State College
Grand Junction, Colorado

Carole A. Zarzyczny, BS
Instructor
Pennsylvania College of Technology
Williamsport, Pennsylvania

Preface

To the Instructor

The sixth edition of *Quick & Easy Medical Terminology* has made learning easier for the students, but has retained all the necessary information. You will quickly notice these new features:

- Quick Tips make the text more readable, while helping students understand what they're reading
- Better differentiation of important concepts (note colored type)
- Lots more practice exercises that include finding word parts in new terms
- A Companion CD that uses animated games for a fun way to review or test

Choose a Text That Has Been Proven to Make Learning Fun and Easy!
First published in 1990, *Quick & Easy Medical Terminology* was quickly recognized as a student-oriented book that provides a working knowledge of medical terms. All of the features that you liked before are retained, and several new features have been added.

Margin Boxes Highlight Special Information!

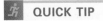 **QUICK TIP**
Leukemia is a disease.
Leukocytosis is
descriptive of the
leukocytes only.

Four types of margin boxes provide helpful information. Reading the text is easy, and the margin boxes give additional information or aid in understanding difficult terms.

Provide a Learning Foundation for Your Students Beyond Memorization
Students will welcome not having to memorize definitions. They will even recognize word parts in unfamiliar terms. The book is written for students who must acquire an understanding of medical terminology in a short time, but it provides skills that students will use for life, enabling them to recognize, comprehend, and write thousands of medical terms.

Use A Text That Adapts Well to a Variety of Classroom Needs.

The book is useful in a short medical terminology course or as self-paced material for anyone pursuing a career in the allied health professions. *Quick & Easy Medical Terminology* can be studied in conjunction with courses in anatomy, physiology, or introductory medical science or in foundation programs for careers in health or medicine. After the first five chapters are completed, you have the advantage of being able to teach chapters 6 to 14 in the order that complements the particular body system being studied.

Incorporate Illustrations from the Text in Classroom Discussion.

The sixth edition provides more illustrations—in full color—to emphasize key terms and to help students understand difficult concepts. Students interact and learn more quickly as they complete the labeling of illustrations. The illustrations are now in PowerPoint format for you to easily access during class time.

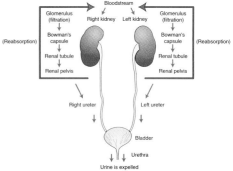

Figure 10-5 Diagram of the process of forming and expelling urine.

Emphasize Resources in the Appendixes to Your Students.

Answers to exercises, an alphabetized glossary of word parts, medical abbreviations, and Spanish translations are only part of the material available in the appendixes. Abbreviations are presented by chapter. An introduction to pharmacology is included, with drug classes and uses added to the Companion CD. Placement of the material in the appendixes is for your convenience and that of your students, whether or not you choose to use the material for a particular class.

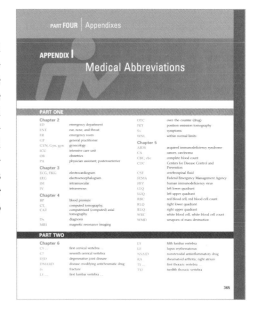

The Companion CD Uses Games to Present Information in a Different Format.

Now more fun than ever, Q&E provides animated games as a refreshing practice for the student, yet the testing mode is still there if you want it! It also has a glossary of terms, animations of physiologic processes and medical procedures, case studies, and pharmacology.

Two Audio CDs Help Students Practice the Pronunciations.
A stream of pronunciations that complement end-of-chapter lists with pauses so that the student can speak, write, or type the terms, provides practice time for students to "listen and learn," pronounce, review, or spell medical terms.

Take Advantage of the Evolve Course Management Platform.
The Evolve companion site provides a course management platform for instructors who want to post course materials online. Elsevier provides hosting and technical support. The student area includes study tips, electronic flashcards, additional exercises and games, links, audio glossaries, and more! The faculty area includes the Instructor's Resource Manual, the computerized test bank, downloads, content updates, Power-Point lecture slides, flashcard masters, and the electronic image collection.

Your Job Is Simpler Because of the TEACH Instructor's Resources.
Classroom Activities, Test Bank, and Image Collection.
Instructors have loved the wealth of testing materials provided in the Instructor's Resource Manual for Quick & Easy Medical Terminology. This edition combines the manual with the TEACH tools in one complete package. Classroom activities and exercises that require students to write and spell terms correctly provide easy-to-use handouts or homework assignments. Chapter tests that include writing terms, multiple choice, spelling, and pronunciation questions, plus midterm or midquarter and final examinations are available for you to use directly or to alter to suit your needs. The entire image collection is now on the Instructor's Evolve site to make your job easier!

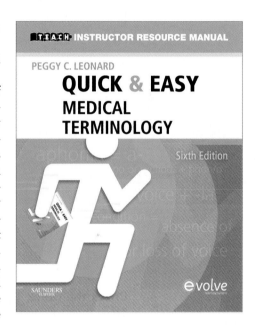

TEACH Lesson Plan Manual Included in the TEACH Instructor Resources!
Available in print or online on the companion Evolve site, the TEACH portion of the manual links all parts of the education package by providing you with customizable lesson plans and lecture outlines based on learning objectives.

Each lesson plan features:
- A three-column format that correlates chapter objectives to content and teaching resources
- Lesson preparation checklists that make planning your class quick and easy
- Critical thinking questions to focus and motivate students
- Teaching resources that cross-reference all of TEACH and Elsevier's curriculum solutions

Each lecture online features:

- PowerPoint slides that present a compelling visual summary of the chapter's main points and key terms
- Practical, concise talking points that complement the slides
- Thought-provoking questions to stimulate classroom discussions
- Unique ideas for moving beyond traditional lectures and getting students involved

 For more information on the benefits of TEACH, visit http://TEACH.elsevier.com or call Faculty Support at 1-800-222-9570.

You can see that you have EVERYTHING YOU NEED for a FABULOUS *Quick & Easy Medical Terminology* **COURSE!**

To the Student

Imagine an easy book that has everything you need. You'll start reading and writing medical terms the first day!

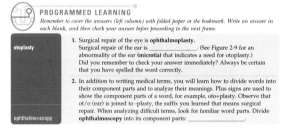

PROGRAMMED LEARNING
Remember to cover the answers (left column) with folded paper or the bookmark. Write an answer in each blank, and then check your answer before proceeding to the next frame.

otoplasty

ophthalmo+scopy

1. Surgical repair of the eye is **ophthalmoplasty.**
   Surgical repair of the ear is _____. (See Figure 2-9 for an abnormality of the ear (**microtia**) that indicates a need for otoplasty.) Did you remember to check your answer immediately? Always be certain that you have spelled the word correctly.

2. In addition to writing medical terms, you will learn how to divide words into their component parts and to analyze their meanings. Plus signs are used to show the component parts of a word, for example, oto+plasty. Observe that ot/o (ear) is joined to -plasty, the suffix you learned that means surgical repair. When analyzing difficult terms, look for familiar word parts. Divide **ophthalmoscopy** into its component parts: _____.

Work at Your Own Pace.

You set the pace! Work on part of a chapter, all of a chapter, or several chapters in one study session. It is important to study chapters 1 through 5 in the order in which they are presented, because these chapters build on the previous material learned. After completing the first five chapters, you may complete chapters 6 through 14 in whatever order you choose, assuming that you are working on your own.

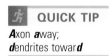

QUICK TIP

Axon **a**way;
dendrites towar**d**

Check the Quick Tips in the Margins.

Three types of Quick Tips provide additional information or help you understand a new term. You'll even be able to understand a term you've never seen before!

Take Advantage of Real-Life Practice Opportunities!

Imagine yourself working in your chosen health care field. The case studies and health reports in this book are just like the ones you will be reading when you are a health care professional! You will be fully prepared to understand the day-to-day medical terminology you will encounter.

MEDICAL REPORT **Mid-City Medical Center**

222 Medical Center Drive   Main City, USA 63017-1000   Phone: (555) 434-0000
                                                           Fax: (555) 434-0001

DIAGNOSIS RECORD/DISCHARGE SUMMARY

Patient: Martha Watkins
Final Diagnosis: Osteoarthritis of the right knee
Secondary Diagnosis: Rheumatoid arthritis; degenerative joint disease left knee
Complications: Postoperative deep vein thrombosis—right lower extremity
Principal Operation(s)/Procedure(s)/Treatment Rendered: Right total knee arthroplasty, posterior stabilized, cemented.
Discharge Instructions: Up ad lib with full weight bearing to right lower extremity. Ambulate with wheeled walker. Home health for physical and occupational therapy 3x week, and nursing visits to monitor incision and medication. Patient to change dry dressing to incision daily.
Medications: Coumadin 5 mg daily
Diet: Regular
Follow-up: Patient to make appointment with Dr. Withers for staple removal in 10 days
Date Admitted: 1/31/2006   **Date Discharged:** 2/05/2006

Dr. John Withers
(Dr. John Withers)

1. osteoarthritis: _____
2. rheumatoid arthritis: _____
3. degenerative joint disease left knee: _____
4. right total knee arthroplasty: _____
5. right lower extremity: _____

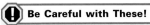

Be Careful with These!

-ist (one who) versus *-iatry* (medical profession or treatment)
-logy (study of) versus *-logist* (one who studies; specialist)
ne/o (new) versus *neur/o* (nerve)
intern (one in postgraduate training) versus *internist* (a physician)

Caution! Helpful Hints Show You How to Distinguish Between Confusing Terms.

Caution boxes help you differentiate terms that look alike, sound alike, or are easily mistaken for something else.

Measure How You Are Doing Before The Test.

Review materials are provided within the chapter, and self-tests help you know if you're ready for the instructor's exam. Always check your answers using Appendix VIII.

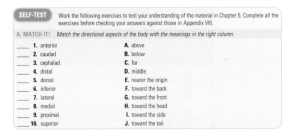

SELF-TEST   Work the following exercises to test your understanding of the material in Chapter 5. Complete all the exercises before checking your answers against those in Appendix VIII.

A. MATCH IT!   *Match the directional aspects of the body with the meanings in the right column.*

____ 1. anterior   A. above
____ 2. caudad   B. below
____ 3. cephalad   C. far
____ 4. distal   D. middle
____ 5. dorsal   E. nearer the origin
____ 6. inferior   F. toward the back
____ 7. lateral   G. toward the front
____ 8. medial   H. toward the head
____ 9. proximal   I. toward the side
____ 10. superior   J. toward the tail

Don't Skip the Companion CD! It's Practice Using Animated Games!

If you're thinking boring, then think again! These games present what you learned in the chapter in a different mode and prepare you for the instructor's exam by challenging you to think quickly in a fun setting. There are also animated illustrations, additional health reports, each chapter's audio glossary, and more.

The Audio CDs Help You Practice Pronunciation and Writing Terms.

The pronunciations for each chapter allow you to listen without clicking on the terms in the end-of-chapter lists. Either repeat the pronunciations as they're given, or write or type them, later checking your spelling in the Q&E Lists at the ends of chapters 2 through 14. You'll quickly discover any terms that you need to review.

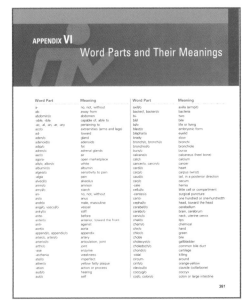

APPENDIX VI
Word Parts and Their Meanings

Use Appendix Material for Abbreviations, Pharmacology, and Other Valuable Resources.

The appendix material provides a means of checking your answers, as well as an alphabetized glossary of word parts, abbreviations, and other helpful resources.

Prepare for the Final Examination with the Useful Materials Provided.

Self-testing for chapters 1 through 14 is provided in Part Three. You can also rework the end-of-chapter reviews and study the tables of word parts within the chapters as preparation for a comprehensive examination of material covered in *Quick & Easy Medical Terminology*.

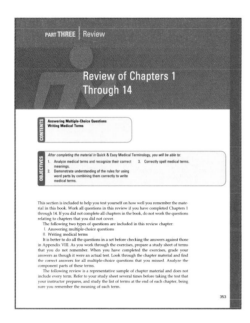

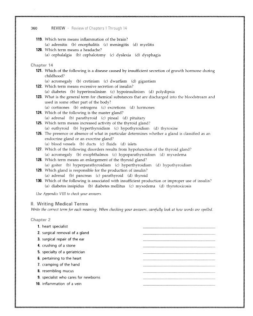

Have Fun As You Take Charge of Your Learning!

This book is written for you! It provides an easy way to learn medical terms and allows you to move at your own pace.

Peggy C. Leonard

Acknowledgments

Special thanks to many individuals who have contributed to making the sixth edition of *Quick & Easy Medical Terminology*. Suggestions from instructors have been incorporated, as well as analyses by an outstanding group of reviewers.

The designer and the illustrator have produced not only an attractive book but one that will greatly enhance the understanding of medical terms. I am also indebted to the companies who have allowed use of illustrations that enhance the written word and bring life to explanations of terms.

The production of this book would not be possible without the producers, editors, proofreaders, and all others who have helped provide a book that I know instructors will enjoy using as they teach students the language of medicine.

Words cannot adequately express my gratitude to Developmental Editor Carolyn Kruse who has provided humor, steadfast encouragement, and herculean efforts during the preparation of many editions of this book, as well as *Building a Medical Vocabulary*.

Peggy Leonard MT, MEd

Contents

Part One   THE BASICS

1   Simplified Medical Language, 1

2   Suffixes and Combining Forms Made Easy, 13

3   Essential Prefixes and More, 51

4   Diagnostic Procedures and Therapeutic Interventions, 78

5   The Body as a Whole, 97

Part Two   BODY SYSTEMS

6   Musculoskeletal System, 133

7   Circulatory System, 165

8   Respiratory System, 191

9   Digestive System, 212

10   Urinary System, 238

11   Reproductive System, 261

12   Integumentary System, 299

13   Nervous System and Psychologic Disorders, 317

14   Endocrine System, 338

Part Three   REVIEW

Review of Chapters 1 Through 14, 353

Part Four   APPENDIXES

I   Medical Abbreviations, 365

II   Finding Medical Abbreviations, 367

III   Pharmacology Overview, 369
      Erinn Kao, PharmD

IV   Spanish Pronunciation of Select Terms, 374

V   Translation of Select Spanish Terms, 378

VI   Word Parts and Their Meanings, 381

VII   English Terms and Corresponding Word Parts, 386

VIII Answers to Exercises, 391

Bibliography, 403

Illustration and Photo Credits, 404

CHAPTER **1**
Simplified Medical Language

CONTENTS

Simplifying Medical Terms
Writing Is Key
Word Parts
Combining Word Parts to Write Terms
Proper Names Are Special

Abbreviations and Pharmacology
Plurals
Pronunciation of Medical Terms
Enhancing Spanish Communication
Self-Test

OBJECTIVES

After completing Chapter 1, you will be able to:

1. Recognize prefixes, suffixes, word roots, and combining forms.
2. Demonstrate understanding of the rules for combining word parts to write medical terms correctly.
3. Identify and distinguish abbreviations from eponyms.
4. Use the rules learned in this chapter to write the singular or plural forms of medical terms.
5. Demonstrate understanding of primary and secondary accent marks.

Simplifying Medical Terms

The great size of a medical dictionary is evidence of the vast number of words in the medical language. Because Latin and Greek are the major sources of medical terms, it is no wonder that some people say, "Medical words look like Greek to me!" Although familiarity with Greek or Latin would simplify the task of learning medical terminology, experience has shown that learning these two languages is not necessary. What is necessary is learning relatively few word parts and recognizing them when you see them in a word. Then you won't have to memorize every new word you encounter.

The material in Chapters 1 through 5 is essential for learning medical terms, because it explains *word building* and teaches you how to divide words into their component parts. Chapters 6 through 14 do not have to be studied in the sequence in which they appear in this book, but they are presented with the assumption that you have learned the material in the first five chapters.

Many word parts are used to form medical terms that pertain to various body systems. For example, *-itis* is a suffix that means "inflammation." Therefore, you will see this word part used in describing various inflammatory conditions that occur throughout the body.

No matter how eager you are to learn medical terminology pertaining to a particular body system, don't skip any of the material in the first five chapters of this book! It is the foundation on which you will base speaking, reading, and writing medical terms correctly.

Writing Is Key

Correct spelling is essential because a misspelled word may have an entirely different meaning. (You are not required to learn specific medical terms in Chapter 1.) In many cases, correct spelling can also help with pronunciation. Starting with Chapter 2, the correct pronunciations are provided at the end of each chapter. Also, use the Companion CD provided in the back of this book or the accompanying audio CDs to listen to pronunciations.*

Writing words helps you to learn faster than if you simply read them, and you will often be asked to write answers. Write an answer whenever you see a blank or a question, and check every answer that you write to see if it is correct. Even when you are sure that you know the answer, check your answer anyway. Sometimes you might misinterpret what you read, and this is an excellent way to check your understanding.

Variety Makes It Fun

Written exercises throughout each chapter get you actively involved. The Self-Test at the end of each chapter helps you know if you have learned the material.

As you study Chapter 1, word parts that make up medical terms are explained first, followed by other forms of communication, such as abbreviations. Plurals and pronunciations are also introduced.

Word Parts

Word Roots and Combining Forms

The *word root* is the main body of a word. All words have a word root, even ordinary words. Word roots are the building blocks for most medical terms. Most medical dictionaries show the origin of terms. If you study these, you will see that many are derived from Greek and Latin words. Look at the examples of word roots and their Greek or Latin origin in Table 1-1. Compound words are sometimes composed of two word roots, as in checkbook (check and book).

Table 1-1 Origin of Word Roots		
Word Root	**Greek or Latin Origin**	**Use in a Word**
lith	*lithos* (G., stone)	lithiasis
psych	*psyche* (G., mind)	psychology
caud	*cauda* (L., tail)	caudal
or	*oris* (L., mouth)	oral

*A pronunciation guide is presented inside the back cover and on the bookmark included with the text.

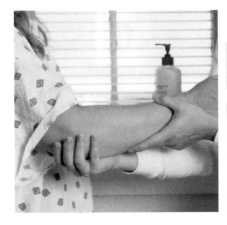

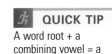

-al, -ous = pertaining to
cutane/o = skin
derm/a = skin

Figure 1-1 Examination of the skin. A patient's skin, the body's largest and most visible organ, can produce valuable information about the patient's health. The scientific name of the skin is dermis, after the Greek term *derma*. The Latin *cutis* also means skin. Both dermal and cutaneous mean pertaining to the skin. Inflammation of the skin is dermatitis.

A vowel, called a *combining vowel,* is often inserted between word roots to make the word easier to pronounce. In the word speed/o/meter, speed/o is a *combining form* that is simply the word root "speed" plus the vowel *o.* A combining form can be recognized in this book by the diagonal slash mark before an ending vowel. (The most frequently used vowel is *o.*) Cardi/o, gastr/o, and oste/o are all combining forms, but so is chol/e. In this book, you will learn the combining forms for word roots.

You will sometimes learn two word roots that have the same meaning. For example, both *dermal* and *cutaneous* mean "pertaining to the skin" (Figure 1-1). As a general rule, Latin roots are used to write words naming and describing structures of the body, whereas Greek roots are used to write words naming and describing diseases, conditions, diagnosis, and treatment. As with most rules, however, there are exceptions.

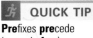

QUICK TIP

A word root + a combining vowel = a combining form.

WRITE IT! | **EXERCISE 1**

Write either WR (for "word root") or CF (for "combining form") in the blanks to identify these word parts.

CF 1. aden/o   CF 3. chol/e   CF 5. or/o

CF 2. carcin/o   WR 4. lith   WR 6. psych

Check your answers with Appendix VIII, Answers to Exercises, in the back of the book.

Prefixes and Suffixes

A word root is usually accompanied by a prefix or a suffix, or sometimes by both. A *prefix* is placed before a word to modify its meaning. When written alone, a prefix is usually followed by a hyphen (e.g., anti-), indicating that another word part follows the prefix to form a complete word.

Example: The prefix a- (meaning "without") joined with febrile (which refers to "fever") yields the term *afebrile,* which means "without fever."

A *suffix* is attached to the end of a word or word root to modify its meaning. Suffixes are joined to combining forms to write nouns (names: the subject of the sentence), adjectives (descriptive words), and verbs (action words). A suffix is usually preceded by a hyphen when the suffix is written alone (e.g., -cyte), indicating that another word part generally precedes it before a complete word can be formed.

QUICK TIP

Prefixes **pre**cede (**c**ome before) **c**ombining **f**orms.

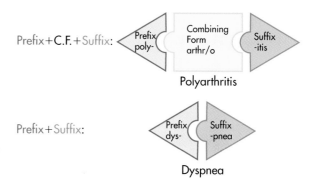

Prefix+C.F.+Suffix:

Polyarthritis

Prefix+Suffix:

Dyspnea

Figure 1-2 Relationship of prefixes, combining forms, and suffixes.

Example: The combining form erythr/o (meaning red) can be joined with the suffix -cyte (meaning cell) to write the term *erythrocyte*, which means a red blood cell (often shortened to red cell).

Occasionally, a word is composed of only a prefix and a suffix (e.g., combining dys- and -pnea). Visualize the relationship of prefixes, combining forms, and suffixes as you study Figure 1-2.

Word Division

Word division is used frequently throughout this book to help you recognize the parts that are used to build a term. For example, the first time you see appendicitis, it may be written as appendic+itis to emphasize its two component parts.

Word roots, combining forms, prefixes, and suffixes are word parts. Learning the meaning of these word parts eliminates the necessity of memorizing each new term you encounter. Do not be concerned with the meanings of the word parts in Chapter 1; you will learn them in subsequent chapters. After writing answers in the blanks, check your answers against the solutions found in Appendix VIII. It is best to work all of a particular exercise before checking your answers. It is also important to confirm your answers before going on to the next exercise. (If you have made a mistake, you do not want to keep repeating it throughout the chapter!)

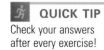 **QUICK TIP**

Check your answers after every exercise!

MATCH IT!

EXERCISE 2

Choose A, B, or C from the right column to classify each of the word parts in the left column.

___A___ **1.** a-
___C___ **2.** cutane/o
___C___ **3.** dermat/o
___A___ **4.** eu-
___B___ **5.** -graphy
___C___ **6.** hydr/o
___B___ **7.** -iasis
___A___ **8.** mal-
___B___ **9.** -pathy
___C___ **10.** phon/o

A. prefix
B. suffix
C. combining form

Check your answers with Appendix VIII, Answers to Exercises.

Combining Word Parts to Write Terms

Remember that when combining forms are written alone, they contain a combining vowel, usually an *o,* as in hepat/o. When medical terms are written, the vowel at the end of a combining form is not always used. The following rule is helpful:

> The combining vowel is used before suffixes that begin with a consonant and before another word root. In other words, drop the combining vowel if the suffix also begins with a vowel (*a, e, i, o,* or *u*).
>
> **Example 1:** When the combining form hepat/o is joined with the suffix -megaly, the combining vowel is used and results in the term *hepatomegaly.* Notice that -megaly begins with a consonant: hepat/o + -megaly = hepatomegaly.
>
> **Example 2:** When the combining form hepat/o is joined with the suffix -itis, the combining vowel is not used and results in the term *hepatitis.* Notice that the *o* is dropped from hepat/o because -itis begins with a vowel: hepat/o + -itis = hepatitis.

Observe use of the previous rule in the following table.

Building Terms with a Combining Form and Suffixes

Combining Form		Suffixes		Term and Meaning
ot/o = ear	+	-itis	=	*otitis,* inflammation of the ear
	+	-logy	=	*otology,* study of the ear
	+	-plasty	=	*otoplasty,* plastic surgery of the ear
	+	-rrhea	=	*otorrhea,* discharge from the ear
	+	-tomy	=	*ototomy,* incision of the ear

There are exceptions to this rule about using the combining vowel, and you will learn these exceptions as you progress through the material.

Most prefixes end with a vowel and may be added to other word parts without change. For example, precancerous, preeruptive, and preoperative result when the prefix pre- is joined with cancerous, eruptive, and operative.

There are exceptions to the rule concerning the use of prefixes. These exceptions are noted when they occur. One exception is *anti-.* When anti- is joined with biotic and coagulant, the terms *antibiotic* and *anticoagulant* result. Often, however, ant- is used when the prefix is joined to a vowel. The term *antacid* results when anti- is joined with acid.

Sometimes two terms are acceptable when a prefix is used to form a new word. *End-* and *endo-* both mean inside. End- is usually joined with word parts beginning with a vowel, as in the term *endarterial.* Common usage, however, has determined whether end- or endo- is used in certain cases. Some terms accept either prefix, as in endoaortitis and endoaortitis. Both terms are acceptable and have identical meanings.

As you learn word parts, you will begin to recognize them within medical terms. You will even be able to know the meaning of many terms by breaking them down into their component parts. Figure 1-3 summarizes examples of using word parts to write and interpret medical terms. Be aware that some terms do not follow the rules you have learned. As you progress through the material, you will find such exceptions noted.

QUICK TIP

Most prefixes do *not* change when added to a word.

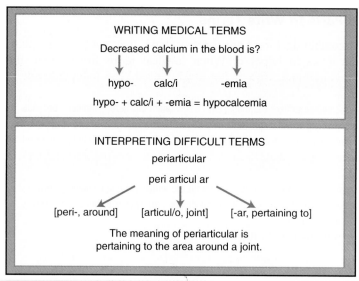

Figure 1-3 Examples of using prefixes, suffixes, and combining forms to write and interpret medical terms.

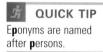

BUILD IT! **EXERCISE 3**

Write terms from these word parts, deciding if you use or drop the combining vowel when present.

1. dys- + -pnea _____ dyspnea
2. enter/o + -ic _____ enteric
3. eu- + -pepsia _____ eupepsia
4. tonsill/o + -itis _____ tonsillitis
5. ur/o + -emia _____ uremia
6. anti- + anxiety _____ antianxiety
7. leuk/o + -cyte _____ leukocyte
8. appendic/o + -itis _____ Appendicitis
9. hyper- + -emia _____ Hyperemia
10. endo- + cardi/o + -al _____ Endocardial

Check your answers with Appendix VIII, Answers to Exercises.

Proper Names Are Special

Eponyms are names for diseases, organs, procedures, or body functions that are derived from the name of a person. A cesarean section, a surgical procedure in which the abdomen and uterus are surgically opened to deliver the infant, is an eponym named after the manner in which Julius Caesar was supposedly born. Parkinson disease and Alzheimer disease are also eponyms.

The word-building rules that you just learned are summarized in Table 1-2.

Abbreviations and Pharmacology

Abbreviations are shortened forms of written words or phrases that are used in place of the whole. For example, MD means "doctor of medicine." However, MD

Table 1-2 Rules for Word Building

Joining of	Rule	Example(s)
Combining forms	The combining vowel is usually retained between combining forms.	gastr/o + enterology = gastroenterology
Combining forms and suffixes	The combining vowel is usually retained when a combining form is joined with a suffix that begins with a consonant.	enter/o + -logy = enterology
	The combining vowel is usually omitted when a combining form is joined with a suffix that begins with a vowel.	enter/o + -ic = enteric
Prefixes and other word parts	Most prefixes require no change when they are joined with other word parts.	peri- + appendicitis = periappendicitis dys- + -pnea = dyspnea

has other meanings, including medical department. Abbreviations include the following:

- Letters (The abbreviation for "shortness of breath" is SOB.)
- Shortened words (The abbreviation stat is short for the Latin *statim,* meaning "at once" or "immediately.")
- *Acronyms,* or words (abbreviations) formed from the initial letters of a compound term (The acronym CABG, pronounced like the vegetable, stands for *coronary artery bypass graft.*)

Using abbreviations and symbols can be dangerous when medications are involved. The Institute for Safe Medications publishes lists of what are considered dangerous abbreviations and recommends that certain terms be written in full because they are easily mistaken for other meanings. For example, especially when written by hand, qn, meaning "nightly" or "at bedtime," can be misinterpreted as qh, which means "every hour." Common abbreviations are presented in this book, but particular caution must be taken in both using and reading abbreviations. Appendixes I and II have alphabetical listings of abbreviations. If a common abbreviation is missing, you may consider checking whether its use is discouraged by the Institute for Safe Medications (www.ismp.org).

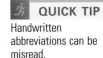

QUICK TIP

Handwritten abbreviations can be misread.

MATCH IT! EXERCISE 4

Choose A or B from the right column to classify the terms in the two left columns as an abbreviation or an eponym.

__A__ **1.** CAD   __A__ **4.** OSHA   **A.** abbreviation

__A__ **2.** D&C   __B__ **5.** Raynaud sign   **B.** eponym

__B__ **3.** Foley catheter

Check your answers with Appendix VIII, Answers to Exercises.

Pharmacology is the study of the preparation, properties, uses, and actions of drugs. Drugs are used in medicine to prevent, diagnose, and treat disease and to relieve pain. Another term for medicines is *pharmaceuticals.* Appendix III provides an overview of pharmacology, and information about drug classes is presented for chapters 2 through 5; pharmacology material for chapters 6 through 14 is found on the Companion CD.

Plurals

Plurals of many medical terms are formed using the rules you may already know, such as simply adding an *s* to the singular term. For example, the plural of abrasion is *abrasions*. Many nouns that end in *s, ch,* or *sh* form their plurals by adding *-es*. For example, the plural of sinus is *sinuses*. Singular nouns that end in *y* preceded by a consonant form their plurals by changing the *y* to *i* and adding *-es*. For example, the plural of allergy is *allergies*.

Use Table 1-3 to learn the rules for forming other plurals of medical terms, but be aware that a few exceptions exist, and that only major rules are included. Also, note that some terms have more than one acceptable plural. Many dictionaries show the plural forms of nouns and can be used as a reference.

CIRCLE IT! **EXERCISE 5**

Circle the correct answer.
1. Which is the plural of atrium? (**atria**, atrion, atriums)
2. Which is the plural of bacillus? (bacilla, **bacilli,** bacilluses)
3. Which is the plural of diagnosis? (**diagnoses**, diagnosises, diagnosus)
4. Which is the plural of larynx? (**larynges**, laryngi, laryngxes)
5. Which is the plural of varix? (**varices,** varixes, varixs)

Check your answers with Appendix VIII, Answers to Exercises.

Pronunciation of Medical Terms

Beginning in Chapter 2, an alphabetical listing near the end of each chapter, the Quick & Easy (Q&E) List, shows the correct spelling of medical terms for each chapter, followed by the phonetic spelling to indicate their pronunciations. It is helpful to look at the term while listening to its pronunciation on the Games Companion CD or audio CDs that are provided.

Pronunciation of most medical terms follows the same rules that govern the pronunciation of all English words. Some general rules and examples to assist you in pronunciation are given in the Pronunciation Guide on the included bookmark and inside the back cover.

Remember that there are exceptions to these rules, and certain terms can have more than one acceptable pronunciation. Also, different pronunciations are often used in different parts of the United States, and certain diseases, disorders, and procedures incorporate proper names, which may be exceptions to English pronunciation.

ⓘ Be Careful with These!

- Drop combining vowels if the suffix begins with a vowel (*example:* ot/o + -itis = otitis).
- Singular words that end in *um* or *on* become *a* when plural. However, words that have the plural ending *ae* use *a* for the singular form. Study the medical terms in Table 1-3 until you can tell the difference.

Table 1-3 Forming Plurals of Nouns with Special Endings

If the Singular Ending Is:	The Plural Ending Is:	Examples	
		Singular	**Plural**
is	es	diagnosis, prognosis, psychosis	diagnoses, prognoses, psychoses
Some words ending in *is* form plurals by dropping the *is* and adding *ides,* as in epididymis and *epididymides.*			
um	a	atrium, ileum, septum, bacterium	atria, ilea, septa, bacteria
us	i	alveolus, bacillus, bronchus	alveoli, bacilli, bronchi
Some singular forms ending in *us* form plurals by dropping the *us* and adding either *era* or *ora,* as in *viscera* and *corpora.* Others form plurals by simply adding *es,* as in *viruses.*			
a	ae	vertebra, patella, petechia	vertebrae, patellae, petechiae
ix	ices	appendix, varix, cervix	appendices, varices, cervices
Through common use, appendixes and cervixes have become acceptable plural forms.			
ex	ices	cortex	cortices
ax	aces	thorax	thoraces (thoraxes also acceptable)
ma	s (or mata)	carcinoma, sarcoma	carcinomas (or carcinomata), sarcomas (or sarcomata)
on	a	protozoon, spermatozoon	protozoa, spermatozoa
Some singular forms ending in *on* form plurals by adding *s,* as in chorion and *chorions.*			
nx	nges	phalanx, larynx	phalanges, larynges

FINDING THE CLUE!

EXERCISE 6

Use a clue to write the correct answers in the blanks. Solve Question 1; each ending letter becomes a clue for the first letter of the next answer.

1. How many syllables does the term ectasis (ek´tə-sis) have? ___three___

2. Using the pronunciation of ectasis in Question 1, which syllable has a primary accent? ___ek___

3. Which syllable has a primary accent in choledochostomy (ko-led-ə-kos´tə-me)? _____

4. Which syllable has a secondary accent in sensibility (sen´´sĭ-bil´ĭ-te)? _____

5. Which syllable has the primary accent in cardiokinetic (kahr´´de-o-kĭ-net´ik)? _____

Check your answers with Appendix VIII.

ESPAÑOL Enhancing Spanish Communication

Spanish translation is given for selected terms beginning in Chapter 2. Appendixes IV and V of *Quick & Easy Medical Terminology* have both English-Spanish and Spanish-English translations, respectively, for easy reference.

Your instructor will set goals pertaining to the needs of your individual class. If you wish to listen to Spanish pronunciation, use http://evolve.elsevier.com/Leonard/quick/.

Spanish vowels invariably have the same sound and must be fully and distinctly pronounced. This does not apply to double vowels. Use the following rules to pronounce vowels:

Spanish Vowel	Pronounce as
a	*a* in mama
e	*a* in day
i	*i* in police
o	*o* in so
u	*u* in rude or *oo* in spool*
y	*e* in see

* The u is generally silent in the syllables que, qui, gue, and gui.

Some consonants have similar sounds in English and Spanish. Only significant differences are noted here. Follow these guidelines to pronounce consonants with different sounds:

Spanish Consonant	Pronounce as
c	sometimes as *k* or *s*
d	sometimes as *th*
g	distinctly different *g*, sometimes *h*
h	not pronounced
j	*h*
ll	blending of *l* and *y*, or simply *y*
ñ	blending of *n* and *y*
q	*k*
r	trilled *r*
rr	strongly trilled *r*
z	*s*

Placement of stress or accent in Spanish terms is simplified by the following general rules:
1. Words ending in a consonant other than *n* or *s* are accented on the last syllable.
2. Words ending in a vowel (or *n* or *s*) are accented on the next-to-last syllable.
3. Words that do not conform to the previous rules must have the written accent over the vowel to be stressed, as in the term *inflamación*. The written accent is also used to distinguish words that are written alike but have different meanings, such as *el* (meaning "the") and *él* ("he").

Phonetic pronunciation is presented with the stressed syllable in uppercase letters, as in inflamación (in-flah-mah-se-ON). In this term, the last syllable is stressed.

SELF-TEST   Work the following exercises to test your understanding of the material in Chapter 1. It is best to do all the exercises before checking your answers against the answers in Appendix VIII.

Don't be concerned about learning the meanings of the word parts for Chapter 1, because all of them are included in subsequent chapters.

A. MATCH IT!   *Choose A, B, or C from the right column to classify the word parts.*

_C_ **1.** bil/i   _A_ **6.** intra-   **A.** prefix
_C_ **2.** crani/o   _A_ **7.** multi-   **B.** suffix
_B_ **3.** -ectomy   _B_ **8.** -oid   **C.** combining form
_C_ **4.** gigant/o   _B_ **9.** -plegia
_B_ **5.** -iatrics   _C_ **10.** spher/o

B. MATCH IT!   *Select A, B, or C from the right column to classify these descriptions (A and B may be used more than once).*

_____ **1.** contains a slash before a vowel when written alone   **A.** prefix
_____ **2.** is attached to the end of a word root to modify its meaning   **B.** suffix
_____ **3.** is followed by a hyphen when written alone   **C.** combining form
_____ **4.** is preceded by a hyphen when written alone
_____ **5.** generally requires no change when joined with other word parts

C. BUILD IT!   *Using the rules you have learned in Chapter 1, combine the word parts to write terms.*

1. hypo- + derm/o + -ic   hypodermic
2. leuk/o + -emia   leukemia
3. melan/o + -oid   melanoid
4. my/o + cardi/o + -al   myocardial
5. thromb/o + -osis   thrombosis

D. WRITE IT!   *Write the plural of these terms.*

1. appendix (two acceptable plurals)   appendices
2. bronchus   bronchti
3. ileum   ilea
4. pharynx   pharynges
5. prognosis   prognoses

Use Appendix VIII to check your Self-Test answers. Pay particular attention to spelling. If most of your answers are correct, you are ready to move on to Chapter 2.

Continued

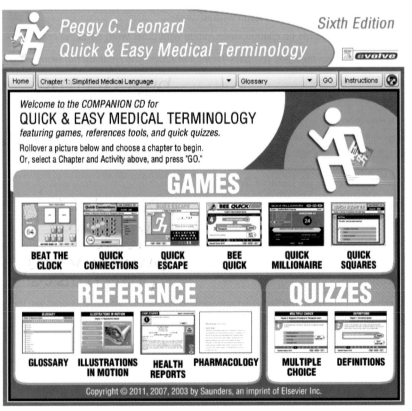 Games on the Games Companion CD in the back of your book provide a fun way to review, but remember that the CD does not replace the Self-Test at the end of each chapter.

- Six games help reassure you that you have learned each chapter's material. Play to "win" a million dollars, make a Quick Escape, or Beat the Clock! Print your scores and prove you are a winner!
- Use the audio glossary of terms from chapters 2 through 14 to check your pronunciation and spelling. The audio terms correspond to the Quick & Easy (Q&E) lists at the end of each chapter beginning with Chapter 2. You can listen, speak the terms, and check the pronunciations while reading the written pronunciations from the list. Or listen, write the terms, and then check your spelling against the chapter Q&E list. The more senses you can use, the easier it will be to learn!
- Illustrations in Motion for chapters 5 through 14 allow you to imagine working in your chosen field, using the medical terminology you have just learned! You will see how medical terms are put into action in real pathologies and actual procedures.
- Case Studies for chapters 6 through 14 build your confidence for recognizing and understanding terms from actual health care reports. Each highlighted term has its definition and audio as a pop-up, so you can read the report and understand what you are reading. To check your understanding, answer the quick questions with each case study.

evolve Visit http://evolve.elsevier.com/Leonard/quick/ for additional review activities, including questions on Spanish medical terms.

CHAPTER 2

Suffixes and Combining Forms Made Easy

CONTENTS

Using Suffixes to Write Words
Suffixes: Medical Specialties and Specialists
Suffixes: Surgical Procedures
Combining Forms for Selected Body Structures
Suffixes: Symptoms or Diagnosis
Miscellaneous Suffixes

Miscellaneous Word Parts
Abbreviations and Pharmacology
Preparing for a Test on This Chapter
Self-Test
Quick & Easy (Q&E) List
Enhancing Spanish Communication

OBJECTIVES

After completing Chapter 2, you will be able to:

1. Write the meanings of Chapter 2 word parts, or match word parts with their meanings.
2. Match medical specialists with the areas in which they specialize.
3. Identify the common medical conditions associated with each specialty.
4. Identify the suffixes for surgical procedures, symptoms, and diagnoses.
5. Identify combining forms for select body structures.
6. Build and analyze medical terms with combining forms and suffixes.
7. Write the correct term when presented with its definition, or match terms with their definitions.
8. Spell medical terms correctly.

Using Suffixes to Write Words

The combining of suffixes with other word parts forms nouns, adjectives, and verbs. You learned in Chapter 1 that when a suffix that begins with a vowel is joined with a combining form, the combining vowel is almost always dropped from the combining form (example: append/o + -ectomy = appendectomy). To help you easily recognize word parts in new terms, word division (example: append+ectomy) will often be used in this text. Dividing words in this manner will help you recognize word parts.

Bold Type

Important! **Bold type** indicates that a term is included in the Quick & Easy (Q&E) list near the end of each chapter and is pronounced on the Companion CD and audio CDs. Examples of bold type are: An **appendectomy** is … or Orthopedics is …

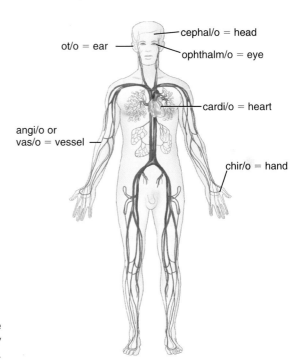

cephal/o = head
ot/o = ear
ophthalm/o = eye
cardi/o = heart
angi/o or vas/o = vessel
chir/o = hand

Figure 2-1 Combining forms. Most terms use combining forms as their foundation. All body structures have corresponding combining forms.

Because it is helpful to know the types of words formed by the use of various suffixes, information on word usage is provided. It is logical that a suffix coincides with how its meaning is used in speech. For example, append+ectomy means surgical removal (-ectomy) of the appendix (append/o). **Appendectomy** is a surgical procedure, and thus it is a noun. From this, we see that the suffix -*ectomy* is used to write nouns.

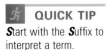

append/o = appendix
-ectomy = surgical removal

To interpret a new word, begin by looking at its ending. If the ending is a suffix, decide its meaning, then go to the beginning of the word and read from left to right, interpreting the remaining elements to develop the full sense of the term.

QUICK TIP
Start with the **S**uffix to interpret a term.

For example, in *appendectomy*, determine the meaning of the suffix -ectomy, then the meaning of the combining form at the beginning of the term, append/o. This method yields surgical removal, appendix. The full meaning of the term is "surgical removal of the appendix."

You will learn many suffixes in this chapter. Although suffixes are emphasized, a limited number of combining forms are also presented. As introduced in Chapter 1, *combining forms* are the foundation of most terms (Figure 2-1), and learning terms is easier and more interesting than only memorizing suffixes. Also, to make it easier, Chapter 2 suffixes are divided into four categories: (1) suffixes used in naming medical specialties and specialists, (2) suffixes used in surgical procedures, (3) suffixes used in symptoms or diagnosis, and (4) miscellaneous suffixes.

Suffixes: Medical Specialties and Specialists

This section introduces several combining forms, as well as a few prefixes and suffixes, that are used in naming specialties and specialists. Study the following suffixes, think of words that you already know that use these suffixes, and mentally prepare a definition of that term using the meaning. For example, the suffix -er may cause you to think of a "doodler." A shortened definition is "one who doodles." The funnier the association, the more likely you are to remember the meaning of the word part.

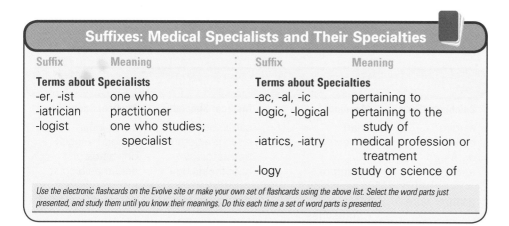

Suffixes: Medical Specialists and Their Specialties

Suffix	Meaning	Suffix	Meaning
Terms about Specialists		**Terms about Specialties**	
-er, -ist	one who	-ac, -al, -ic	pertaining to
-iatrician	practitioner	-logic, -logical	pertaining to the study of
-logist	one who studies; specialist	-iatrics, -iatry	medical profession or treatment
		-logy	study or science of

Use the electronic flashcards on the Evolve site or make your own set of flashcards using the above list. Select the word parts just presented, and study them until you know their meanings. Do this each time a set of word parts is presented.

MATCH IT!

EXERCISE 1

Match the suffixes in the left column with their meaning in the right column (a choice may be used more than once).

E 1. -ac   A. medical profession or treatment
B 2. -er   B. one who
D 3. -iatrician   C. one who studies; specialist
A 4. -iatry   D. practitioner
E 5. -ic   E. pertaining to
B 6. -ist   F. study or science of
C 7. -logist
F 8. -logy

Check your answers with Appendix VIII, Answers to Exercises, in the back of the book.

The term *medicine* has several meanings, including "a drug" or "a remedy for illness." A second meaning of medicine is "the art and science of diagnosis, treatment, and prevention of disease."

Family practice is a medical specialty that encompasses several branches of medicine and coordinates health care for all members of a family. A family practice physician often acts as the primary health care provider, referring complex disorders to other specialists. The family practice physician has largely replaced the concept of a general practitioner (GP).

Internal medicine is a nonsurgical specialty of medicine that deals specifically with the diagnosis and treatment of diseases of the internal structures of the body. The specialist is called an **internist**.

It is important not to confuse internist with the term *intern*. An intern in many clinical programs is any immediate postgraduate trainee. A physician intern is in

QUICK TIP

Family practice physicians don't specialize, but treat all illnesses.

-ist = one who
Think of "florist" or "balloonist."

postgraduate training, learning medical practice under supervision before being licensed as a physician. An internist, however, is a licensed medical specialist.

Study the following combining forms associated with the medical specialties, and also learn the titles of the specialists. Think of people you know who either see this specialist or need to see each specialist, and you will remember the terms better.

Combining Forms for Selected Medical Specialties

Combining Form	Meaning	Medical Specialty	Medical Specialist
cardi/o	heart	cardiology	cardiologist
crin/o	to secrete	endocrinology	endocrinologist
dermat/o	skin	dermatology	dermatologist
esthesi/o	feeling or sensation	anesthesiology	anesthesiologist
gastr/o, enter/o	stomach, intestines*	gastroenterology	gastroenterologist
ger/a, ger/o, geront/o	elderly	geriatrics	geriatrician
gynec/o	female	gynecology	gynecologist
immun/o	immune	immunology	immunologist
ne/o, nat/o	new, birth	neonatology	neonatologist
neur/o	nerve	neurology	neurologist
obstetr/o	midwife	obstetrics	obstetrician
onc/o	tumor	oncology	oncologist
ophthalm/o	eye	ophthalmology	ophthalmologist
orth/o, ped/o	orth/o, straight ped/o, child†	orthopedics	orthopedist, orthopedic surgeon
ot/o, laryng/o	ear, larynx	otolaryngology	otolaryngologist
path/o	disease	pathology	pathologist
ped/o	child†	pediatrics	pediatrician
psych/o	mind	psychiatry	psychiatrist
radi/o	radiation (or radius)	radiology	radiologist
rheumat/o	rheumatism	rheumatology	rheumatologist
rhin/o	nose	rhinology	rhinologist
ur/o	urinary tract (or urine)	urology	urologist

Use the electronic flashcards on the Evolve site or make your own set of flashcards using the above list. Select the word parts just presented, and study them until you know their meanings.

*enter/o *sometimes refers specifically to the small intestine.*
†ped/o *sometimes means "foot."*

FIND IT!

EXERCISE 2

Find the combining form in each of these terms. Write the combining form as well as its meaning.

		Combining Form	Meaning
1.	cardiology	cardi/o	heart
2.	dermatology	dermat/o	skin
3.	gynecology	gynec/o	female
4.	immunology	immun/o	immune
5.	neurology	neur/o	nerve
6.	oncology	onc/o	tumor
7.	ophthalmology	~~opth~~ ophthalm/o	eye
8.	pathology	path/o	disease
9.	psychiatry	psych/o	mind
10.	radiology	radi/o	radiation, radius
11.	rhinology	rhin/o	nose
12.	urology	ur/o	urinary tract/ urine

Check your answers with Appendix VIII, Answers to Exercises.

WRITE IT!

EXERCISE 3

Write the meaning of these combining forms.

1.	crin/o	to secrete
2.	enter/o	intestines
3.	esthesi/o	feeling or sensation
4.	gastr/o	stomach
5.	ger/o	elderly
6.	laryng/o	larynx
7.	nat/o	birth
8.	ne/o	new
9.	obstetr/o	midwife
10.	orth/o	straight
11.	ot/o	ear
12.	ped/o	child, foot

Check your answers with Appendix VIII, Answers to Exercises.

Now use these combining forms with the suffixes you learned earlier to explore some new medical terms. One of the learning methods that you will be using in this book is known as *programmed learning*. Programmed learning begins with what you already know and teaches new concepts by the progressive introduction of new information or ideas. In some ways, it is similar to using a computer program, because it tells you immediately if you are right and allows you to learn at your own speed. The primary difference is that here you write your answers in the blanks provided. It is a proven and easy way to learn medical terminology.

PROGRAMMED LEARNING

Write down the answers as you work through the following programmed learning section. Details about how to use programmed learning are presented in the information below.

1. The left column is the answer column, which should be covered. Use the bookmark provided on the side cover, or fold a piece of paper lengthwise and position it so that it covers only the answer column.

   In programmed learning, each block of information preceded by a number is called a *frame.* This is the first frame of this chapter. Within most frames, there will be a blank in which to write an answer. After writing your answer in the blank, check to see if it is correct by sliding the bookmark down so that the answer column is uncovered.

   left   By the information presented here, you know that the answer is located in the _____ column of each frame. (Write an answer in the blank.)

2. You are using the programmed learning method. A block of information with a number is called a _____. Whenever you see frames, you **frame** will recognize that you are learning by the programmed method.

   Always check your answer immediately. If your answer is incorrect, look back at previous frames to determine where you went wrong. You are now ready to put this information to use.

3. You may already know some of the terms that are associated with the medical specialties. If you do not recognize the combining forms used in the following frames, look back at the listing that you just studied. For example, the study of the heart and its function is **cardio+logy.** A physician who **cardiologist** specializes in diseases of the heart is a _____.

   Cardiac (*cardi/o,* heart + *-ac,* pertaining to) means "pertaining to the heart."

4. Combine derm/a and -al to write a term that means "pertaining to the skin": **dermal** _____.

   Dermato+logic and **dermato+logical** also refer to the skin. Whether one chooses to say dermatologic or dermatological depends on one's preference. Both -ic and -al mean "pertaining to." Many adjectives accept either -ic or -al. The ending -ical makes use of both suffixes.

5. A person with acne problems or skin allergies would be treated by a **dermatologist. Dermatology** is the medical specialty concerned with the **skin** diagnosis and treatment of diseases of the _____.

6. **Gyneco+logy** (GYN, Gyn, gyn) is devoted to treating diseases of the female reproductive organs, including the breasts. A physician who specializes in the **gynecologist** treatment of females is a _____.

7. Many gynecologists also specialize in obstetrics. **Obstetrics** deals with pregnancy, labor, delivery, and immediate care after childbirth; however, obstetr/o means midwife. Midwives assisted women during childbirth before obstetrics developed as a medical specialty. Physicians who specialize in obstetrics are **obstetricians.** Two adjectives, **obstetric** and **obstetrical,** mean **pertaining** _____ to obstetrics.

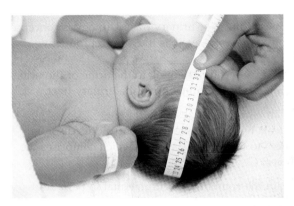

-logy = science of
nat/o = birth
ne/o = new

Figure 2-2 Measuring the head of a newborn.
This is the appropriate placement of the measuring tape to obtain the head circumference of a newborn. Neonatology focuses on care of the newborn.

neonatologist

8. **Neo+nato+logy** is the branch of medicine that specializes in the care of newborns, infants from birth to 28 days of age. Newborns are given a physical examination after birth, including weight, length, and head circumference measurements (Figure 2-2). A physician who specializes in neonatology is a _____.

practitioner

9. **Ped+iatrics** is devoted to the treatment of children. Diseases of children are often quite different from diseases encountered later in life.
The combining form for child is ped/o. Pediatric means pertaining to children. The suffix -iatrician, which means _____, is used to write the name of the physician who specializes in pediatrics. A **pediatrician** specializes in the development and care of infants and children and in the treatment of their diseases.

ophthalmologist

10. **Ophthalmo+logy** is the branch of medicine that specializes in the study, diagnosis, and treatment of disorders of the eye. Write the name of the specialist in ophthalmology by combining ophthalm/o and -logist: _____. **Ophthalmic, ophthalmologic,** and **ophthalmological** mean pertaining to the eye.

11. An **oto+logist** specializes in **otology,** the study of the ear, including the diagnosis and treatment of its diseases and disorders. Physicians who specialize in ear, nose, and throat disorders are ear, nose, and throat (ENT) specialists. The combining form ot/o means ear, and laryng/o means larynx (voice box). **Oto+laryngo+logy** refers to the branch of medicine dealing with diseases and disorders of the ears, nose, throat, and nearby structures. An

otolaryngology

otolaryngologist is a physician who practices _____. **Ot+ic** means pertaining to the ear.

12. **Rhino+logy** specializes in the diagnosis and treatment of disorders involving the nose. Write the name of the physician who specializes in rhinology: _____.

rhinologist

urologist

13. The combining form ur/o means urine or urinary tract. Urology is concerned with the urinary tract in both genders, as well as the male reproductive system. A specialist in **urology** is a _____.
Urologic, urological, and **urinary** mean pertaining to the urine or the urinary system. A urologic examination is an examination of the urinary tract.

neurology

14. A **neuro+logist** is a physician who specializes in _____, the field of medicine that deals with the nervous system and its disorders. In many words, neur/o refers to the nervous system, which comprises the brain, spinal cord, and nerves.

rheumatologist

15. Almost all words that contain the combining form rheumat/o pertain to **rheumatism. Rheumato+logy** is the branch of medicine that deals with rheumatic disorders. Rather than just one disease, rheumatism is any of a variety of disorders marked by inflammation, degeneration, and other problems of the connective tissues, especially the joints and related structures. A specialist in rheumatology is a _____.
   Ancient Greeks believed that one's health was determined by the mixture of "humors," or certain fluids within the body. The word *rheum* meant "a watery discharge"; rheumatism was thought to be caused by a flowing of humors in the body and was thus named.

immunologist

16. **Immuno+logy** represents one of the most rapidly expanding areas of science, and immun/o is the combining form for immune. This branch of science involves assessment of the patient's immune defense mechanism against disease and the many associated diseases. The immune mechanism includes the natural defenses that protect the body from diseases and cancer, but it is also involved in *allergies*, excessive reactions to common and often harmless substances in the environment.
   The immunology specialist is an _____. In some cases, immunology is combined with the identification and treatment of allergies.

endocrinologist

17. The **endocrine** glands secrete chemical messengers called *hormones* into the bloodstream. These hormones play an important role in regulating the body's metabolism. The prefix *endo-* means "inside." The suffix *-crine*, from the combining form crin/o, means "to secrete." Glands that secrete hormones into the bloodstream are endocrine glands.
   The science of the endocrine glands and the hormones they produce is **endocrinology.** A specialist in endocrinology is an _____.

radiologist

18. The combining form radi/o means radiation (sometimes radi/o is used to mean *radius*, a bone of the forearm, but usually it refers to radiation). **Radio+logy** is the use of various forms of radiation (e.g., x-rays) in the diagnosis and treatment of disease. The physician who specializes in radiology is a diagnostic imaging specialist, called a _____.
Two terms that mean pertaining to radiology are **radiologic** and **radiological.**

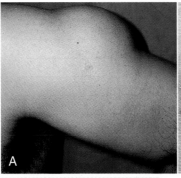
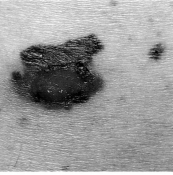

melan/o = black
-oma = tumor

Figure 2-3 Two types of tumors. A, Benign tumor, a lipoma, which consists of mature fat cells. **B,** Malignant melanoma, a type of skin cancer. Benign and malignant tumors have different characteristics; however, definite diagnosis is possible by microscopic study of the cells of a suspicious tumor.

oncologist

19. **Onco+logy,** a rapidly changing specialty, involves the study of malignancy. The combining form *onc/o* means "tumor." Oncology is particularly concerned with malignant tumors and their treatment. **Malignant** means "tending to become worse, spread, and cause death." *Cancer* refers to any of a large group of diseases that are characterized by the presence of malignant cells.
    A specialist who practices oncology is an _____.

neoplasm

20. The word *tumor* is used in different ways. It sometimes means a swelling or enlargement, but it often refers to a spontaneous new growth of tissue that forms an abnormal mass. This latter definition is also called a **neoplasm.** A **benign** tumor is not cancerous, so it does not spread to other parts of the body. Benign is the opposite of malignant (Figure 2-3). Write the term you just learned that means a spontaneous new growth of tissue: _____.

gastroenterology

21. **Gastro+entero+logy** is the study of diseases affecting the gastrointestinal tract, including the stomach and intestines. Write the name of this specialty that deals with the stomach and intestines: _____.
    Gastr+ic means pertaining to the stomach. A physician who specializes in gastric and intestinal disorders is a **gastroenterologist.**

geriatrician

22. Three combining forms *ger/a, ger/o,* and *geront/o* mean "old age" or "the aged." The scientific study of all aspects of the aging process and issues encountered by older persons is **gerontology.** The branch of medicine that deals with the problems of aging and the diseases of elderly persons is **geriatrics.** A physician who specializes in gerontology is a _____.

The selection of the correct combining form may be confusing. Common usage determines which term is proper. Practice will help you remember.

Write terms using these words parts.

1. cardi/o + -ac   cardiac
2. gynec/o + -logic   gynecologic
3. obstetr/o + -ics   obstetrics
4. ne/o + nat/o + -logy   neonatology
5. ophthalm/o + -ic   ophthalmic
6. ot/o + laryng/o + -logy   otolaryngology
7. rheumat/o + -logist   rheumatologist
8. endo- + -crine   endocrine
9. onc/o + -logist   oncologist
10. gastr/o + enter/o + -logist   gastroenterologist

Check your answers with Appendix VIII, Answers to Exercises.

path/o = disease

Pathology is the general study of the characteristics, causes, and effects of disease. *Cellular* pathology is the study of cellular changes in disease. *Clinical* pathology is the study of disease by the use of laboratory tests and methods. A medical **pathologist** usually specializes in either clinical or *surgical* pathology. A clinical pathologist is especially concerned with the use of laboratory methods in clinical diagnosis.

Tissues and organs that are removed in surgery are sent to the surgical pathology laboratory. The physician who studies those tissues and organs to determine the cause of disease is a surgical pathologist.

The terms **pathologic** and **pathological** mean "morbid" or "pertaining to a condition that is caused by or that involves a disease process."

The term *surgery* is derived from a Greek word that means "handwork." Surgery includes several branches of medicine that treat disease, injuries, and deformities by manual or operative procedures (Figure 2-4). Surgery also

an- = no
esthesi/o = feeling
-logy = science of

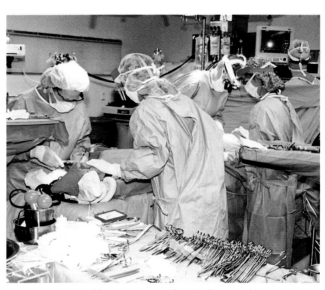

Figure 2-4 **Surgery.** Surgeons are assisted by nurses, technologists, and persons specialized in anesthesiology.

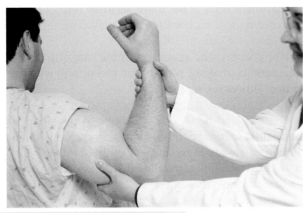

-ist = specialist
orth/o = straight
ped/o = child

Figure 2-5 Orthopedist examining a patient. Orthopedics is a branch of medicine that specializes in the prevention and correction of disorders of the muscular and skeletal systems of the body.

refers to the work performed by a surgeon or the place where surgery is performed.

General surgery deals with all types of surgical procedures. There are many other surgical specialties, such as those dealing exclusively with the head and neck, hand, and urinary system. A **neurosurgeon** specializes in surgery of the nervous system. Neurosurgery is surgery involving the brain, spinal cord, or peripheral nerves.

neur/o = nerve

Ortho+ped+ics is a branch of surgery that deals with the preservation and restoration of the bones and associated structures. The specialist is called an **ortho+ped+ist**, or orthopedic surgeon (Figure 2-5). The orthopedist originally straightened children's bones and corrected deformities. Today an orthopedist specializes in disorders of the bones and associated structures in people of all ages.

orth/o = straight
ped/o = child

An+esthesio+logy is the branch of medicine concerned with the administration of anesthetics and their effects. The physician who administers anesthetics during surgery is an **anesthesiologist**. The prefix *an-* means no, not, or without. Although the literal interpretation of anesthesiology is "the study of no feeling," you need to remember that it is the branch of medicine concerned with the administration of drugs that produce a loss of feeling.

An **an+esthetist** is not a physician but is trained in administering anesthetics. An **anesthetic** is a drug or agent that is capable of producing an+esthes+ia, or loss of sensation or feeling. Anesthetic also means pertaining to anesthesia.

Anesthetics are classified as local or general according to their action. *Local* anesthetics affect a local area only, rather than the entire body. *General* anesthetics act on the brain and cause loss of consciousness.

Some people mistakenly associate anesthesia with normal sleep. A sleeping person can be awakened and normal awareness immediately restored, unlike someone who has been given a general anesthetic.

There are many other areas in which physicians specialize. Emergency medicine deals with very ill or injured patients who require immediate medical treatment. The emergency department is commonly called the "ER" (emergency room), but emergency department (ED) is the more accurate term. On arrival, patients are often prioritized according to their need for treatment. The method of sorting according to the patients' needs for care is called **triage.**

Hospital+ists are physicians who specialize in the care of patients who are staying in the hospital, sometimes making rounds for physicians who are on vacation or choose to stay in their offices seeing patients.

Psych+iatry is a medical specialty that deals with the causes, treatment, and prevention of mental, emotional, and behavioral disorders. A physician who specializes in psychiatry is a **psychiatrist.** Clinical psycho+logy is concerned with the diagnosis, treatment, and prevention of a wide range of personality and behavioral disorders. One who is trained in this area is a clinical psychologist. Clinical psychology is not a branch of medicine but a branch of psychology.

psych/o = mind

Physicians who specialize in the care of patients in intensive care are **intensivists.** The intensive care unit (ICU) is a place in the hospital that contains sophisticated monitoring devices and equipment for patients requiring close monitoring and care by specially trained personnel.

Preventive medicine is the branch of medicine involving the prevention of disease and methods for increasing the abilities of the patient and community to resist disease and prolong life. A physician or scientist who studies the incidence, prevalence, spread, prevention, and control of disease in a community or a specific group of individuals is an **epidemiologist.** An epidemic attacks several people in a region at the same time. In a hospital, physicians who specialize in **epidemiology** may have the responsibility of directing infection control programs.

Some physicians specialize in sports medicine, involving the prevention, diagnosis, and treatment of sports-related injuries. Physicians are often assisted by a **therapist,** a person with special skills who is trained in one or more areas of health care. A specialist in **forensic medicine** deals with the legal aspects of health care. Aerospace medicine is concerned with the effects of living and working in an artificial environment beyond the Earth's atmosphere and the forces of gravity.

Work the following reviews to test your understanding of the medical specialists.

MATCH IT!
EXERCISE 5

Match the medical specialists with the areas in which they specialize.

D **1.** anesthesiologist   A children
I **2.** dermatologist   B disease in general
H **3.** geriatrician   C ear, nose, and throat
E **4.** gynecologist   D feeling or sensation
G **5.** neonatologist   E females
F **6.** neurologist   F nervous system
J **7.** oncologist   G newborns
C **8.** otolaryngologist   H older persons
B **9.** pathologist   I skin
A **10.** pediatrician   J tumors

Check your answers with Appendix VIII, Answers to Exercises.

WRITE IT!

EXERCISE 6

Write the specialty associated with these conditions or situations.

1. heart attack — cardiology
2. interpreting a radiograph — radiology
3. deficiency of the immune system — immunology
4. hormonal deficiency — endocrinology
5. nosebleed — rhinology
6. miscarriage — obstetrics
7. irritable bowel disease — gastroenterology
8. urinary infection — urology
9. broken wrist — orthopedics
10. rheumatoid arthritis — rheumatology

Suffixes: Surgical Procedures

A list of suffixes pertaining to surgical procedures follows. Commit the meanings of these suffixes to memory. It is necessary to take some time now to memorize the suffixes and their meanings; this can be done in several ways. One way is to read each suffix, its meaning, and its *word association* (a familiar word associated with the suffix). Also, think of words you may know that can help you to remember the meaning. After you have studied the list for a few minutes and think you know it, use flashcards, or cover the column that contains the meanings and word associations, and then check to make sure that you know each meaning.

All the suffixes in the surgical procedures list form nouns when combined with other word parts.

Suffixes: Surgical Procedures

Suffix	Meaning	Word Association
-centesis	surgical puncture to aspirate or remove fluid	**Amniocentesis** is puncture of the amnion for removing fluid for study or administering treatment to the fetus (Figure 2-6).
-ectomy	excision (surgical removal or cutting out)	Appendectomy is **excision** of the appendix.
-lysis	process of loosening, freeing, or destroying	This suffix is also used in nonsurgical words to mean destruction or dissolving, as in **hemolysis.**
-pexy	surgical fixation (fastening in a fixed position)	**Mastopexy** is plastic surgery that fastens breasts in a fixed position to correct sagging.
-plasty	surgical repair	Plastic is derived from the same word root as -plasty. Plastic surgery repairs, restores, and reconstructs body structures. **Mammoplasty** is plastic surgery of the breast and is done for a variety of reasons.
-rrhaphy	suture (uniting a wound by stitches)	This suffix is not generally used in everyday language, but **angiorrhaphy** means **suture** of a blood vessel.
-scopy	visual examination with a lighted instrument (not always a surgical procedure)	**Microscopy** is visual examination of very small objects with a magnifying instrument **(microscope).** The suffix -scope means the instrument. Micro- means small.

Suffixes: Surgical Procedures—Cont'd

Suffix	Meaning	Word Association
-stomy	formation of an opening	A **tracheostomy** is a surgical procedure that forms a new opening into the trachea (windpipe).
-tome	an instrument used for cutting	A **microtome** is an instrument used for cutting thin sections of tissue for microscopic study.
-tomy	incision (cutting into tissue)	A **tracheotomy** is an **incision** of the trachea through the skin and muscles in the neck that overlie the **trachea** (windpipe).
-tripsy	surgical crushing	**Lithotripsy** is surgical crushing of a calculus (stone) (Figure 2-7)

Use the electronic flashcards on the Evolve site or make your own set of flashcards using the above list. Select the word parts just presented, and study them until you know their meanings.

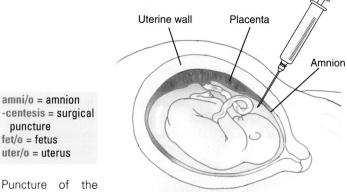

amni/o = amnion
-centesis = surgical puncture
fet/o = fetus
uter/o = uterus

Figure 2-6 Amniocentesis. Puncture of the amniotic sac is done to remove fluid for study of the fetal cells.

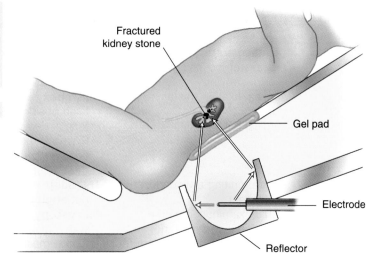

-ary, -eal = pertaining to
corpor/o = body
extra- = outside
lith/o = stone (calculus)
-tripsy = surgical crushing
urin/o = urine or urination

Figure 2-7 Lithotripsy, crushing of a stone (calculus). Extracorporeal shock wave lithotripsy, illustrated here, is used to crush certain urinary tract stones. Extracorporeal means outside the body. The reflector focuses a high-energy shock wave on the stone. The stone disintegrates into particles and is passed in the urine. Originally, lithotripsy referred only to the surgical technique of crushing the stone with an instrument.

MATCH IT!

EXERCISE 7

Match the suffixes in the right column with their meanings in the left column.

J	1. instrument used for cutting	A. -centesis
G	2. instrument used for viewing	B. -ectomy
B	3. excision	C. -lysis
I	4. formation of an opening	D. -pexy
K	5. incision	E. -plasty
C	6. process of destroying	F. -rrhaphy
L	7. surgical crushing*	G. -scope
D	8. surgical fixation	H. -scopy
A	9. surgical puncture	I. -stomy
E	10. surgical repair	J. -tome
F	11. suture	K. -tomy
H	12. visual examination with an instrument	L. -tripsy

* Specifically means crushing and not "destruction by other means."

Combining Forms for Selected Body Structures

You already know combining forms for several body structures used earlier to name the medical specialists. Additional combining forms are presented in the following list. This list is not intended to be complete. Many combining forms are presented in later chapters, which discuss major body systems. You should commit the following list to memory because subsequent chapters assume that you have learned these combining forms. Practice learning the material here in the same manner as you learned the list of suffixes pertaining to surgical procedures.

Read the term, its meaning, and its word association. When you think you know the material, use flashcards, or cover the two columns on the right, and try to recall the meaning of each combining form. These combining forms will be used shortly to study medical terminology in more detail and to learn how to build words. Read on!

Combining Forms for Selected Body Structures

Combining Form	Meaning	Word Association
aden/o	gland	**Adenoids** were so named because they resembled or were thought to be glands.
angi/o	vessel	An **angiogram** is an x-ray film of blood vessels filled with a contrast medium.
append/o, appendic/o	appendix	An appendectomy is excision of the appendix.
bi/o	life or living	**Biology** is the science of life and living things.
blephar/o	eyelid	**Blepharoptosis** is the drooping of the upper eyelid.
cerebr/o,* encephal/o	brain	**Cerebral** palsy is paralysis caused by a brain defect. **Encephalitis** is inflammation of the brain.
chir/o	hand	Writer's cramp is a type of **chirospasm**.

Continued

Combining Forms for Selected Body Structures—cont'd

Combining Form	Meaning	Word Association
col/o	colon or large intestine	Coloscopy is visual examination of the colon, but the term **colonoscopy** is more commonly used.
cutane/o, derm/a, dermat/o	skin	**Cutaneous** means pertaining to the skin. A dermatologist is a specialist who treats diseases of the skin. Dermabrasion removes small scars, tattoos, or fine wrinkles from the skin.
faci/o	face	**Facial** pertains to the face.
hepat/o	liver	**Hepatitis** is an inflammatory condition of the liver.
mamm/o, mast/o	breast	**Mammography** is the use of x-rays to diagnose breast diseases. Mastectomy is surgical removal of the breast.
muscul/o, my/o	muscle	A person with well-developed muscles is **muscular.** **Myalgia** is muscle pain.
myel/o	bone marrow or spinal cord	**Myelopathy** has two meanings: any disease of the spinal cord or any disease of the bone marrow.
oste/o	bone	**Osteoarthritis** is a common type of arthritis of older persons, in which one or more joints undergo degenerative changes, but named to include both bones and joints.
pulm/o, pulmon/o, pneum/o,† pneumon/o	lungs	**Pulmonary** means pertaining to the lungs. **Pneumonia** is a lung condition. **Pneumatic** means pertaining to air or gas.
tonsill/o	tonsil	**Tonsillitis** is inflammation of the tonsils.
trache/o	trachea (windpipe)	A tracheostomy is an operation that forms a new opening into the trachea.
vas/o	vessel; **ductus deferens‡**	**Vasectomy** is the removal of all or a segment of the vas deferens and is a form of male contraception.

Use the electronic flashcards on the Evolve site or make your own set of flashcards using the above list. Select the word parts just presented, and study them until you know their meanings.

*cerebr/o sometimes means **cerebrum,** the main portion of the brain.
†pneum/o sometimes means air or gas.
‡Also called vas deferens, excretory duct of the testicle.*

CIRCLE IT!   EXERCISE 8

Circle the correct answer.

1. Which combining form means vessel? (aden/o, angi/o, chir/o, faci/o)
2. Which combining form means bone? (bi/o, blephar/o, myel/o, oste/o)
3. Which combining form means brain? (cutane/o, encephal/o, faci/o, vas/o)
4. Which combining form means breast? (cerebr/o, mast/o, pneumon/o, pulm/o)
5. Which combining form means skin? (derm/a, hepat/o, mamm/o, my/o)

Check your answers with Appendix VIII, Answers to Exercises.

Write the combining form, suffix, and their meanings for these new terms (Question 1 is done as an example). A short definition is provided for each term.

Term/Meaning	Combining Form	Suffix
1. **colopexy** surgical fixation of the colon to the abdominal wall	*col/o, colon*	*-pexy, surgical fixation*
2. **adenectomy** excision of a gland	*aden/o, gland*	*-ectomy, excision*
3. **colostomy** opening of some portion of the large intestine onto abdominal surface	*col/o, large intestine*	*-stomy, formation of an opening*
4. **coloscopy** visual examination of the colon with a lighted instrument	*col/o, colon*	*-scopy, visual exam*
5. **mastectomy** removal of one or both breasts	*mast/o, breast*	*-ectomy, excision*
6. **mastitis** inflammation of the breast	*mast/o, breast*	*-itis, inflammation*
7. **mastopexy** surgical fixation of the breasts	*mast/o, breast*	*-pexy, surgical fixation*
8. **neurectomy** partial or total excision of a nerve (partial or total is implied)	*neur/o, nerve*	*-ectomy, excision*
9. **neurolysis** destruction of nerve tissue or loosening of adhesions surrounding a nerve	*neur/o, nerve*	*-ectomy, excision*
10. **neuroplasty** surgical repair of a nerve or nerves	*neur/o, nerve*	*-plasty, surgical repair*

Check your answers with Appendix VIII, Answers to Exercises.

A colostomy is an opening of some portion of the large intestine onto the abdominal surface. This type of surgery is performed when solid waste (feces) cannot be eliminated through the normal opening because of some pathologic condition.

col/o = colon
-stomy = formation of an opening
-pexy = surgical fixation

Colopexy is a surgical procedure in which the colon is sutured (surgically fixed, sewn, or otherwise attached) to the abdominal wall. The term *suture* has several meanings: the act of uniting a wound by stitches, the material used in closing a wound with stitches, or the stitch made to secure the edges of a wound. If you study anatomy, you will learn that suture also refers to a type of joint in which the opposed surfaces are closely united, as in the skull.

Mastectomy may be performed when cancer of the breast is present. A breast biopsy is often done when a suspicious lump is found in the breast. A **biopsy** is excision of a small lump for microscopic examination, usually performed to establish a diagnosis (bi/o means life or living). The biopsy can be performed with a needle (needle biopsy) or by excision of the suspicious lump (**lumpectomy**).

mast/o = breast
-ectomy = excision

Mammoplasty is plastic surgery of the breast and is done for a variety of reasons. Reduction mammoplasty is done to reduce the size of the breasts, whereas **augmentation mammoplasty** increases the size of the breasts (Figure 2-8).

-mamm/o = breast
-plasty = surgical repair

Figure 2-8 Augmentation mammoplasty. This surgical procedure to enlarge the breasts is achieved by inserting envelopes filled with silicone gel (shown here) or saline beneath normal breast tissue or beneath the muscle of the chest. The incision below the breast causes the least obvious scarring of several approaches that may be taken.

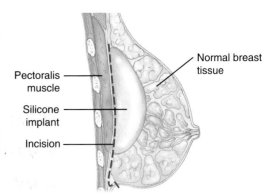

Pectoralis muscle
Normal breast tissue
Silicone implant
Incision

mamm/o = breast
-plasty = surgical repair

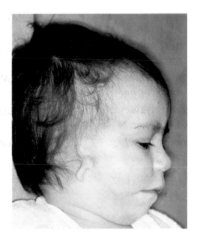

-ia = condition
micro- = small
ot/o = ear
-plasty = surgical repair

Figure 2-9 Microtia. This example shows the unusual size that results from underdevelopment of the external ear. Otoplasty, reconstructive surgery of the ear, is generally performed before the child reaches school age.

PROGRAMMED LEARNING

Remember to cover the answers (left column) with folded paper or the bookmark. Write an answer in each blank, and then check your answer before proceeding to the next frame.

otoplasty	1. Surgical repair of the eye is **ophthalmoplasty.** Surgical repair of the ear is _____. (See Figure 2-9 for an abnormality of the ear **(microtia)** that indicates a need for otoplasty.) Did you remember to check your answer immediately? Always be certain that you have spelled the word correctly.
ophthalmo+scopy	2. In addition to writing medical terms, you will learn how to divide words into their component parts and to analyze their meanings. Plus signs are used to show the component parts of a word, for example, oto+plasty. Observe that ot/o (ear) is joined to -plasty, the suffix you learned that means surgical repair. When analyzing difficult terms, look for familiar word parts. Divide **ophthalmoscopy** into its component parts: _____.

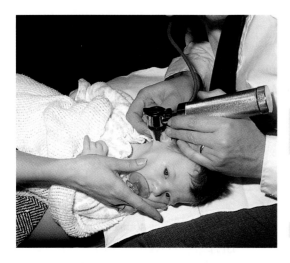

ot/o = ear
-scope = instrument used for viewing
-scopy = visual examination

Figure 2-10 Otoscopy. An otoscope is used to visually examine the eardrum.

otoscopy	3. You learned that -scopy means visual examination. Ophthalmoscopy means examination of the eye. Visual examination of the ear is _____. These examinations are often called **otoscopic** and **ophthalmoscopic** examinations. (The child in Figure 2-10 is undergoing otoscopy with an **otoscope.**) The instrument used in ophthalmoscopy is an **ophthalmoscope.**
skin	4. Cutane+ous means pertaining to the _____.
pertaining	5. In the previous frame, -ous is a suffix that means _____ to. (It can also mean "characterized by.")
skin	6. **Dermato+plasty** is surgical repair of the _____. This is skin grafting or transplantation of living skin to cover defects caused by injury, surgery, or disease.
dermatome	7. Use derm/a to write a term that means "an instrument used to incise the skin": _____.*
encephalotome	8. Use encephal/o to write a word that means an instrument for incising brain tissue: _____.
cerebrotomy	9. Two words that mean incision of the brain are **encephalotomy** and _____.
ophthalmoplasty	10. Surgical repair of the eye is _____.
angioplasty	11. Use angi/o to write a word that means surgical repair of vessels (blood vessels, in this case): _____.
angiorrhaphy	12. Use angio+plasty as a model to write a word that means suture of a vessel (especially a blood vessel): _____.

*Most anatomy books give a different meaning for dermatome. For terminology purposes, just be aware that dermatome has a second meaning.

angiectomy	13. Use the last word you wrote as a model to form a word that means excision or cutting out of a blood vessel: _____.
appendectomy	14. Use append/o to write a word that means removal of the appendix: _____.
tonsillectomy	15. Write a word that means excision of the tonsils: _____.
puncture	16. The **amnion** is the thin transparent membrane that surrounds the fetus (unborn child). Amnio+centesis is surgical _____ of the amnion.
hepatic	17. Use -ic to write a word that means pertaining to the liver: _____.
my/o	18. Muscular means pertaining to muscle or describes someone with well-developed muscles. You also need to remember another combining form for muscle, which is _____.
myel/o	19. A combining form that means either bone marrow or the spinal cord is _____.
lungs	20. Pulm/o, pulmon/o, and pneum/o mean _____.

See how easy it is to learn new words using the programmed method! You are already writing impressive medical terms.

BUILD IT!

EXERCISE 10

Use -plasty to write terms for these meanings.

1. surgical repair of a vessel _vasoplasty_
2. surgical repair of the breast _mastoplasty_
3. surgical repair of the ear _ophthalmoplasty_
4. surgical repair of the eye _otoplasty_
5. surgical repair of the skin _derm dermaplasty_

BUILD IT!

EXERCISE 11

Combine the word parts to write terms.

1. excision of the appendix: append/o + -ectomy _appendectomy_
2. instrument for incising brain tissue: encephal/o + -tome _encephalotome_
3. instrument for viewing the eye: ophthalm/o + -scope _ophthalmoscope_
4. pertaining to the ear: ot/o + -ic _otic_
5. removal of the tonsils: tonsill/o + -ectomy _tonsillectomy_
6. surgical fixation of the colon: col/o + -pexy _colopexy_
7. suture of a vessel: angi/o + -rrhaphy _angiorrhaphy_
8. visual examination of the ear: ot/o + -scopy _otoscopy_

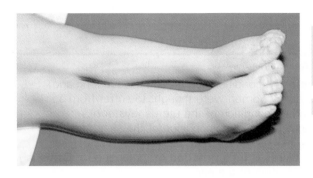

-edema = swelling
-ic = pertaining to
lymph/o = lymph, lymphatics
lymphat/o = lymphatics

Figure 2-11 Lymphedema. This particular type of edema of the right lower limb and foot is caused by obstructed lymphatic vessels. It is sometimes an inherited trait, but the cause is not always known.

Suffixes: Symptoms or Diagnosis

Symptoms and diagnosis are frequently used terms, but they are sometimes used inaccurately. You will study both terms more in depth in Chapter 4. *A symptom is a health change as perceived by the patient, and diagnosis is the identification of a disease or condition by scientific evaluation.* Several important suffixes pertain to symptoms and diagnosis.

Commit the following suffixes and their meanings to memory. Remember to read each suffix, its meaning, and the word association presented. Be certain that you are familiar with this information before proceeding to Exercises 12 and 13.

Suffixes: Symptoms or Diagnosis

Suffix	Meaning	Word Association
-algia, -dynia	pain	**Neuralgia** is pain along the course of a nerve. Both **otodynia** and **otalgia** mean pain in the ear.
-cele	**hernia** (protrusion of all or part of an organ through wall of cavity that contains it)	An **encephalocele** is a hernia of the brain through an opening in the skull.
-ectasia, -ectasis	**dilatation** (dilation, enlargement or stretching of a structure or part)	**Angiectasis** means dilation of a blood or lymph vessel. **Neurectasia** is stretching of a nerve.
-edema	swelling	**Edema** is a word that means the presence of abnormally large amounts of fluid in the tissues; it is usually applied to an accumulation of excessive fluid in the subcutaneous tissues, resulting in swelling (Figure 2-11). **Lymphedema** is an abnormal accumulation of tissue fluid brought about by lymphatic vessel disruption.
-emesis	vomiting	**Emesis** is a word that means vomiting.
-emia	condition of the blood	**Bacteremia** is the presence of bacteria in the blood.

Continued

Suffixes: Symptoms or Diagnosis—cont'd

Suffix	Meaning	Word Association
-ia, -iasis	condition	**Hysteria** is a condition so named because long ago hysterical women were thought to suffer from a disturbed condition of the uterus (hyster/o). **Psoriasis** is a disease condition of the skin marked by itchy lesions (from Greek *psora,* "itch").
-itis	inflammation	**Appendicitis** is **inflammation** of the appendix. **Otitis** is inflammation of the ear.
-lith	stone or calculus	Another name for a gallstone is **cholelith.**
-malacia	soft, softening	**Osteomalacia** is softening of the bones.
-mania	excessive preoccupation	In **kleptomania,** an excessive preoccupation leads to stealing on impulse.
-megaly	enlargement	You may be more familiar with mega-. Both mega- and megal- mean large, as in megalopolis, a large city, and megaton, a large explosive force.
-oid (forms adjectives and nouns)	resembling	**Mucoid** means similar to or resembling mucus. **Paranoid** means resembling **paranoia,** a psychotic disorder characterized by delusions of persecution.
-oma	tumor	**Carcinoma** is cancer, or a cancerous tumor.
-osis	condition (often an abnormal condition; sometimes an increase)	**Neurosis** is a nervous condition (disorder) that is not caused by a demonstrable structural change.
-pathy	disease	The suffix -pathy is derived from the same source as many words that contain path/o; for example, **pathogenic** organisms can cause disease.
-penia	deficiency	**Calcipenia** means a deficiency of calcium.
-phobia	abnormal fear	**Phobia** means an obsessive, irrational fear of a specific object, activity, or a physical situation, such as fear of heights. "Hydrophobia" is an obsolete term for rabies.*
-ptosis	prolapse (sagging)	**Ptosis** means sagging. It also refers to drooping or sagging eyelids.
-rrhage, -rrhagia	excessive bleeding or hemorrhage	**Hemorrhage** is abnormal internal or external bleeding.
-rrhea	flow or discharge	A urethral or vaginal discharge is a primary feature of **gonorrhea.**
-rrhexis	rupture	**Cardiorrhexis** literally means "ruptured heart." One might think of a lover's broken heart, but cardiorrhexis is a pathologic condition in which the heart ruptures.
-spasm	twitching, cramp	**Spasm** means involuntary and sudden movement or convulsive muscular contraction. When contractions are strong and painful, they are often called "cramps."
-stasis	stopping, controlling	**Stasis** means slowing or stopping.

Use the electronic flashcards on the Evolve site or make your own set of flashcards using the above list. Select the word parts just presented, and study them until you know their meanings.

*A viral disease transmitted to humans by the bite of an infected animal, rabies was given the name hydrophobia after it was observed that stricken animals avoided water, as though they had a fear of it. Actually, rabid animals avoid water because they cannot swallow as a result of the paralysis caused by the virus.

MATCH IT!
EXERCISE 12

Match the suffixes in the right column with their meanings in the left column.

E **1.** condition   A. -algia
J **2.** controlling   B. -cele
C **3.** dilatation   C. -ectasis
I **4.** enlargement   D. -emesis
H **5.** excessive preoccupation   E. -iasis
B **6.** hernia   F. -itis
F **7.** inflammation   G. -malacia
A **8.** pain   H. -mania
G **9.** softening   I. -megaly
D **10.** vomiting   J. -stasis

CIRCLE IT!
EXERCISE 13

Circle the correct answer to complete each sentence.

1. The suffix -penia means (resembling, condition, (deficiency,) rupture).
2. The suffix -rrhexis means (resembling, (rupture,) preoccupation, cramp).
3. The suffix -oid means (flow, hemorrhage, (resembling,) condition).
4. The suffix -phobia means ((abnormal fear,) excessive preoccupation, deficiency, stopping).
5. The suffix -ptosis means (disease, fear, (prolapse,) decreased).
6. The suffix that means tumor is (-oid, (-oma,) -osis, -rrhagia).
7. The suffix meaning disease is ((-pathy,) -penia, -phobia, -ptosis).
8. The suffix that means flow or discharge is (-rrhage, (-rrhea,) -rrhexis, -penia).
9. Several of the suffixes that you learned are also words. One suffix that means cramp or twitching and that can also stand alone as a word is (ptosis, phobia, (spasm,) stasis).
10. Excessive bleeding is represented by the suffix (-rrhea, (-rrhage,) -rrhexis, -pathy).

PROGRAMMED LEARNING

Remember to cover the answers (left column) with folded paper or the bookmark. Write an answer in each blank, and then check your answer before proceeding to the next frame.

inflammation	**1.** In studying the suffixes pertaining to symptoms or diagnosis, you learned that -itis means _____.
ophthalmitis	**2.** The combining form for eye is ophthalm/o. Write a word that means inflammation of the eye: _____.
appendicitis	**3.** Using the combining form appendic/o (meaning appendix), write a word that means inflammation of the appendix: _____. (See how easy it is to write medical terms using this method!)

pain	4. When analyzing the term neur+algia, we see that it is derived from neur/o (meaning nerve) and the suffix -algia. Neur+algia means _____ along a nerve.
pain	5. **Ophthalm+algia** is _____ of the eye.
hernia	6. The Suffixes: Symptoms or Diagnosis list contains a word meaning "protrusion of all or part of an organ through the wall of the cavity that normally contains it." This word is _____.
-cele	7. The suffix that means hernia is _____.
hernia (or herniation)	8. An encephalo+cele is _____ of the brain through an opening in the skull. (This is also called a cerebral hernia.)
hernia	9. Gastr/o means stomach. A **gastro+cele** is a _____ of the stomach.
vomiting	10. **Hyper+emesis** means excessive _____. Hyper- means excessive or above normal.
vomiting	11. **Hemat+emesis** is _____ of blood. Hemat/o means blood.
prolapse	12. The word ptosis means sag or prolapse. Blepharo+ptosis is _____ of the eyelid. Blephar/o means eyelid.
-rrhagia	13. The suffix -rrhage means excessive bleeding. Another suffix for forming words to indicate hemorrhage is _____.
bleeding	14. **Ophthalmo+rrhagia** is hemorrhage or excessive _____ from the eye.
discharge	15. Another suffix beginning with a double *r* is -rrhea. In the sexually transmitted disease gono+rrhea, -rrhea refers to the heavy _____ that is characteristic of the disease.
rupture	16. Cardi/o means heart. Cardio+rrhexis is _____ of the heart.
ophthalmorrhexis	17. Using ophthalm/o and the suffix for rupture, write a word that means rupture of the eyeball: _____. Translated literally, the word means rupture of the eye.
chirospasm	18. Chir/o means hand. The word that means cramping of the hand is _____. This is sometimes called "writer's cramp."
angiectasis	19. Using angi/o, write a word that means dilation of a blood or lymph vessel: _____.
softening	20. Osteo+malacia is a disease marked by increased _____ of the bone (oste/o means bone).
preoccupation	21. You have probably heard of the word pyromaniac. **Pyro+mania** is excessive _____ with fire. **Pyromaniacs** enjoy watching or setting fires (pyr/o means fire).

pyrophobia	22. Add another suffix to pyr/o to form a word that means abnormal fear of fire: _____.
enlargement	23. **Cardio+megaly** is _____ of the heart.
resembling	24. Muc/o means mucus. Muc+oid means _____ mucus.
tumor	25. Carcinoma is a synonym for cancer. Carcin+oma is a cancerous growth or malignant _____.
skin	26. **Dermat+itis** is inflammation of the _____. It is evidenced by itching, redness, and various skin lesions (Figure 2-12)
condition	27. The suffix -osis means condition, but it sometimes implies a disease or abnormal increase. **Dermat+osis** is a skin _____. (Specifically, a dermatosis is any skin condition in which inflammation is not necessarily a symptom.)
dermatitis	28. A skin condition involving inflammation is called _____.
disease	29. Another suffix you learned that means disease is -pathy. **Ophthalmo+pathy** refers to any _____ of the eye.
	30. Perhaps you are familiar with the word **phlebitis,** which means inflammation of a vein. Add another suffix to phleb/o to write a word that means "controlling the flow of blood in a vein by means of compression":
phlebostasis	_____.
deficiency	31. Calci+penia means a _____ of calcium in body tissues and fluids.
condition	32. Lith/o is a combining form that means stone or calculus. **Lith+iasis** is a _____ in which a stone or calculus is present.

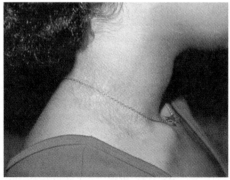

dermat/o = skin
-itis = inflammation

Figure 2-12 Dermatitis. This example of allergic dermatitis is caused by the metal nickel and usually results from contact with jewelry, metal clasps, or coins. Other types of allergic dermatitis may be caused by contact with poison ivy, other metals, or chemicals, including latex, dyes, and perfumes.

WRITE IT!
EXERCISE 14

Write terms for these meanings.
1. inflammation of a vein — _phlebitis_
2. inflammation of the appendix — _appendicitis_
3. inflammation of the ear — _otitis_
4. inflammation of the eye — _ophthalmitis_
5. inflammation of the skin — _dermatitis_

BUILD IT!
EXERCISE 15

Combine the word parts to write terms.
1. cramping of the hand: chir/o + -spasm — _chirospasm_
2. dilation of a vessel: angi/o + -ectasis — _angiectasis_
3. excessive preoccupation with fire: pyr/o + -mania — _pyromania_
4. hemorrhage from the eye: ophthalm/o + -rrhagia — _ophthalmorrhagia_
5. herniation of the brain: encephal/o + -cele — _encephalocele_
6. herniation of the stomach: gastr/o + -cele — _gastrocele_
7. skin condition lacking inflammation: dermat/o + -osis — _dermatosis_
8. pain along a nerve: neur/o + -algia — _neuralgia_
9. painful eye: ophthalm/o + -algia — _ophthalmalgia_
10. prolapse of the eyelid: blephar/o + -ptosis — _blepharoptosis_
11. rupture of the heart: cardi/o + -rrhexis — _cardiorrhexis_
12. vomiting of blood: hemat/o + -emesis — _hematemesis_

Miscellaneous Suffixes

Commit the following list of suffixes and their meanings to memory. Some important suffixes have been omitted, but they will be presented with their associated combining forms in subsequent chapters.

Miscellaneous Suffixes		
Suffix	**Meaning**	**Use in Sentence**
-able, -ible	capable of, able to	(adjective) Preventable means "capable of being prevented." Illegible describes writing that is not capable of being read.
-ac, -al, -an, -ar, -ary, -eal, -ic, -ive, -tic	pertaining to	(adjective) Cardiac, **thermal, median, alveolar, salivary, peritoneal, lymphatic, invasive,** and **nephrotic** mean pertaining to the heart, heat, middle, alveoli, saliva, peritoneum, lymphatic system, invasion, and kidney, respectively.
-ase	enzyme	(noun) **Lactase** is an enzyme that breaks down lactose.
-eum, -ium	membrane	(noun) The **peritoneum** lines the abdominal cavity. The membrane that lines the heart is **endocardium.**
-ia, -ism	condition or theory	(noun) **Synergism** is a condition in which two agents, such as medications, produce a greater effect than the total effects of each agent alone.

Miscellaneous Suffixes—cont'd

Suffix	Meaning	Use in Sentence
-iac	one who suffers	(noun) A **hemophiliac** is one who suffers from (is afflicted by) **hemophilia.**
-opia	vision	(noun) **Diplopia** is double vision.
-ose	sugar	(noun) **Lactose** is a sugar found in milk.
-ous	pertaining to or characterized by	(adjective) **Cancerous** means pertaining to cancer.
-y	state or condition	(noun) **Atrophy** is a condition of wasting away of a cell, tissue, organ, or part.

Use the electronic flashcards on the Evolve site or make your own set of flashcards using the above list. Select the word parts just presented, and study them until you know their meanings.

WRITE IT!

EXERCISE 16

Write the meaning of each underlined suffix. (Some meanings may have more than one word; e.g., the first answer is "capable of.")

1. coagul**able**   capable of
2. derm**al**   pertaining to
3. gluc**ose**   sugar
4. lact**ase**   enzyme
5. neuro**logist**   one who studies; specialist
6. ot**ic**   pertaining to
7. periton**eum**   membrane
8. synerg**ism**   condition/theory
9. oto**logist**   one who
10. tonsill**ar**   pertaining to

PROGRAMMED LEARNING

Remember to cover the answers (left column) with folded paper or the bookmark. Write an answer in each blank, and then check your answer before proceeding to the next frame.

studies

1. You have learned that -ist means one who and that -logist means one who _____. The suffixes -ist and -logist are both used to form nouns. The suffix -logist is derived from log/o, meaning knowledge or study, and from -ist, but -logist is used so frequently that it is more convenient to learn the suffix form. The suffix -logist often refers to a specialist. In medicine, a specialist is a person who has advanced education and training in one area of practice, such as internal medicine, dermatology, or cardiology.

specialist

2. A patho+logist is a _____ in pathology, the medical specialty that studies the nature and cause of disease.

pertaining	3. Log/o is combined with -y so often that we learn -logy as a suffix form that means "the study of." Whether pathology is divided as patho+logy or patho+log+y, the meaning is the same. Patho+log+ic means _____ to pathology or disease. (Pathological is another term that means the same as pathologic, but pathologic is the preferred form.)
pertaining	4. A neurologist treats neural disorders. **Neur+al** means _____ to the nerves or nervous system.
pertaining	5. Many suffixes mean pertaining to, and you will have an opportunity to practice using them as you progress through the material. You learned earlier that mamm/o means breast. **Mamm+ary** is an adjective that means _____ to the breast.
enzyme	6. **Enzymat+ic** (occasionally enzym+ic) means pertaining to enzymes, substances that facilitate chemical reactions. The suffix that means enzyme is -ase. By its suffix, we know that lact+ase has something to do with an _____.
lactase	7. Lact/o means milk. Lact+ase is an enzyme that acts on a sugar called lactose that is present in milk. Enzymes are usually named by adding -ase to the combining form of the substance on which they act. Translated literally, lact+ose means milk sugar. The enzyme that acts on lactose is called _____.
fat	8. Lip/o means fat. Fats are also called **lipids**, which should help you to remember the combining form. **Lip+ase** is an enzyme that breaks down _____.
amylase	9. Amyl/o means starch. Write the term that means an enzyme that breaks down starch: _____.
starch	10. The suffix for destruction is -lysis. **Amylo+lysis** is the destruction (digestion) of _____. In amylolysis, starch is broken down into sugar.
sugar	11. Glyc/o means sugar. **Glyco+lysis** is the breaking down of _____, which is accomplished by enzymes. These enzymes are named according to the specific sugar on which they act. Sucrase is an enzyme that acts on sucrose, common table sugar.
protease	12. Protein/o or prote/o means protein. Two words that mean "an enzyme that breaks down protein" are **proteinase** and _____. The breaking down or digestion of proteins is **proteo+lysis.** Proteins, as well as most substances we eat, must be broken down chemically before they can be absorbed by the body.

Miscellaneous Word Parts

You have learned several additional word parts in this chapter. If you do not recognize their meanings in the following list, commit them to memory before proceeding.

Reminder: **Bold type** indicates that a term is included in the Quick & Easy List and is pronounced on the Companion CD and audio CDs.

Miscellaneous Word Parts

Word Part	Meaning	Word Association
amyl/o	starch	Amylase is an enzyme that breaks down starch.
glyc/o	sugar	In **hypoglycemia** the blood sugar level is too low.
hemat/o	blood	Hematemesis is the vomiting of blood.
lact/o	milk	Milk is secreted by a woman during **lactation.**
lip/o	fat	Lipids are fats or fatlike substances.
lith/o	stone	Lithology is the study of rocks.
micro-	small	A microscope is an instrument used to view small (microscopic) objects.
muc/o	mucus	Generally, **mucous** membranes secrete **mucus.**
prote/o, protein/o	protein	**Proteinuria** is an excess of proteins in urine.
pyr/o	fire	Pyromaniacs enjoy setting fires or seeing fires burn.

Use the electronic flashcards on the Evolve site or make your own set of flashcards using the above list. Select the word parts just presented, and study them until you know their meanings.

FINDING THE CLUE!

EXERCISE 17

Use a clue to write the correct answers in the blanks. Solve Question 1; each ending letter becomes the clue for the first letter of the next answer.

1. Lip/o means fats or _fatlike substances_.
2. Lith/o means _stone_.
3. Inflammation of the brain is _encephalitis_.
4. Amyl/o means _starch_.
5. Vomiting of blood is _Hematesis_.
6. Micro- means _small_.
7. The combining form for stone is _lith/o_.

Abbreviations and Pharmacology

Selected abbreviations are presented in Appendixes I and II. See Appendix III for pharmacologic terms; your Companion CD presents drugs and their uses for Chapters 6-14.

Preparing for a Test on This Chapter

Study the Word Lists

Review all lists of word parts and their meanings, using the flashcards you prepared or the flashcards on the Evolve site. Review the cards several times before the test.

Practice with the Self-Test
Work the Self-Test. The review helps you know if you have learned the material. After completing all sections of the review, check your answers with those in Appendix VIII. Additional questions and games are also provided on the Companion CD.

 Be Careful with These!

-ist (one who) versus *-iatry* (medical profession or treatment)
-logy (study of) versus *-logist* (one who studies; specialist)
ne/o (new) versus *neur/o* (nerve)
intern (one in postgraduate training) versus *internist* (a physician)

Use the Games on the Companion CD
The games on the Companion CD are fun! They don't feel like testing, yet help you prepare for the test. The CD does not replace the Self-Test at the end of each chapter.

Practice with the List of Medical Terms
While looking at the terms listed at the end of each chapter, listen to the pronunciations on the Companion CD. Look closely at the spelling, and be sure that you know its meaning. If you can't recall its meaning, reread the frames that pertain to the term. (The index in the back of the book may help you locate the page on which the term appears.) Once you've mastered the chapter, you may want to use the audio CDs to test your recognition and spelling of terms.

Check the Evolve site
Visit http://evolve.elsevier.com/Leonard/quick/ for additional review activities, including questions on Spanish medical terms.

SELF-TEST Work the following exercises to test your understanding of the material in Chapter 2. Complete all the exercises before checking your answers against the answers in Appendix VIII.

A. FIND IT! *Find the combining forms and suffixes and write their meanings (the first is done as an example).*

1. amylolysis ___amyl/o (starch) + -lysis (destruction)___
2. appendicitis *append/o (appendix) + -itis (inflammation)*
3. blepharoptosis *blephar/o (eyelid) + -ptosis (prolapse; sagging)*
4. dermatologist *dermat/o (skin) + -logist (one who studies; specialist)*
5. lipase *lip/o (fat) + -ase (enzyme)*
6. mucoid *muc/o (mucus) + -oid (resembling)*
7. neuroplasty *neur/o (nerve) + -plasty (surgical repair)*
8. ophthalmorrhagia *ophthalm/o (eye) + -rrhagia (hemorrhage)*
9. otic *ot/o (ear) + -ic (pertaining to)*
10. tonsillectomy *tonsill/o (tonsil) + -ectomy (excision)*

SELF-TEST   (cont'd)

B. WRITE IT!   *Write the meanings of the underlined word parts in each of these terms.*

1. adenoid — gland
2. dermatosis — skin
3. cardiology — study or science of
4. chirospasm — hand
5. colopexy — surgical fixation
6. lactose — sugar
7. mammoplasty — breast
8. neural — nerve
9. ophthalmoscope — eye
10. osteomalacia — softening

C. FINDING THE CLUE!   *Use a clue to write terms for these descriptions. Solve Question 1; each ending letter becomes the clue for the first letter of the next answer.*

1. pertaining to the eye — ophthalmic
2. heart specialists — cardiologists
3. cramp or twitching — spasm
4. opposite of benign — malignant
5. method for sorting patients in an emergency — triage
6. inflammation of the brain — encephalitis
7. surgically sew — suture
8. surgical removal — excision
9. tumor — neoplasm
10. any disease of the bone marrow — myelopathy

D. MATCH IT!   *Match the medical specialists with the areas in which they specialize.*

B	1. anesthesiologist	A. children
K	2. dermatologist	B. drugs that produce loss of feeling or sensation
F	3. endocrinologist	C. ear, nose, and throat
J	4. geriatrician	D. eyes
E	5. gynecologist	E. females
H	6. neurologist	F. hormones and the glands that secrete them
L	7. oncologist	G. mental, emotional, and behavioral disorders
D	8. ophthalmologist	H. nervous system
C	9. otolaryngologist	I. nose
A	10. pediatrician	J. older persons
G	11. psychiatrist	K. skin
I	12. rhinologist	L. tumors

SELF-TEST   (cont'd)

E. CIRCLE IT!   *Circle the one correct answer (a, b, c, or d) for each question.*

1. Which term means the abnormal accumulation of fluid in the tissue and results in swelling?
   (a) dilatation   (b) edema   (c) emesis   (d) ptosis
2. Which of the following terms is a condition in which a calculus is present?
   (a) diplopia   (b) lithiasis   (c) neurotripsy   (d) pathology
3. Which branch of medicine specializes in the study of the nature and cause of disease?
   (a) cardiology   (b) dermatology   (c) pathology   (d) urology
4. Which of the following terms means pertaining to the ear?
   (a) dermatologic   (b) neural   (c) ophthalmic   (d) otic
5. Which of the following terms means an enzyme that breaks down starches?
   (a) adipose   (b) amylase   (c) lipase   (d) lipid
6. What does mastopexy mean?
   (a) enlarged breasts   (b) inflammation of the breast   (c) surgical fixation of the breast
   (d) surgical removal of a breast
7. Which of the following terms means excision of a small piece of living tissue for microscopic examination?
   (a) biopsy   (b) emesis   (c) ptosis   (d) stasis
8. Which term means pertaining to the skin?
   (a) blepharal   (b) cutaneous   (c) hernia   (d) suture
9. Which of the following terms means pain along the course of a nerve?
   (a) neuralgia   (b) neurocele   (c) neuroplasty   (d) neurosis
10. Which term means stretching of a structure?
    (a) dilatation   (b) ptosis   (c) prolapse   (d) spasm
11. A 65-year-old man has a history of heart problems. Which type of specialist should he see for care of his heart condition?
    (a) cardiologist   (b) endocrinologist   (c) laryngologist   (d) orthopedist
12. Cynthia is pregnant. Which type of specialist should she see to care for her during her pregnancy, labor, and delivery?
    (a) gerontologist   (b) obstetrician   (c) orthopedist   (d) otologist
13. Which term means a person who is not a physician, but is trained in administering drugs that cause a loss of feeling?
    (a) anesthesiologist   (b) anesthesist   (c) anesthetics   (d) anesthetist
14. Which of the following physicians specializes in the diagnosis and treatment of newborns through the age of 28 days?
    (a) geriatrician   (b) gynecologist   (c) neonatologist   (d) urologist
15. John suffers from persistent digestive problems. To which specialist in disorders of the stomach and intestine is John referred?
    (a) gastroenterologist   (b) immunologist   (c) rheumatologist   (d) toxicologist
16. Sally injures her arm while ice skating. The emergency department physician orders an x-ray examination. Which type of physician is a specialist in interpreting x-ray images?
    (a) gynecologist   (b) ophthalmologist   (c) plastic surgeon   (d) radiologist
17. Sally's x-ray image reveals a fractured radius, one of the bones of her forearm. Dr. Bonelly, a bone specialist, puts a cast on Sally's arm. Which type of specialist is Dr. Bonelly?
    (a) dermatologist   (b) orthopedist   (c) otologist   (d) rhinologist
18. Which physician specializes in diagnosis of disease using clinical laboratory results?
    (a) clinical pathologist   (b) gastroenterologist   (c) internist   (d) surgical pathologist

SELF-TEST   (cont'd)

F. WRITE IT!   *Write one word for each of the following meanings.*

1. enzyme that breaks down starch   *amylase*
2. examination of the eye   *ophthalmoscopy*
3. incision of the trachea   *tracheotomy*
4. inflammation of the appendix   *appendicitis*
5. inflammation of the ear   *otitis*
6. pertaining to a nerve   *neural*
7. removal of the tonsils   *tonsillectomy*
8. skin specialist   *dermatologist*
9. surgical crushing of a stone   *lithotripsy*
10. surgical removal of a breast   *mastectomy*

G. SPELL IT!   *Circle all incorrectly spelled terms, and write their correct spelling.*

1. adenectomy
2. ~~chirospazm~~   *chirospasm*
3. ~~incizion~~   *incision*
4. mammoplasty
5. trachea

Use Appendix VIII to check your answers, paying particular attention to spelling.

Quick & Easy (Q&E) List

Use the Companion CD or audio CDs to review the terms presented in Chapter 2.
Look closely at the spelling of each term as it is pronounced.

adenectomy (**ad´´ə-nek´tə-me**)
adenoids (**ad´ə-noids**)
alveolar (**al-ve´ə-lər**)
amniocentesis (**am´´ne-o-sen-te´sis**)
amnion (**am´ne-on**)
amylase (**am´ə-lās**)
amylolysis (**am´´ə-lol´ə-sis**)
anesthesiologist (**an´´əs-the´´ze-ol´ə-jist**)
anesthesiology (**an´´əs-the´´ze-ol´ə-je**)
anesthetic (**an´´əs-thet´ik**)
anesthetist (**ə-nes´thə-tist**)
angiectasis (**an´´je-ek´tə-sis**)
angiectomy (**an´´je-ek´tə-me**)
angiogram (**an´je-o-gram´´**)
angioplasty (**an´je-o-plas´´te**)
angiorrhaphy (**an´´je-or´ə-fe**)

appendectomy (**ap´´en-dek´tə-me**)
appendicitis (**ə-pen´´dĭ-si´tis**)
atrophy (**at´rə-fe**)
augmentation mammoplasty (**awg´´men-ta´shən**
    mam´o-plas´´te)
bacteremia (**bak´´tər-e´me-ə**)
benign (**bə-nīn´**)
biology (**bi-ol´ə-je**)
biopsy (**bi´op-se**)
blepharoptosis (**blef´´ə-rop-to´sis**)
calcipenia (**kal´´sĭ-pe´ne-ə**)
cancerous (**kan´sər-əs**)
carcinoma (**kahr´´sĭ-no´mə**)
cardiac (**kahr´de-ak**)
cardiologist (**kahr´´de-ol´ə-jist**)
cardiology (**kahr´´de-ol´ə-je**)

continued

cardiomegaly (kahr˝de-o-meg´ə-le)
cardiorrhexis (kahr˝de-o-rek´sis)
cerebral (sə-re´brəl, ser´ə-brəl)
cerebrotomy (ser˝ə-brot´ə-me)
cerebrum (ser´ə-brəm, sə-re´brəm)
chirospasm (ki´ro-spaz˝əm)
cholelith (ko´lə-lith)
colonoscopy (ko˝lən-os´kə-pe)
colopexy (ko´lo-pek˝se)
coloscopy (ko-los´ko-pe)
colostomy (kə-los´tə-me)
cutaneous (ku-ta´ne-əs)
dermal (dur´məl)
dermatitis (dur˝mə-ti´tis)
dermatologic (dur˝mə-to-loj´ik)
dermatological (dur˝mə-to-loj´ĭ-kəl)
dermatologist (dur˝mə-tol´o-jist)
dermatology (dur˝mə-tol´o-je)
dermatome (dur´mə-tōm)
dermatoplasty (dur´mə-to-plas˝te)
dermatosis (dur˝mə-to´sis)
dilatation (dil˝ə-ta´shən)
diplopia (dĭ-plo´pe-ə)
ductus deferens (duk´təs def´ər-enz)
edema (ə-de´mə)
emesis (em´ə-sis)
encephalitis (en-sef˝ə-li´tis)
encephalocele (en-sef´ə-lo-sēl˝)
encephalotome (en-sef´ə-lə-tōm)
encephalotomy (en-sef˝ə-lot´ə-me)
endocardium (en˝do-kahr´de-um)
endocrine (en´do-krīn, en´do-krin)
endocrinologist (en˝do-krĭ-nol´ə-jist)
endocrinology (en˝do-krĭ-nol´ə-je)
enzymatic (en˝zi-mat´ik)
epidemiologist (ep˝ĭ-de˝me-ol´ə-jist)
epidemiology (ep˝ĭ-de˝me-ol´ə-je)
excision (ek-sizh´ən)
facial (fa´shəl)
forensic medicine (fə-ren´zik med´ĭ-sin)
gastric (gas´trik)
gastrocele (gas´tro-sēl)
gastroenterologist (gas˝tro-en˝tər-ol´ə-jist)
gastroenterology (gas˝tro-en˝tər-ol´ə-je)
geriatrician (jer˝e-ə-trish´ən)
geriatrics (jer˝e-at´riks)

gerontology (jer˝on-tol´ə-je)
glycolysis (gli-kol´ə-sis)
gonorrhea (gon˝o-re´ə)
gynecologist (gi˝nə-kol´ə-jist, jin˝ə-kol´ə-jist)
gynecology (gi˝nə-kol´ə-je, jin˝ə-kol´ə-je)
hematemesis (he˝mə-tem´ə-sis)
hemolysis (he-mol´ə-sis)
hemophilia (he˝mo-fil´e-ə)
hemophiliac (he˝mo-fil´e-ak)
hemorrhage (hem´ə-rəj)
hepatitis (hep´ə-ti´tis)
hernia (hur´ne-ə)
hospitalist (hos´pĭ-tal-ist)
hyperemesis (hi˝pər-em´ə-sis)
hypoglycemia (hi˝po-gli-se´me-ə)
hysteria (his-ter´e-ə)
immunologist (im˝u-nol´ə-jist)
immunology (im˝u-nol´ə-je)
incision (in-sizh´ən)
inflammation (in˝flə-ma´shən)
intensivist (in-ten´sĭ-vist)
internist (in-tur´nist)
invasive (in-va´siv)
kleptomania (klep˝to-ma´ne-ə)
lactase (lak´tās)
lactation (lak-ta´shən)
lactose (lak´tōs)
lipase (lip´ās, li´pās)
lipids (lip´ids)
lithiasis (lĭ-thi´ə-sis)
lithotripsy (lith´o-trip˝se)
lumpectomy (ləm-pek´tə-me)
lymphatic (lim-fat´ik)
lymphedema (lim˝fə-de´mə)
malignant (mə-lig´nənt)
mammary (mam´ər-e)
mammography (mə-mog´rə-fe)
mammoplasty (mam´o-plas˝te)
mastectomy (mas-tek´tə-me)
mastitis (mas-ti´tis)
mastopexy (mas´to-pek-se)
median (me´de-ən)
microscope (mi´kro-skōp)
microscopy (mi-kros´kə-pe)
microtia (mi-kro´shə)
microtome (mi´kro-tōm)

mucoid (mu´koid)
mucous (mu´kəs)
mucus (mu´kəs)
muscular (mus´ku-lər)
myalgia (mi-al´jə)
myelopathy (mi´´ə-lop´ə-the)
neonatologist (ne´´o-na-tol´ə-jist)
neonatology (ne´´o-na-tol´ə-je)
neoplasm (ne´o-plaz-əm)
nephrotic (nə-frot´ik)
neural (noor´əl)
neuralgia (nŏŏ-ral´jə)
neurectasia (noor´´ək-ta´zhə)
neurectomy (nŏŏ-rek´tə-me)
neurologist (nŏŏ-rol´ə-jist)
neurology (nŏŏ-rol´ə-je)
neurolysis (nŏŏ-rol´ĭ-sis)
neuroplasty (noor´o-plas´´te)
neurosis (nŏŏ-ro´sis)
neurosurgeon (noor´´o-sur´jən)
obstetric (ob-stet´rik)
obstetrical (ob-stet´rĭ-kəl)
obstetrician (ob´´stə-trĭ´shən)
obstetrics (ob-stet´riks)
oncologist (ong-kol´ə-jist)
oncology (ong-kol´ə-je)
ophthalmalgia (of´´thəl-mal´jə)
ophthalmic (of-thal´mik)
ophthalmitis (of´´thəl-mi´tis)
ophthalmologic (of´´thəl-mə-loj´ik)
ophthalmological (of´´thal-mə-log´ĭ-kəl)
ophthalmologist (of´´thəl-mol´ə-jist)
ophthalmology (of´´thəl-mol´ə-je)
ophthalmopathy (of´´thəl-mop´ə-the)
ophthalmoplasty (of-thal´mo-plas´´te)
ophthalmorrhagia (of-thal´´mo-ra´je-ə)
ophthalmorrhexis (of-thal´´mo-rek´sis)
ophthalmoscope (of-thal´´mə-skōp)
ophthalmoscopic (of-thal´´mo-skop´ik)
ophthalmoscopy (of´´thəl-mos´kə-pe)
orthopedics (or´´tho-pe´diks)
orthopedist (or´´tho-pe´dist)
osteoarthritis (os´´te-o-ahr-thri´tis)
osteomalacia (os´´te-o-mə-la´shə)
otalgia (o-tal´je-ə)
otic (o´tik)

otitis (o-ti´tis)
otodynia (o´´to-din´e-ə)
otolaryngologist (o´´to-lar´´ing-gol´ə-jist)
otolaryngology (o´´to-lar´´ing-gol´ə-je)
otologist (o-tol´ə-jist)
otology (o-tol´ə-je)
otoplasty (o´to-plas´´te)
otoscope (o´to-skōp)
otoscopic (o´´to-skop´ik)
otoscopy (o-tos´kə-pe)
paranoia (par´´ə-noi´ah)
paranoid (par´ə-noid)
pathogenic (path-o-jen´ik)
pathologic (path´´o-loj´ik)
pathological (path´´o-loj´ĭ-kəl)
pathologist (pə-thol´ə-jist)
pathology (pə-thol´ə-je)
pediatrician (pe´´de-ə-trĭ´shən)
pediatrics (pe´´de-at´riks)
peritoneal (per´´ĭ-to-ne´əl)
peritoneum (per´´ĭ-to-ne´əm)
phlebitis (flə-bi´tis)
phlebostasis (flə-bos´tə-sis)
phobia (fo´be-ə)
pneumatic (noo-mat´ik)
pneumonia (noo-mo´ne-ə)
protease (pro´te-ās)
proteinase (pro´tēn-ās)
proteinuria (pro´´te-nu´re-ə)
proteolysis (pro´´te-ol´ĭ-sis)
psoriasis (sə-ri´ə-sis)
psychiatrist (si-ki´ə-trist)
psychiatry (si-ki´ə-tre)
ptosis (to´sis)
pulmonary (pool´mo-nar´´e)
pyromania (pi´´ro-ma´ne-ə)
pyromaniac (pi´´ro-ma´ne-ak)
pyrophobia (pi´´ro-fo´be-ə)
radiologic (ra´´de-o-loj´ik)
radiological (ra´´de-o-loj´ĭ-kəl)
radiologist (ra´´de-ol´ə-jist)
radiology (ra´´de-ol´ə-je)
rheumatism (roo´mə-tiz-əm)
rheumatologist (roo´´mə-tol´ə-jist)
rheumatology (roo´´mə-tol´ə-je)
rhinologist (ri-nol´ə-jist)

continued

rhinology (ri˝nol´ə-je)
salivary (sal´ĭ-var-e)
spasm (spaz´əm)
stasis (sta´sis)
suture (soo´chər)
synergism (sin´ər-jizm)
therapist (ther´ə-pist)
thermal (thur´məl)
tonsillectomy (ton˝sĭ-lek´tə-me)
tonsillitis (ton˝sĭ-li´tis)

trachea (tra´ke-ə)
tracheostomy (tra˝ke-os´tə-me)
tracheotomy (tra˝ke-ot´ə-me)
triage (tre-ahzh´, tre´ahzh)
urinary (u´rĭ-nar˝e)
urologic (u˝ro-loj´ik)
urological (u˝ro-loj´ĭ-kəl)
urologist (u-rol´ə-jist)
urology (u-rol´ə-je)
vasectomy (və-sek´tə-me)

 Don't forget the games on the Companion CD and http://evolve.elsevier.com/Leonard/quick/ for additional review, including questions on Spanish medical terms.

ESPAÑOL Enhancing Spanish Communication

English	Spanish (pronunciation)
aged	envejecido (en-vay-hay-SEE-do)
anesthetic	anestésico (ah-nes-TAY-se-co)
appendix	apéndice (ah-PEN-de-say)
benign	benigno (bay-NEEG-no)
biopsy	biopsia (be-OP-see-ah)
bladder	vejiga (vay-HEE-gah)
blood	sangre (SAHN-gray)
body	cuerpo (coo-ERR-po)
bone	hueso (oo-AY-so)
brain	cerebro (say-RAY-bro)
breasts	senos (SAY-nos)
burn	quemadura (kay-mah-DOO-rah)
calcium	calcio (CAHL-se-o)
calculus	cálculo (CAHL-coo-lo)
cancer	cáncer (CAHN-ser)
child	niña (NEE-nya), niño (NEE-nyo)
clot	coágulo (co-AH-goo-lo)
disease	enfermedad (en-fer-may-DAHD)
ear	oreja (o-RAY-hah)
edema	hidropesía (e-dro-pay-SEE-ah)
enzyme	enzima (en-SEE-mah)
eye	ojo (O-ho)
eyelid	párpado (PAR-pah-do)
face	cara (CAH-rah)
fear	miedo (me-AY-do)
feces	excremento (ex-cray-MEN-to)

English	Spanish (pronunciation)
fetus	feto (**FAY-to**)
fire	fuego (**foo-AY-go**)
fluid	fluido (**floo-EE-do**)
gland	glándula (**GLAN-doo-lah**)
glucose	glucosa (**gloo-CO-sah**)
gynecology	ginecología (**he-nay-co-lo-HEE-ah**)
hand	mano (**MAH-no**)
heart	corazón (**co-rah-SON**)
heat	calor (**cah-LOR**)
hemorrhage	hemorragia (**ay-mor-RAH-he-ah**)
hernia	hernia (**AYR-ne-ah**), quebradura (**kay-brah-DOO-rah**)
instrument	instrumento (**ins-troo-MEN-to**)
intestine	intestino (**in-tes-TEE-no**)
joint	articulación (**ar-te-coo-lah-se-ON**), coyuntura (**co-yoon-TOO-rah**)
kidney	riñón (**ree-NYOHN**)
malignant	maligno (**mah-LEEG-no**)
membrane	membrana (**mem-BRAH-nah**)
microscope	microscopio (**me-cros-CO-pe-o**)
milk	leche (**LAY-chay**)
mind	mente (**MEN-te**)
mucus	moco (**MO-co**)
muscle	músculo (**MOOS-coo-lo**)
nerve	nervio (**NERR-ve-o**)
pain	dolor (**do-LOR**)
pathology	patología (**pah-to-lo-HEE-ah**)
prolapse	prolapso (**pro-LAHP-so**)
psychiatry	psiquiatría (**se-ke-ah-TREE-ah**)
psychology	psicología (**se-co-lo-HEE-ah**)
pulse	pulso (**POOL-so**)
radiation	radiación (**rah-de-ah-se-ON**)
rupture	ruptura (**roop-TOO-rah**)
saliva	saliva (**sah-LEE-vah**)
skin	piel (**pe-EL**)
spasm	espasmo (**es-PAHS-mo**)
starch	almidón (**al-me-DON**)
stomach	estómago (**es-TOH-mah-go**)
surgeon	cirujano,-a (**se-roo-HAH-no,-na**)
surgery	cirugía (**se-roo-HEE-ah**)
swelling (to swell)	hinchar (**in-CHAR**)
throat	garganta (**gar-GAHN-tah**)
tonsil	tonsila (**ton-SEE-lah**), amígdala (**ah-MEEG-dah-lah**)

English	Spanish (pronunciation)
trachea	tráquea **(TRAH-kay-ah)**
urinary system	sistema urinario **(sis-TAY-mah oo-re-NAH-re-o)**
urology	urología **(oo-ro-lo-HEE-ah)**
uterus	útero **(OO-tay-ro)**
vein	vena **(VAY-nah)**
vessel	vaso **(VAH-so)**
vision	visión **(ve-se-ON)**
vomiting	vómito **(VO-me-to)**
water	agua **(AH-goo-ah)**

CHAPTER 3

Essential Prefixes and More

CONTENTS

How Prefixes Are Used to Form Words
Prefixes: Numbers or Quantity
Prefixes: Position or Direction
Miscellaneous Prefixes
Recognizing Prefixes in Terms
Using Prefixes to Write Terms

Combining Forms for Colors
Combining Forms and Related Suffixes
Miscellaneous Combining Forms
Self-Test
Q&E List
Enhancing Spanish Communication

OBJECTIVES

After completing Chapter 3, you will be able to:

1. Write the meaning of Chapter 3 word parts, or match word parts with their meanings.
2. Use prefixes for numbers, quantities, position, and direction to write medical terms.
3. Use combining forms for colors to write medical terms.
4. Identify and combine word parts correctly, and use clues to write medical terms.
5. Write the correct term when presented with its definition or match terms with their definitions.
6. Build and analyze medical terms with Chapter 3 word parts.
7. Spell medical terms correctly.

How Prefixes Are Used to Form Words

Prefixes are emphasized in this chapter, although you are already familiar with many of them. Several new combining forms and suffixes are also introduced.

Instead of only memorizing lists of prefixes, you will learn to combine them with other word parts. Learning new terms will help you remember the prefixes that are presented.

A *prefix* is placed before a word to modify its meaning. Most prefixes, including those ending with a vowel, can be added to the remainder of the word without change. Exceptions are noted. Prefixes are grouped here as follows: (1) prefixes used in numbers or quantity, (2) prefixes used in position or direction, and (3) miscellaneous prefixes.

Prefixes: Numbers or Quantity

Many of the prefixes in the following table are used in everyday language. Common words are given to help you associate prefixes with their meanings. Commit their meanings to memory.

Prefixes: Numbers or Quantity

Prefix	Meaning	Word Association
Specific Numbers		
mono-, uni-	one	A *monorail* is a single rail that serves as a track for a wheeled vehicle. A *monocular* scope has one eyepiece.
		A *unicorn* has one horn, and a *unicycle* has one wheel.
bi-, di-	two	A *bicycle* has two wheels.
		Carbon dioxide contains two atoms of oxygen.
tri-	three	A *tricycle* has three wheels.
quad-, quadri-, tetra-	four	*Quadruplets* are four offspring born at one birth.
		Quadriplegia is paralysis of all four extremities (arms and legs).
		A *tetrahedron* is a solid figure having four faces.
centi-	one hundred, one-hundredth	*Centigrade* is a measurement of temperature that is divided into one hundred degrees, with 0 degrees representing the freezing point and 100 degrees representing the boiling point.
		A *centimeter* is one-hundredth of a meter.
milli-	one-thousandth	A *millimeter* is one-thousandth of a meter.
Quantities		
diplo-	double	**Diplopia** means double vision (two images of a single object are seen).
hemi-, semi-	half, partly	Each of Earth's *hemispheres* is half of the Earth.
		A *semipermeable* membrane is one that allows the passage of some substances but prevents the passage of others (Figure 3-1).
hyper-	excessive, more than normal	*Hyperactive* means excessively active. **Hyperglycemia** means an above-normal amount of sugar in the blood.
hypo-	under, less than normal	**Hypodermic** means under or beneath the skin.
		Hypoglycemia is a condition characterized by a below-normal amount of sugar in the blood.
multi-, poly-	many	A *multitude* means many or several. *Multipurpose* means serving many purposes.
		Polyunsaturated fats have many unsaturated chemical bonds. *Polysaccharides* are complex carbohydrates generally composed of many molecules of simpler sugars.
nulli-	none	The word *null* means having no value, amounting to nothing, or equal to zero.
pan-	all	**Pandemic** means occurring throughout (i.e., affecting all) the population of a country, people, or the world.
primi-	first	*Primary* means standing first in rank or importance.
super-, ultra-	excessive	**Supervitaminosis** is a condition resulting from excessive ingestion (swallowing or taking by mouth) of vitamins.
		Ultraviolet (UV) describes light beyond the visible spectrum at its violet end. UV rays cause sunburn and skin tanning but are also used in the diagnosis and treatment of disease (Figure 3-2).

Use the electronic flashcards on the Evolve site or make your own set of flashcards using the above list. Select the word parts just presented, and study them until you know their meaning. Do this each time a set of word parts is presented.

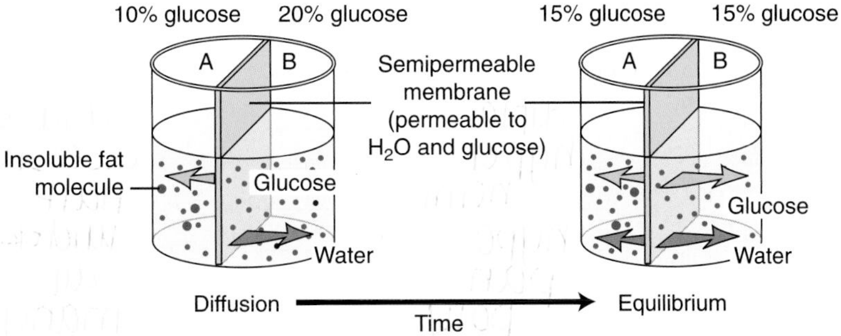

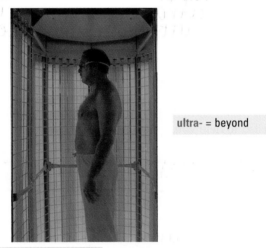

10% glucose   20% glucose   15% glucose   15% glucose

Semipermeable
membrane
(permeable to
H₂O and glucose)

Insoluble fat
molecule
Glucose
Water

Glucose
Water

Diffusion ──────────→ Equilibrium
Time

Figure 3-1 Semipermeable membrane. Some particles in a fluid move from an area of higher concentration to an area of lower concentration, but other particles cannot move across the membrane because of size, charge, or solubility.

ultra- = beyond

Figure 3-2 Ultraviolet therapy. Patient receiving treatment for a skin disorder.

MATCH IT!

EXERCISE 1

Match the prefixes in the left column with their meaning in the right column (a choice may be used more than once).

B 1. bi-
B 2. di-
E 3. centi-
F 4. milli-
A 5. mono-
D 6. quad-
C 7. tri-
A 8. uni-

A. one
B. two
C. three
D. four
E. one hundred or 1/100
F. 1/1000

Use Appendix VIII, Answers to Exercises, to check all your answers to the exercises in Chapter 3.

Find the prefix in each of these terms. Write each prefix and its meaning.

		Prefix	Meaning
1.	diplopia	*diplo*	*double*
2.	hyperglycemia	*hyper*	*excessive*
3.	hemisphere	*hemi*	*Half*
4.	hypodermic	*hypo*	*under*
5.	pandemic	*pan*	*all*
6.	polysaccharides	*poly*	*many*
7.	primary	*prim*	*first*
8.	quadriplegic	*quad*	*four*
9.	semipermeable	*semi*	*partly*
10.	supervitaminosis	*super*	*excessive*
11.	tetrahedron	*tetra*	*four*
12.	ultraviolet	*ultra*	*excessive*

Prefixes: Position or Direction

Commit the meanings of the prefixes in the following table to memory. Familiar words are also listed to help you remember the prefixes.

Prefixes: Position or Direction		
Prefix	**Meaning**	**Word Association**
ab-	away from	*Abduct* means to carry away by force or to draw away from a given position.
ad-	toward	In drug *addiction* (now called chemical dependency), one is "drawn toward" a habit-forming drug. In other words, one has a compulsive physiologic need for a certain drug.
ante-, pre-	before in time or in place	An *anteroom* is an outer room that is generally entered before a more important room. **Prerenal** pertains to the area in front of (literally, "before in place") the kidney.
circum-, peri-	around	The *perimeter* is the outer boundary or the line that is drawn around the outside of an area. The *circumference* is the line that is drawn around a circle.
dia-	through	The *diameter* passes through the center of a circle.
ecto-, ex-, exo-, extra-	out, without, away from	To *export* is to carry or send away to another place. The skeletons of some animals, such as insects, are on the outer surface and are called *exoskeletons*. *Extranuclear* means outside a nucleus.
en-, end-, endo-	inside	*Enclose* means to close up inside something, hold in, or include. **Endotracheal** means within the trachea.
epi-	above, on	An *epitaph* is often inscribed on the tombstone or above the grave of the person buried there.

Prefixes: Position or Direction—cont'd

Prefix	Meaning	Word Association
hypo-, infra-, sub-	beneath, under	*Hypodermic* means pertaining to the area below the skin. A **subcutaneous** injection places a small amount of medication below the skin layer into the subcutaneous tissue. Four types of hypodermic injections are shown in Figure 3-3.
inter-	between	An *interval* is a space of time between events.
intra-	within	*Intracollegiate* activities are those within a college or engaged in by members of a college. See Figure 3-3 for explanations of the terms **intramuscular, intradermal,** and **intravenous.**
meso-, mid-	middle	The **mesoderm** is the middle of three tissue layers that form during the development of an embryo.
para-	near, beside, or abnormal	Two *parallel* lines run beside each other.

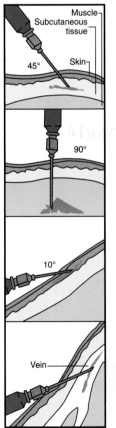

A, A subcutaneous injection places a small amount (0.5-2 mL) of medication below the skin layer into the subcutaneous tissue. The needle is inserted at a 45-degree angle.

B, An intramuscular injection deposits medication into a muscular layer. As much as 3 to 5 mL may be administered in one injection, and depending on the size of the patient, a needle 1 to 3 inches in length is used.

C, An intradermal injection places very small amounts into the outer layers of the skin with a short, fine-gauge needle. This type of injection is often used to test allergic reactions.

D, An intravenous injection is used to administer medications directly into the bloodstream for immediate effect. A few milliliters of medication, or much larger amounts given over a long period, may be administered after venipuncture of the selected vein has been performed.

-al, -ar, -ous = pertaining to
derm/a, cutane/o = skin
intra- = within
muscul/o = muscle
sub- = below or under
ven/o = vein

Figure 3-3 Using prefixes in naming types of injections. Note how the prefixes sub- and intra- are added to terms and used to describe the correct position of the needle: **A,** subcutaneous; **B,** intramuscular; **C,** intradermal; **D,** intravenous.

Prefixes: Position or Direction—Cont'd

Prefix	Meaning	Word Association
per-	through or by	To *perspire* is to excrete fluid through the pores of the skin.
post-	after, behind	To *postdate* is to assign a date to something after the date it actually occurred, such as when one postdates a check. **Postnasal** means lying or occurring behind the nose.
retro-	behind, backward	*Retroactive* means extending back to a prior time or condition. *Retrospection* means looking backward in time or surveying the past.
super-, supra-	above, beyond	*Supernormal* is beyond normal human powers. A **suprarenal** gland is situated above each kidney.
sym-, syn-	joined, together	A **syndrome** is a set of symptoms that occur together and collectively characterize a particular disease or condition. In *symbiosis*, two organisms of different species beneficially live together (coexist).
trans-	across	A **transdermal** drug is one that can be absorbed through (or across) unbroken skin, such as the nitroglycerin patch to relieve *angina pectoris*, chest pain caused by heart disease (Figure 3-4).

WRITE IT!
EXERCISE 3

Write answers in the blank lines to complete the sentences. (Although an answer may require more than one word, it is represented by one blank line.)

1. The prefix ab- means _away from_, but ad- means _toward_.
2. Postnasal pertains to the region _behind_ the nose.
3. Two prefixes that have opposite meanings are endo- and ecto-, which mean _inside_ and _out_, respectively.
4. Inter- means _Between_, and intra- means _within_.
5. Suprarenal glands are located _above_ each kidney.

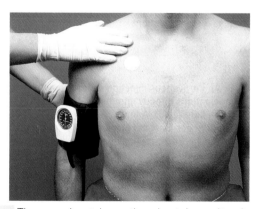

-al = pertaining to
derm/a = skin
trans- = across

Figure 3-4 Transdermal drug delivery. The round patch on the chest is a nitroglycerin patch. The patient also has a blood pressure cuff on his right arm.

FIND IT!

EXERCISE 4

Find the prefix in each of these terms. Write each prefix and its meaning.

		Prefix	Meaning
1.	circumference	circum-	Around
2.	diameter	dia-	through
3.	exoskeleton	exo-	out
4.	endotracheal	endo-	inside
5.	epitaph	epi-	above
6.	hypodermic	Hypo-	beneath
7.	mesoderm	meso-	middle
8.	perimeter	peri-	through/by Around
9.	perspire	per-	through/by
10.	prerenal	pre-	Before
11.	retroactive	retro-	Behind, backward
12.	subcutaneous	sub-	under
13.	supernormal	super-	Above
14.	syndrome	syn-	together
15.	transdermal	trans-	ACROSS

Miscellaneous Prefixes

The following list contains additional prefixes that you should commit to memory. Their meanings should be easy to remember because many of them are used in every-day language.

Note that some prefixes have more than one meaning and may pertain to two classifications, such as position and time. Two examples are ante- and post-, which you also saw in the prefixes related to position.

Miscellaneous Prefixes

Prefix	Meaning	Word Association
Related to Time		
ante-, pre-, pro-	before	**Antepartum** means before childbirth.
		Premarital means existing or occurring before marriage.
		Proactive involves taking action before an anticipated event.
post-	after or behind	**Postpartum** means after childbirth.
Related to Size		
macro-, mega-, megalo-	large or great	**Macroscopic** structures are large enough to be seen by the naked eye.
		A *megalith* is a very large stone.
		Megalomania is an abnormal mental state characterized by delusions of greatness.
micro-	small	A **microscope** is used to view very small objects.

Continued

Miscellaneous Prefixes—cont'd		
Prefix	Meaning	Word Association
Related to Negation		
a-, an-	no, not, without	*Rule:* Use a- before a consonant. Use an- before a vowel and often the letter h. **Asymptomatic** means without symptoms. *Anesthesia* means without feeling.
in-	not or inside (in)	*Inconsistent* means not consistent. *Inhale* means "to breathe in."
Related to Description		
anti-, contra-	against	An *antiperspirant* acts against perspiration. A **contraceptive** acts against or prevents conception (the beginning of pregnancy). (The *i* in anti- is sometimes dropped before a vowel.)
brady-	slow	**Bradycardia** means a decreased pulse rate, but its literal translation is "a slow heart condition."
dys-	bad, difficult	Reading is very difficult when one has **dyslexia.** This disorder is thought to be an inability to organize written symbols.
eu-	good, normal	**Euthanasia** is "mercy killing," thought by some to be a good, painless death when a person has a terminal, intolerably painful condition.
mal-	bad	*Maladjusted* means poorly or badly adjusted.
pro-	favoring, supporting	To *prolong* is to make something longer; in other words, to support making it longer.
tachy-	fast	**Tachycardia** means an increased pulse rate, but its literal translation is "a fast heart condition."

MATCH IT! EXERCISE 5

Match the prefixes in the left column with their meanings in the right column (a choice may be used more than once).

B **1.** dys-   A. good, normal
E **2.** tachy-   B. bad
F **3.** brady-   C. not
D **4.** anti-   D. against
C **5.** in-   E. fast
B **6.** mal-   F. slow
C **7.** a-
D **8.** contra-
A **9.** eu-
C **10.** an-

Recognizing Prefixes in Terms

You are now ready to recognize prefixes in terms. Several words in the following exercises contain prefixes that you have learned.

Write the prefix and its meaning for these new terms (Question 1 is done as an example). A short definition is provided for each term.

Term/Meaning	Prefix	Meaning
1. **bradyphasia** slowness of speech	*brady-*	*slow*
2. **tachyphasia** fast speech	tachy-	fast
3. **hypothyroidism** decreased activity of the thyroid gland	hypo-	under
4. **hyperthyroidism** increased activity of the thyroid gland	hyper-	excessive
5. **incontinence** not having **continence***	in-	not
6. **malabsorption** poor absorption	mal-	bad
7. **antacid** acts against acidity, especially an agent acting against acidity in digestive tract	an-	no, not, without
8. **incompatible** not capable of uniting; not compatible	in-	not or inside
9. **dysphonia** weak voice	dys-	bad, difficult
10. **contraindication** any condition that renders some particular form of treatment improper	contra-	against
11. **anticonvulsive** agent that suppresses convulsions	anti-	against
12. **para-appendicitis** inflammation of tissue adjacent to or near the appendix	para-	near, beside
13. **parathyroids** small glands that lie near the thyroid gland, sometimes embedded within the gland	para-	near, beside
14. **hyposecretion** less-than-normal secretion	hypo-	beneath, under
15. **hypersecretion** greater-than-normal secretion	hyper-	greater than normal
16. **euthyroid** pertaining to a normal (or normally functioning) thyroid gland	eu-	good, normal
17. **hypoparathyroidism** insufficient secretion of parathyroid glands	hypo-	beneath, under
18. **hyperparathyroidism** excessive activity of parathyroid glands	hyper-	excessive

* **Continence** is the ability to refrain from yielding to the urge to defecate or urinate.

Complete the sentences by writing in the blank a word or words that correspond to the underlined prefix.

1. **Unilateral** means ____one____ side of the body only.
2. **Primigravida** refers to a woman who is pregnant for the ____first____ time.
3. Translated literally, **hemiplegia** means paralysis of ____half____ of the body. In this case, it means one side of the body.
4. A **tripara** is a woman who has had ____three____ pregnancies that resulted in viable offspring. This can be viewed as births of live offspring but does not reflect the result of multiple births.
5. **Bifocal** means having ____two____ focal distances. In eyeglasses, the upper part of the lens is generally used for distant vision and the lower section for near vision.
6. A **nullipara** is a woman who has borne ____no[ne]____ children.
7. **Semiconscious** is being ____partly____ aware of one's surroundings.
8. **Multicellular** means composed of ____many____ cells.
9. **Polydipsia** literally means ____many____ thirsts. It actually means excessive thirst.
10. Quadriplegia is paralysis of all ____four____ extremities.
11. **Mononuclear** describes a cell that has how many nuclei? ____one____
12. The term **hypocalcemia** indicates something about the amount of calcium in the blood. It means that the amount of calcium is ____less than normal____.
13. Translated literally, **macrocephaly** means ____large____ head. It actually means excessive size of the head.
14. **Hyperlipemia** means having an ____excessive____ amount of fat in the blood.
15. Multiple sclerosis is a chronic, progressive disease of the central nervous system characterized by destruction of the myelin sheaths of neurons (nerve cells). The damaged myelin sheaths deteriorate to scleroses (scler/o means hard), hardened scars, or plaques. The disorder is called multiple **sclerosis** because of the ____many____ scleroses formed on the neurons.
16. **Microorganisms** are ____small____ living organisms, usually microscopic, such as bacteria, rickettsiae, viruses, molds, yeasts, and protozoa.

Using Prefixes to Write Terms

Learn new terms by writing prefixes in the blank spaces in the next exercise. After you complete it, you will study additional combining forms in three groups: (1) combining forms that pertain to colors, (2) combining forms that have the same root as several common suffixes, and (3) miscellaneous combining forms.

Write a word in each blank space to complete the terms in this exercise.

1. Small flaps on certain valves of the heart are called *cusps.* If two flaps are present, the valve is called a **bicuspid** valve. If ___three___ flaps are present, the valve is called a **tricuspid** valve.

2. A muscle that draws a body part away from the midline of the body is called an **abductor.** An **adductor** is a muscle that draws a body part ___toward___ the axis or midline of the body.

3. **Dermal** refers to the skin. Write a word that refers to a procedure that is performed through (literally, across) the skin: ___transdermal___.

4. **Dysphasia** is ___difficulty___ or impairment in speech.

5. Use a prefix with -kinesia to write a word that means an abnormal condition characterized by slowness of all voluntary movement: ___bradykinesia___.

6. **Aerobic** means living only in the presence of oxygen; living without ___oxygen___ is **anaerobic.**

7. Esthesia means feeling or sensation; partial or complete loss of sensation is ___anesthesia___.

8. **Febrile** refers to a fever; ___without___ fever is **afebrile.**

9. Hydrous means containing water; without or lacking ___water___ is **anhydrous.**

10. **Symptomatic** means of the nature of a symptom or concerning a symptom; "___without___ symptoms" defines *asymptomatic.*

WRITE IT! EXERCISE 8

Combining Forms for Colors

Commit the combining forms for colors and their meanings in the following list to memory. Again, word association (familiar words derived from the same root) is included to facilitate learning the word parts.

Combining Forms for Colors		
Combining Form	**Meaning**	**Word Association**
alb/o, albin/o, leuk/o (leuc/o)	white	An **albino** is an individual with congenital absence of pigment in the skin, hair, and eyes. The skin and hair appear white because of lack of pigment (Figure 3-5). The Latin term *alba* means white.
		Leukemia is a malignant disease of the blood-forming organs characterized by a marked increase in the number of **leukocytes** (white blood cells). There are also immature leukocytes.

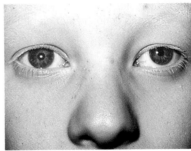

albin/o = white
-ism = condition, theory, or process
melan/o = black

Figure 3-5 Albinism. Note the white hair and pale skin of this condition, which is characterized by partial or total lack of melanin pigment in the body.

Combining Forms for Colors—cont'd

Combining Form	Meaning	Word Association
chlor/o	green	Chlorophyll is the green pigment contained in chloroplasts in the leaves of plants and is the reason that plants are green.
cyan/o	blue	Deficiency of oxygen in the blood can cause a condition called **cyanosis,** a slightly bluish, slatelike skin discoloration (Figure 3-6).
erythr/o	red	**Erythrocytes** are red blood cells.
melan/o	black	A **melancholy** person is sad. In ancient times, people thought the bodies of melancholy persons produced a black bile that caused sadness. A melanoma is a malignant skin cancer (see Figure 2-3, *B,* p. 21).
xanth/o	yellow	Xanthophyll is a yellow pigment in plants.
		A condition called **jaundice** is often associated with a yellow appearance in the patient; however, it is derived from French and does not use xanth/o as a combining form. Jaundice is characterized by a yellowish discoloration of the skin, mucous membranes, and white outer part of the eyeballs (Figure 3-7).

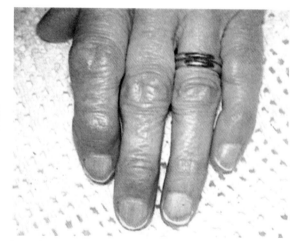

cyan/o = blue
-osis = condition, disease, or increase

Figure 3-6 Cyanosis. This bluish discoloration of the skin is caused by a deficiency of oxygen in the blood. Cyanosis is generally not as obvious as it is in this patient.

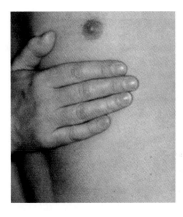

Figure 3-7 Jaundice. Note the contrast in the examiner's hand and the yellow discoloration of the skin of a patient with an acute liver disorder.

WRITE IT!
EXERCISE 9

Write the meaning of each underlined word part in the blank spaces.

1. <u>erythr</u>o<u>cyt</u>osis   <u>Red</u>   ; <u>condition</u>
2. <u>xanth</u>osis   <u>yellow</u>   ; <u>condition</u>
3. <u>melan</u>oma   <u>black</u>   ; <u>tumor</u>
4. <u>leuk</u>o<u>derma</u>   <u>white</u>   ; <u>skin</u>
5. <u>chlor</u>opia   <u>green</u>   ; <u>vision</u>
6. <u>albin</u>ism   <u>white</u>   ; <u>condition, theory</u>
7. <u>cyan</u>otic   <u>Blue</u>   ; <u>pertaining to</u>

Combining Forms and Related Suffixes

Several combining forms have related suffixes that are frequently used in writing medical terms. Commit the following list to memory. All these suffixes are used to form nouns, with the exception of those ending in -ic and -tic. (The suffixes -genic, -lytic, -phagic, and -trophic are used to form adjectives, words that modify or describe nouns. The suffix -ic can also be used to form words with several of the combining forms presented.)

Select Combining Forms and Related Suffixes

Combining Form	Suffixes	Meaning
cyt/o	-cyte	cell
gen/o		beginning, origin (sometimes genes)
	-genic	produced by or in
	-genesis	producing or forming

Continued

Select Combining Forms and Related Suffixes—cont'd

Combining Form	Suffixes	Meaning
gram/o		to record
	-gram	a record
	-graph	instrument for recording
	-graphy	process of recording
kinesi/o		movement
	-kinesia, -kinesis	movement, motion
leps/o	-lepsy	seizure
lys/o		destruction, dissolving
	-lysin	that which destroys
	-lysis	process of destroying
	-lytic*	capable of or producing destruction
malac/o		soft, softening
	-malacia	abnormal softening
megal/o		large, enlarged
	-megaly	enlargement
metr/o		measure, uterine tissue
	-meter	instrument used to measure
	-metry	process of measuring
path/o	-pathy	disease
phag/o		eat, ingest
	-phagia, -phagic, -phagy	eating, swallowing
phas/o	-phasia	speech
pleg/o	-plegia	paralysis
schis/o, schiz/o, schist/o	-schisis	split, cleft
scler/o		hard
	-sclerosis	hardening
scop/o		to examine, to view
	-scope	instrument used for viewing
	-scopy	process of examining visually
troph/o	-trophic, -trophy	nutrition

* Careful! Note the change in s to t in the spelling of -lytic.

Write a word in each blank to complete these sentences. Several new word parts are introduced in this exercise.

WRITE IT! **EXERCISE 10**

1. An **electro+cardio+gram** (electr/o, electricity; cardi/o, heart) is a record (tracing) of the electrical impulses of the heart. **Electrocardiography** is the ___process___ of recording the electrical impulses of the heart, and an **electrocardiograph** is the ___instrument___ used (Figure 3-8). The abbreviation for electrocardiogram is ECG (also EKG, from the German term).
2. A **micro+scope** is an instrument for viewing small objects that must be magnified so they can be studied. **Microscopy** is the ___process___ of viewing things with a microscope.
3. **Hemo+lysis** (hem/o, blood; lysis, destruction) is the destruction of red blood cells that results in the liberation of **hemoglobin,** a red pigment in the cells. The term for a substance that causes hemolysis is ___hemolysin___. **Hemolyze** is a verb that means to destroy red blood cells and cause them to release hemoglobin. **Hemolytic** substances cause hemolysis and are known as **hemolysins.**
4. Cephal/o means head. **Cephalo+metry** is measurement of the dimensions of the head. A device or instrument for measuring the head is a ___cephalometer___.
5. A **carcino+gen** is a substance or agent that produces cancer. The production or origin of cancer is called ___carcinogenesis___. A **carcinogenic** substance causes ___cancer___.
6. **Ophthalmo+pathy** is any ___disease___ of the eye.
7. **Dys+trophic** muscle deteriorates because of defective nutrition or metabolism. A **dystrophy** is any disorder caused by defective metabolism or ___nutrition___.
8. A **phago+cyte** (phag/o, eat or ingest; cyte, cell) is a cell that can ingest and destroy particulate substances such as bacteria. Ingest means to ___eat___.
9. **Tele+kinesis** is the concept of controlling ___movement___ of an object by the powers of the mind.

Write the meaning of each underlined word part. A brief definition is provided for each term.

WRITE IT! **EXERCISE 11**

Term	Meaning of Word Part	Meaning of Term
1. kinesio<u>therapy</u>	movement	treatment through movement
2. osteo<u>malacia</u>	softening	softening of bone
3. dys<u>phagia</u>	swallowing	difficulty swallowing
4. cardio<u>megaly</u>	enlargement	enlarged heart
5. arterio<u>sclerosis</u>	hardening	hardening of the arteries
6. <u>phago</u>cyte	ingest	cell that ingests
7. a<u>phasia</u>	speech	inability to speak
8. quadri<u>plegia</u>	paralysis	paralysis of all four limbs
9. <u>schizo</u>phrenic	split	psychosis with distortions of reality
10. dys<u>kinesia</u>	movement	difficulty moving
11. <u>megalo</u>cyte	large	large cell
12. rachi<u>schisis</u>	split	split spine (spina bifida)

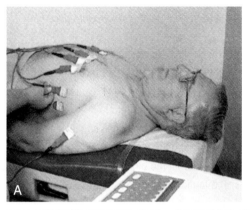

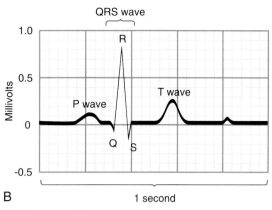

cardi/o = heart
electr/o = electric
-gram = a record
-graph = recording instrument
-graphy = process of recording

Figure 3-8 Electrocardiography. A, Patient undergoing electrocardiography, the making of graphic records produced by electrical activity of the heart muscle. The instrument, an electrocardiograph, is shown. The electrical impulses that are given off by the heart are picked up by electrodes (sensors) and conducted into the electrocardiograph through wires. **B,** An enlarged section of the tracing called an electrocardiogram, or ECG. It represents the heart's electrical impulses, which are picked up and conducted to the electrocardiograph by electrodes or leads connected to the body. The pattern of the graphic recording indicates the heart's rhythm and other actions. The normal ECG is composed of the labeled parts shown in the drawing. Each labeled segment represents a different part of the heartbeat.

Miscellaneous Combining Forms

Commit the following combining forms to memory.

Miscellaneous Combining Forms		
Combining Form	**Meaning**	**Word Association**
aer/o	air	*Aeroplane* is the British spelling of airplane.
blast/o	embryonic form	The names of early **(embryonic)** forms have -blast endings. For example, embryonic bone cells are **osteoblasts.**
cancer/o, carcin/o	cancer	A **carcinoma** is a cancerous tumor.
cephal/o	head	**Cephalic** means pertaining to the head.
cry/o	cold	**Cryotherapy** uses cold temperatures to treat certain conditions.
crypt/o	hidden	A *cryptic* remark has a hidden meaning. A cryptogram is a message written in code, so it has a hidden meaning.
dips/o	thirst	*Polydipsia* means excessive thirst.

Combining Form	Meaning	Word Association
	Miscellaneous Combining Forms—cont'd	
electr/o	electricity	Electr/o will be easy to remember because the combining form is contained in its meaning, electricity.
fibr/o	fiber	**Fibrous** means containing, consisting of, or resembling fiber.
hist/o	tissue	**Histocompatibility** is a measure of the compatibility of tissue of a donor and recipient.
myc/o	fungus	**Mycology** is a branch of botany that deals with fungi (plural of fungus).
narc/o	stupor	**Narcotics** are so named because they produce insensibility or stupor.
necr/o	dead	**Necrosis** is localized tissue death in response to disease or injury.
optic/o, opt/o	vision	**Optical** pertains to vision. An **optometrist** tests the eyes to measure visual acuity and prescribes corrective lenses, if necessary.
pharmac/o	drugs, medicine	Medicines are dispensed at a *pharmacy*.
phon/o	voice	We hear someone's voice when we speak with that person by *phone*.
phot/o	light	Photography produces images on a film by the action of radiant energy, especially light.
py/o	pus	**Pyogenic** means "pus producing."
therm/o	heat	*Thermal* clothing is designed to prevent loss of body heat.
top/o	position, place	*Topography* is often concerned with the making of maps or charts to show relative positions and elevations of a particular place or region.
trache/o	trachea (windpipe)	*Endotracheal* means within or through the trachea.

PROGRAMMED LEARNING

Remember to cover the answers (left column) with folded paper or the bookmark. Write an answer in each blank, and then check your answer before proceeding to the next frame.

large (enlarged)	1. You have learned that megalo- means _____.
large	2. A megalo+cyte is a _____ cell. (This term usually refers to an extremely large red blood cell.)
red	3. You learned earlier that erythr/o means red. Translated literally, an erythro+cyte is a _____ cell. (This is an abbreviated way of saying red blood cell, a blood cell that carries oxygen.)
leukocyte	4. With erythro+cyte as a model, use leuk/o to write a word that means white cell (or white blood cell): _____.

cytoscopy

5. Combine cyt/o and the suffix that means process of visually examining to form a new word that means examination of cells: _____. (Congratulations if you answered this correctly. You can see that you really are learning medical terms. You might even have written a word that you've never seen before!)

cytology

6. Write a word that means the study of cells: _____.

black

7. A melan+oma, one type of skin cancer, is a malignant pigmented mole or tumor (see Figure 2-3, *B*). Translated literally, a melanoma is a _____ tumor. Carcin+oma is a synonym for cancer. The combining form carcin/o means cancer, and -oma means tumor.

cancer

8. Carcino+gens are agents that cause _____.

psychogenesis

9. Change psycho+genic to a word that means the origin and development of the mind, or the formation of mental traits: _____.

origin

10. **Litho+genesis** is the _____ of stones, or calculi. A **calculus** is an abnormal concretion that forms within the body, such as a kidney stone.

dissolving (or destruction)

11. **Litho+lysis** means _____ of stones. Large amounts of water can sometimes dissolve small stones in the bladder. A common surgical procedure crushes small stones using an instrument called a **lithotrite** or, more recently, using ultrasonic energy from a source outside the body.

stones

12. **Lith+iasis** is a condition marked by the formation of _____.

sugar

13. **Glyco+lysis** is the breaking down of sugar by an enzyme in the body. In Chapter 2 you learned that glyc/o means _____. Most sugars that we consume are converted to **glyco+gen** and stored for future conversion into glucose, which is used for performing work. Sugars and starches (carbohydrates) are important in providing the body with energy. Glucose is the most important carbohydrate in metabolism because cells use glucose for energy.

14. **Lipids** are fats that are used by our bodies to store energy on a long-term basis. Fats also act as insulation against cold. You learned previously that lip/o means fat. A **lip+oma** is a benign tumor composed of

fat (fatty)

_____ tissue (see Figure 2-3, *A*, p. 21).

destruction

15. Remembering that -lysis means dissolving or destruction, **electro+lysis** is _____ using an electric current. Electrolysis is sometimes used to remove unwanted hair.

electro-encephalo-graphy

16. An **electro+encephalo+gram** (EEG) is a record produced by the electrical impulses of the brain. The process of recording the electrical impulses of the brain is _____ (see Figure 3-9).

electro-encephalograph

17. Now write the name of the instrument used in electroencephalography: _____.

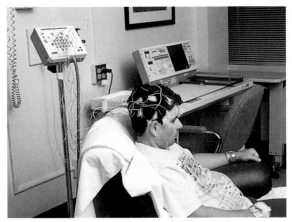

electr/o = electricity
encephal/o = brain
-graph = process of recording

Figure 3-9 Electroencephalography. Electrodes are attached to various areas of the patient's head. The patient generally remains quiet with closed eyes during the procedure. In certain cases, prescribed activities may be requested.

cephalometer

18. The combining form, encephal/o, is derived from en- (meaning inside) and cephal/o (meaning head). Cephalo+metry is measurement of the head. Change the suffix to write a word that means an instrument used to measure the head: _____.

light

19. Photo+graphy is the process of making images on sensitized material (film) by exposure to light or other radiant energy. What we call a photograph is actually a "photogram," but the picture is commonly called a photograph. Translated literally, **photo+phobia** is abnormal fear of _____. It means unusual sensitivity of the eyes to light. A person with measles may experience photophobia.

fear

20. Necro+phobia is abnormal _____ of death or dead bodies.

dead

21. Translated literally, necr+osis means a _____ condition. Necrosis is the death of areas of tissue or bone surrounded by healthy tissue.

fire

22. Pyro+phobia is abnormal fear of fire. You can see from the term pyrophobia that pyr/o means _____.

fire

23. Pyro+mania is abnormal preoccupation with _____. A **pyromaniac** derives pleasure from seeing or setting fires.

fever

24. A **pyro+gen** is any substance that produces fever. In this new term, the meaning is implied. In an infection, pyrogenic bacteria produce or cause _____ in their *host*, the individual who is harboring the bacteria. **Pyrogenic** means producing fever.

producing

25. Using pyro+genic as a model, pyo+genic means _____ pus.

pus

26. Pyo+derma is any acute, inflammatory disease of the skin in which _____ is produced.

study	27. **Histo+logy** is the _____ of the structure, function, and composition of tissues.
histologist	28. Write a word that means one who specializes in histology: _____.
tissue	29. **Histo+logic** means pertaining to _____.
tissue	30. Histologic compatibility refers to _____ that is suitable for transplantation to another individual.
stupor	31. A **narco+tic** is a drug that produces insensibility or _____.
stupor	32. **Narco+lepsy** is a chronic ailment that consists of recurrent attacks of drowsiness and _____, or sleep.
seizure	33. You probably have heard of **epi+lepsy,** a brain disorder characterized by sudden, brief attacks of altered consciousness, motor activity, or sensory phenomena. Convulsive seizures are the most common form of these attacks, and this is the basis for the term epilepsy. The suffix -lepsy means _____.
thirst	34. **Poly+dips+ia** is a condition characterized by excessive _____. Translated literally, polydipsia means many thirsts.
place	35. The term *ectopic* results when ecto- is joined with top/o and -ic (note the omission of the syllable *to*). In an **ectopic** pregnancy, the embryo is implanted outside the uterus. In other words, the embryo is implanted outside the usual _____.
straight	36. **Ortho+pnea** is a condition in which breathing is possible only when the person is sitting in an upright, or _____, position (-pnea refers to breathing).
vision	37. An **optic+ian** specializes in the translation, filling, and adapting of prescriptions, products, and accessories for _____.
heat	38. **Hyper+therm+ia** is a serious condition in which the body temperature is greatly elevated because of retention of body _____.
hidden	39. **Crypt+orchid+ism** is a developmental defect in which the testicles remain in the abdominal cavity. Because the testes cannot be seen, they might be considered _____; thus the name cryptorchidism.
fiber	40. **Fibr+in** is the essential portion of a blood clot. By its name, we know that fibrin has the characteristic of a _____.

FIND IT IN NEW TERMS!

EXERCISE 12

Write the combining form and its meaning for these new terms. A short definition is provided for each term.

Term/Meaning	Combining Form(s)	Meaning of Combining Form(s)
1. **aerosol** suspension of fine particles in a gas or in the air	aer/o	AIR
2. **aphonia** absence or loss of voice	phon/o	voice
3. **carcinogenesis** origin of cancer	carcin/o	cancer
4. **cryosurgery** destruction of tissue by extremely cold temperatures	cry/o	cold
5. **electrosurgery** surgery performed with high-frequency electric current	electr/o	electricity
6. **erythroblast** embryonic form of red blood cell	erythr/o	red
7. **lithotripsy** surgical crushing of a stone	lith/o	stone
8. **mycodermatitis** skin inflammation caused by fungus	myc/o	fungus
9. **necrotic** pertaining to the death of tissue	necr/o	dead
10. **pharmacotherapy** use of drugs to treat disease	pharmac/o	drugs
11. **psychogenic** originating in the mind	psycho	mind
12. **pyogenesis** formation of pus	py/o	pus

⊘ Be Careful with These!

in- *(not)* versus in- *(inside)*
infra- (under) versus intra- (within)
pro- (before) versus pro- (favoring, supporting)
py/o (pus) versus pyr/o (fire)

Opposites
ab- (away from) versus ad- (toward)
ante-, pre- (before) versus post- (after)
en-, end-, endo- (inside) versus ecto-, exo-, extra- (outside)
hyper- (more than normal) versus hypo- (less than normal)
macro- (large) versus micro- (small)
nulli- (none) versus pan- (all)
super-, supra- (above) versus hypo-, infra-, sub- (below)

SELF-TEST Work the following exercises to test your understanding of the material in Chapter 3. It is best to do all the exercises before checking your answers against the answers in Appendix VIII.

A. MATCH IT! *Match the word parts and the meanings in the right column.*

F	1. blast/o	A.	after
D	2. cry/o	B.	bad
H	3. crypt/o	C.	before
J	4. kinesi/o	D.	cold
E	5. lys/o	E.	destruction
I	6. macro-	F.	embryonic form
B	7. mal-	G.	fast
A	8. post-	H.	hidden
C	9. pro-	I.	large
G	10. tachy-	J.	movement

B. MATCH IT! *Match the terms in the left column with the colors suggested by the combining form.*

E	1. albinism	A.	black
C	2. chloroplast	B.	blue
B	3. cyanosis	C.	green
D	4. erthyrocyte	D.	red
A	5. melancholy	E.	white
F	6. xanthophyll	F.	yellow

C. FINDING THE CLUE! *Use a clue to write terms for these descriptions. Solve Question 1; each ending letter becomes the clue for the first letter of the next answer.*

1. pertaining to the presence of air or oxygen _____

2. stone _____

3. partially aware of one's surroundings _____

4. beneath the skin _____

5. pertaining to a location above a kidney _____

6. type of body fat _____

7. double vision _____

8. suspension of fine particles in a gas or air _____

9. presence of a stone _____

10. having a symptom or indication of a disease; sick _____

SELF-TEST (cont'd)

D. CIRCLE IT! *Choose the one correct response (a, b, c, or d) for each question.*

1. Which term means a white blood cell?
(a) chlorocyte   (b) erythrocyte   (c) leukocyte   (d) melanocyte

2. Which of the following means recording the electrical impulses of the brain?
(a) electroencephalogram   (b) electroencephalograph   (c) electroencephalography   (d) electroencephology

3. Which term means a substance that causes cancer?
(a) cancerous   (b) carcinogen   (c) carcinogenic   (d) carcinogenesis

4. Which term means an inflammation of the skin caused by a fungus?
(a) cutaneous   (b) dermatology   (c) dermatosis   (d) mycodermatitis

5. Which term means destruction of red blood cells resulting in the liberation of hemoglobin?
(a) hemolysin   (b) hemolysis   (c) hemolytic   (d) hemostasis

6. Which term means able to live without oxygen?
(a) aerobic   (b) aerosol   (c) anaerobic   (d) a-aerobic

7. What does bradycardia mean?
(a) decreased blood pressure   (b) decreased pulse rate   (c) increased blood pressure
(d) increased pulse rate

8. What is the term for any condition that renders some particular line of treatment improper?
(a) antipathology   (b) contraindication   (c) continence   (d) incontinence

9. Which of the following specifically means a cell that can ingest and destroy particulate substances?
(a) erythrocyte   (b) leukocyte   (c) melanocyte   (d) phagocyte

10. Which term means a fever-producing agent?
(a) pyoderma   (b) pyogen   (c) pyrogen   (d) pyrophobia

E. WRITE IT! *Write one-word terms for these meanings.*

1. difficult or weak voice   _____
2. malignant pigmented tumor   _____
3. increased amount of lipids in the blood   _____
4. composed of many cells   _____
5. excessive thirst   _____
6. increased pulse rate   _____
7. inside the trachea   _____
8. measurement of the head   _____
9. paralysis of one side of the body   _____
10. slowness of all body movement   _____

F. SPELL IT! *Circle all incorrectly spelled terms, and write their correct spelling.*

1. intramuscular   _____
2. distrofy   _____
3. ophthalmology   _____
4. oncolytik   _____
5. sindrome   _____

Use Appendix VIII to check your answers, paying particular attention to spelling.

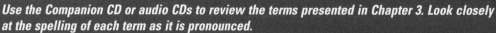

Q&E List
Use the Companion CD or audio CDs to review the terms presented in Chapter 3. Look closely at the spelling of each term as it is pronounced.

abductor (**ab-duk´tor**)
adductor (**ă-duk´tor**)
aerobic (**ār-o´bik**)
aerosol (**ār´o-sol´´**)
afebrile (**a-feb´ril**)
albinism (**al´bĭ-niz-əm**)
albino (**al-bi´no**)
anaerobic (**an´´ə-ro´bik**)
anhydrous (**an-hi´drəs**)
antacid (**ant-as´id**)
antepartum (**an´´te-pahr´təm**)
anticonvulsive (**an´´te-, an´´ti-kən-vul´siv**)
aphasia (**ə-fa´zhə**)
aphonia (**a-fo´ne-ə**)
arteriosclerosis (**ahr-tēr´´e-o-sklə-ro´sis**)
asymptomatic (**a´´simp-to-mat´ik**)
bicuspid (**bi-kus´pid**)
bifocal (**bi-fo´kəl, bi´fo-kəl**)
bradycardia (**brad´´e-kahr´de-ə**)
bradyphasia (**brad´´ĭ-fa´zhə**)
calculus (**kal´ku-ləs**)
carcinogen (**kahr-sin´ə-jen**)
carcinogenesis (**kahr´´sĭ-no-jen´ə-sis**)
carcinogenic (**kahr´´sin-o-jen´ik**)
carcinoma (**kahr´´sĭ-no´mə**)
cardiomegaly (**kahr´´de-o-meg´ə-le**)
cephalic (**sə-fal´ik**)
cephalometer (**sef´ə-lom´ə-tər**)
cephalometry (**sef´ə-lom´ə-tre**)
chloropia (**klor-ōp´e-ə**)
continence (**kon´tĭ-nəns**)
contraceptive (**kon´´trə-sep´tiv**)
contraindication (**kon´´trə-in´´dĭ-ka´shən**)
cryosurgery (**kri´´o-sur´jər-e**)
cryotherapy (**kri´´o-ther´ə-pe**)
cryptorchidism (**krip-tor´kĭ-diz´´əm**)
cyanosis (**si´´ə-no´sis**)
cyanotic (**si´´ə-not´ik**)
cytology (**si-tol´ə-je**)
cytoscopy (**si-tos´kə-pe**)
dermal (**dur´məl**)
diplopia (**dĭ-plo´pe-ə**)
dyskinesia (**dis´´kĭ-ne´zhə**)

dyslexia (**dis-lek´se-ə**)
dysphagia (**dis-fa´je-ə**)
dysphasia (**dis-fa´zhə**)
dysphonia (**dis-fo´ne-ə**)
dystrophic (**dis-tro´fik**)
dystrophy (**dis´trə-fe**)
ectopic (**ek-top´ik**)
electrocardiogram (**e-lek´´tro-kahr´de-o-gram´´**)
electrocardiograph (**e-lek´´tro-kahr´de-o-graf´´**)
electrocardiography (**e-lek´´tro-kahr´´de-og´rə-fe**)
electroencephalogram (**e-lek´´tro-en-sef´ə-lo-gram´´**)
electroencephalograph (**e-lek´´tro-ən-sef´ə-lo-graf´´**)
electroencephalography (**e-lek´´tro-ən-sef´´ə-log´rə-fe**)
electrolysis (**e´´lek-trol´ə-sis**)
electrosurgery (**e-lek´´tro-sur´jər-e**)
embryonic (**em´´bre-on´ik**)
endotracheal (**en´´do-tra´ke-əl**)
epilepsy (**ep´ĭ-lep´´se**)
erythroblast (**ə-rith´ro-blast**)
erythrocyte (**ə-rith´ro-sīt**)
erythrocytosis (**ə-rith´´ro-si-to´sis**)
euthanasia (**u´´thə-na´zhə**)
euthyroid (**u-thi´roid**)
febrile (**feb´ril**)
fibrin (**fi´brin**)
fibrous (**fi´brəs**)
glycogen (**gli´ko-jən**)
glycolysis (**gli-kol´ə-sis**)
hemiplegia (**hem´´e-ple´jə**)
hemoglobin (**he´mo-glo´´bin**)
hemolysin (**he-mol´ə-sin**)
hemolysis (**he-mol´ə-sis**)
hemolytic (**he´´mo-lit´ik**)
hemolyze (**he´mo-līz**)
histocompatibility (**his´´to-kəm-pat´´ĭ-bil´ĭ-te**)
histologic (**his´´to-log´ik**)
histologist (**his-tol´ə-jist**)
histology (**his-tol´ə-je**)
hyperglycemia (**hi´´pər-gli-se´me-ə**)
hyperlipemia (**hi´´pər-li-pe´me-ə**)
hyperparathyroidism (**hi´´pər-par´´ə-thi´roid-iz-əm**)
hypersecretion (**hi´´pər-se-kre´shən**)
hyperthermia (**hi´´pər-thur´me-ə**)

hyperthyroidism (hi˝pər-thi´roid-iz-əm)
hypocalcemia (hi˝po-kal-se´me-ə)
hypodermic (hi˝po-dur´mik)
hypoglycemia (hi˝po-gli-se´me-ə)
hypoparathyroidism (hi˝po-par˝ə-thi´roid-iz-əm)
hyposecretion (hi˝po-sə-kre´shən)
hypothyroidism (hi˝po-thi´roid-iz-əm)
incompatible (in˝kəm-pat´ĭ-bəl)
incontinence (in-kon´tĭ-nəns)
intradermal (in˝trə-dur´məl)
intramuscular (in˝trə-mus´ku-lər)
intravenous (in˝trə-ve´nəs)
jaundice (jawn´dis)
kinesiotherapy (kĭ-ne˝se-o-ther´ə-pe)
leukemia (loo-ke´me-ə)
leukocyte (loo´ko-sīt)
leukoderma (loo˝ko-dur´mə)
lipid (lip´id)
lipoma (lip-o´mə)
lithiasis (lĭ-thi´ə-sis)
lithogenesis (lith˝o-gen´ə-sis)
litholysis (lĭ-thol´ĭ-sis)
lithotripsy (lith´o-trip˝se)
lithotrite (lith´o-trīt)
macrocephaly (mak˝ro-sef´ə-le)
macroscopic (mak˝ro-skop´ik)
malabsorption (mal˝əb-sorp´shən)
megalocyte (meg´ə-lo-sīt˝)
megalomania (meg˝ə-lo-ma´ne-ə)
melancholy (mel´ən-kol˝e)
melanoma (mel˝ə-no´mə)
mesoderm (mez´o-, me´zo-dərm)
microorganism (mi˝kro-or´gən-iz-əm)
microscope (mi´kro-skōp)
microscopy (mi-kros´kə-pe)
mononuclear (mon˝o-noo´kle-ər)
multicellular (mul˝tĭ-sel´u-lər)
mycodermatitis (mi˝ko-der˝mə-ti´tis)
mycology (mi-kol´ə-je)
narcolepsy (nahr´ko-lep˝se)
narcotic (nahr-kot´ik)
necrophobia (nek˝ro-fo´be-ə)
necrosis (nə-kro´sis)
necrotic (nə-krot´ik)
nullipara (nə-lip´ə-rə)

ophthalmopathy (of˝thəl-mop´ə-the)
optical (op´tĭ-kəl)
optician (op-tish´ən)
optometrist (op-tom´ə-trist)
orthopnea (or˝thop-ne´ə)
osteoblast (os´te-o-blast˝)
osteomalacia (os˝te-o-mə-la´shə)
pandemic (pan-dem´ik)
para-appendicitis (par˝ə-ə-pen˝dĭ-si´tis)
parathyroids (par˝ə-thi´roids)
phagocyte (fa´go-sīt)
pharmacotherapy (fahr˝mə-ko-ther´ə-pe)
photophobia (fo˝to-fo´be-ə)
polydipsia (pol˝e-dip´se-ə)
postnasal (pōst-na´zəl)
postpartum (pōst-pahr´təm)
prerenal (pre-re´nəl)
primigravida (pri˝mĭ-grav´ĭ-də)
psychogenesis (si˝ko-jen´ə-sis)
psychogenic (si˝ko-jen´ik)
pyoderma (pi˝o-dur´mə)
pyogenesis (pi˝o-jen´ə-sis)
pyogenic (pi˝o-jen´ik)
pyrogen (pi´ro-jən)
pyrogenic (pi˝ro-jen´ik)
pyromania (pi˝ro-ma´ne-ə)
pyromaniac (pi˝ro-ma´ne-ak)
pyrophobia (pi˝ro-fo´be-ə)
quadriplegia (kwod˝rĭ-ple´jə)
rachischisis (ra˝kis´kĭ-sis)
schizophrenic (skit˝so-, skiz˝o-fren´ik)
sclerosis (sklə-ro´sis)
semiconscious (sem˝e-kon´shəs)
subcutaneous (sub˝ku-ta´ne-əs)
supervitaminosis (soo˝pər-vi˝tə-min-o´sis)
suprarenal (soo˝prə-re´nəl)
symptomatic (simp˝to-mat´ik)
syndrome (sin´drōm)
tachycardia (tak˝ĭ-kahr´de-ə)
tachyphasia (tak˝e-fa´zhə)
transdermal (trans-dur´məl)
tricuspid (tri-kus´pid)
tripara (trip´ə-rə)
unilateral (u˝nĭ-lat´ər-əl)
xanthosis (zan-tho´sis)

 Don't forget the games on the Companion CD and http://evolve.elsevier.com/Leonard/quick/ for additional review, including questions on Spanish terms.

ESPAÑOL Enhancing Spanish Communication

English	Spanish (pronunciation)
Colors	**Los Colores**
black	negro (**NAY-gro**)
blue	azul (**ah-SOOL**)
gray	gris (**grees**)
green	verde (**VERR-day**)
orange	anaranjado (**ah-nah-ran-HAH-do**), naranjado (**nah-ran-HAH-do**)
pink	rosa (**RO-sah**)
red	rojo (**ROH-ho**)
white	blanco (**BLAHN-co**)
yellow	amarillo (**ah-mah-REEL-lyo**)
Additional Terms	**Mas Vocabulario**
acidity	acidez (**ah-se-DES**)
breathing	respiración (**res-pe-rah-se-ON**)
childbirth	parto (**PAR-to**)
consciousness	conciencia (**con-se-EN-se-ah**)
creams	creamas (**CRAY-mahs**)
defecate	evacuar (**ay-vah-coo-AR**)
destruction	destrucción (**des-trooc-se-ON**)
electricity	electricidad (**ay-lec-tre-se-DAHD**)
epilepsy	epilepsia (**ay-pe-LEP-se-ah**)
esophagus	esófago (**ay-SO-fah-go**)
fainting	languidez (**lan-gee-DES**)
fatigue	fatiga (**fah-TEE-gah**)
fever	fiebre (**fe-AY-bray**)
fiber	fibra (**FEE-brah**)
head	cabeza (**cah-BAY-sah**)
hypodermic	hipodérmico (**e-po-DER-me-co**)
injection	inyección (**in-yec-se-ON**)
injury	daño (**DAH-nyo**)
leukemia	leucemia (**lay-oo-SAY-me-ah**)
life	vida (**VEE-dah**)
light	luz (**loos**)
movement	movimiento (**mo-ve-me-EN-to**)
narcotic	narcótico (**nar-CO-te-co**)
nose	nariz (**nah-REES**)
optician	óptico (**OP-te-co**)
oxygen	oxígeno (**ok-SEE-hay-no**)
paralysis	parálisis (**pah-RAH-le-sis**)
seizure	ataque (**ah-TAH-kay**)

English	Spanish (pronunciation)
speech	habla **(AH-blah)**, lenguaje **(len-goo-AH-hay)**
thirst	sed **(sayd)**
urinate	orinar **(oo-re-NAR)**
voice	voz **(vos)**
weakness	debilidad **(day-be-le-DAHD)**
wound	lesión **(lay-se-ON)**

CHAPTER 4

Diagnostic Procedures and Therapeutic Interventions

CONTENTS

Signs and Symptoms in Diagnosis
Basic Examination Procedures
Common Diagnostic Tests and Procedures
Diagnostic Radiology

Radiation and Other Therapeutic Interventions
Self-Test
Q&E List
Enhancing Spanish Communication

OBJECTIVES

After completing Chapter 4, you will be able to:

1. Identify the difference between signs and symptoms.
2. List the vital signs and the four basic examination procedures.
3. Match diagnostic terms with their meanings.
4. Match therapeutic interventions with their meanings.

5. Write the meanings of Chapter 4 word parts, or match word parts with their meanings.
6. Build and analyze medical terms with Chapter 4 word parts.
7. Spell medical terms correctly.

Signs and Symptoms in Diagnosis

Diagnosis is the identification of a disease or condition by a scientific evaluation of physical signs, symptoms, history, tests, and procedures. **Prognosis** means the predicted outcome of a disease.

A disease is often described as acute or chronic. **Acute** means having a short and relatively severe course. The opposite of acute is **chronic**, meaning that the disease exists over a long time.

Signs are objective, or definitive, evidence of an illness or disordered function that are perceived by an examiner, such as fever, a rash, or evidence established by radiologic or laboratory testing. **Symptoms** are subjective evidence as perceived by the patient, such as pain.

Diagnostic terms are used to describe the signs and symptoms of disease as well as the tests used to establish a diagnosis. The tests include clinical studies (e.g., measuring blood pressure), laboratory tests (e.g., determination of blood gases), and **radio+logic** studies, which relate to the use of radiation (e.g., chest x-ray image). Laboratory (lab) tests, ranging from simple to sophisticated studies, identify and quantify substances to evaluate organ functions or establish a diagnosis. Various body fluids are collected and sent to the laboratory for testing, most often blood and urine. In addition, fluids are collected from various body cavities or wounds. A small sample or part taken from the body to represent the nature of the whole is called a *specimen*.

When the body is in a healthy state, it functions normally, and the physical and chemical characteristics of the body substances are generally within a certain accept-able range, known as the *normal range*. The abbreviation WNL, meaning "within normal limits," is sometimes used to describe the results of a laboratory test. When a pathologic condition exists, changes take place within the body and may cause an alteration in the physical and chemical characteristics of body substances, as evidenced by abnormal laboratory values or results.

WRITE IT! **EXERCISE 1**

Write terms for these meanings.

1. descriptive of a disease with a short, relatively severe course   *acute*
2. descriptive of a disease that exists over a long period   *chronic*
3. identification of a disease or condition by scientific evaluation   *diagnosis*
4. predicted outcome of a disease   *prognosis*

Use Appendix VIII, Answers to Exercises, to check all your answers to the exercises throughout Chapter 4.

MATCH IT! **EXERCISE 2**

Choose A or B from the right column to classify the items in the left column as a sign or a symptom.

A **1.** blood pressure reading   **A.** sign
A **2.** definitive evidence of a disease   **B.** symptom
B **3.** subjective evidence perceived by a patient
B **4.** itching
A **5.** rash

Basic Examination Procedures

Basic examinations are performed to assess the patient's condition. Vital signs are measured and recorded for most patients. Vital signs are the measurements of pulse rate, respiration rate, and body temperature.

The **pulse** is the rhythmic expansion of an artery that occurs as the heart beats; it may be felt with a finger. The pulse results from the expansion and contraction of an artery as blood is forced from the heart (Figure 4-1). The pulse rate is the count of the heartbeats per minute. A normal pulse rate in a resting state is 60 to 100 beats per minute.

The **respiration** (or respiratory) rate is the number of breaths per minute. The rise and fall of the patient's chest is observed while counting the number of breaths and noting the ease with which breathing is accomplished.

Body temperature can be measured through several routes, including the mouth, the rectum, under the armpit, and the external opening of the ear canal. Thermo+meters are instruments used to measure temperature. Originally, a ther-mometer consisted of a sealed glass tube, marked in degrees Celsius or Fahrenheit, and contained a liquid such as mercury. The liquid rises or falls as it expands or contracts according to changes in temperature. Electronic measurement of body

QUICK TIP
Caution: Although sometimes included, blood pressure is not strictly a vital sign.

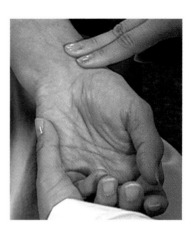

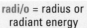
radi/o = radius or
radiant energy

Figure 4-1 Assessment of the radial pulse. The pulse is an intermittent throbbing sensation felt when the fingers are pressed against an artery such as the radial artery. Radi/o sometimes means radiant energy, but in this case it is used to mean *radius,* a bone of the forearm, for which the artery is named.

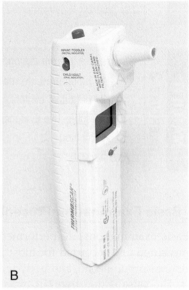

-al = pertaining to
or/o = mouth
rect/o = rectum
therm/o = heat

Figure 4-2 Devices for electronic temperature measurement. A, Thermometer for measuring temperature orally, rectally, or under the arm. **B,** Tympanic membrane thermometer that uses a probe placed in the ear.

therm/o = heat
(also used to
write terms about
temperature)
-meter = instrument
used to measure

temperature has reduced the time required for accurate readings. Some devices for electronic temperature measurement have a probe that is covered by a disposable sheath and placed under the tongue with the mouth tightly closed, in the rectum, or under the arm with the arm held close to the body (Figure 4-2). The **tympanic thermometer** has a specially designed probe tip that is placed at the external opening of the ear canal.

Blood pressure is the pressure exerted by the circulating volume of blood on the walls of the arteries and veins and on the chambers of the heart. Indirect measurement of blood pressure is made with a stethoscope and a blood pressure cuff. The readings generally consist of two numbers expressed as a fraction, with the first number representing the maximum pressure on the artery and the second number representing the amount of pressure that still exists when the heart is relaxed (in other words, not contracting). The standard unit of measurement is millimeters of mercury (mm Hg). For example, a healthy young person has a blood pressure of approximately 120/80 mm Hg. The higher reading is the **systolic pressure**, and the lower reading is the **diastolic pressure** (Figure 4-3).

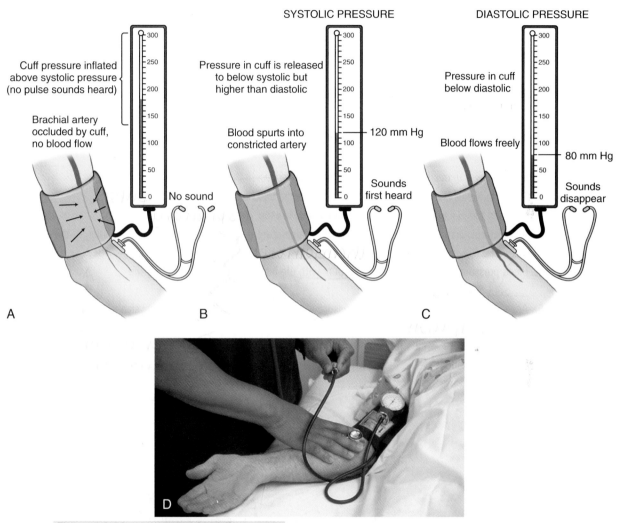

Figure 4-3 Measurement of blood pressure. A, B, C, Drawings of the mercury manometer apparatus, an older method of measuring blood pressure, facilitate the understanding of blood pressure readings. In **A,** no sounds are heard because the pressure in the cuff is higher than the systolic pressure. In **B,** the first sound heard (a systolic pressure of 120 mm Hg) is noted. In **C,** the last sound heard (80 mm Hg) represents the diastolic pressure. This example represents a normal blood pressure reading of 120/80 mm Hg (the height of mercury in a graduated column on the blood pressure apparatus). **D,** A common indirect measurement of blood pressure using a blood pressure cuff and a stethoscope. The pulse sounds heard through the stethoscope result from blood flow in the artery. Systolic pressure is caused by ventricular contraction. Diastolic pressure occurs when the ventricles relax. After rapid inflation of the blood cuff and slow deflation of it, the first pulse sound heard represents the systolic pressure. As the pressure is slowly released, the last sound heard represents the diastolic pressure.

The history and physical examination are important parts of a patient's medical record. The following four techniques are useful in the physical examination:

- **Inspection.** The examiner uses the eyes and ears to observe and listen to the patient.
- **Palpation.** The examiner feels the texture, size, consistency, and location of certain body parts with the hands (Figure 4-4, *A*).
- **Percussion.** The examiner taps the body with the fingertips or fist to evaluate the size, borders, and consistency of internal organs and to determine the amount of fluid in a body cavity (Figure 4-4, *B*).
- **Auscultation.** The examiner listens for sounds within the body to evaluate the heart, blood vessels, lungs, intestines, or other organs, or to detect the fetal heart sound. Auscultation is performed most frequently with a stethoscope (Figure 4-4, *C*). A **stethoscope** is basically an instrument consisting of two earpieces connected by flexible tubing; the diaphragm is placed against the patient's skin to hear sounds within the body.

steth/o = chest
-scope = instrument used for viewing

WRITE IT! **EXERCISE 3**

Write an answer in each blank to complete these sentences.

1. The rhythmic expansion of an artery that occurs as the heart beats is called the ___pulse___.
2. Counting the number of breaths per minute measures the ___respiratory___ rate.
3. An electronic instrument that measures body temperature by placing the probe at the opening of the external ear is called a tympanic ___thermometer___.
4. Blood pressure is represented as a fraction, with the higher reading representing the ___systolic___ pressure.
5. Application of the fingers with light pressure to the surface of the body during physical examination is called ___palpation___.
6. Tapping the body with the fingertips or fist during physical examination is ___percussion___.
7. Listening for sounds within the body using a stethoscope is called ___Auscultation___.

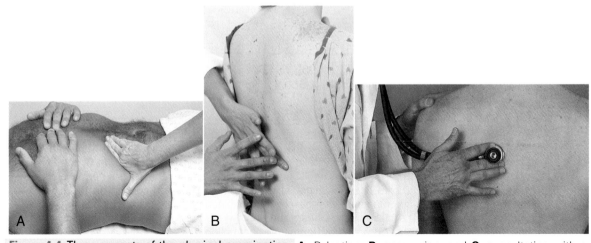

Figure 4-4 Three aspects of the physical examination. A, Palpation; **B,** percussion; and **C,** auscultation with a stethoscope help in assessing the internal organs.

Common Diagnostic Tests and Procedures

The diagnostic process helps determine a patient's health status. You have already studied several tests and procedures that aid in this process. Laboratory analyses of blood, urine, and stool specimens, along with diagnostic radiology (presented in the next section), assist the physician in establishing a diagnosis.

You have already learned several combining forms and associated suffixes that are used in terms pertaining to diagnostic procedures, such as gram/o, metr/o, and scop/o (meaning to record, measure, and examine, respectively).

BUILD IT!   EXERCISE 4

Write terms for these diagnostic instruments and procedures, which you studied in Chapter 3.

1. instrument used to record the electrical impulses of the heart   *electrocardiograph*
2. recording the electrical impulses of the heart (see Figure 3-8, p. 66)   *electrocardiography*
3. the record produced in electrocardiography   *electrocardiogram*
4. measurement of the dimensions of the head (see Figure 2-2, p. 19)   *cephalometry*
5. instrument used to examine the eye   *ophthalmoscope*
6. examination of the eye with an ophthalmoscope (Figure 4-5)   *ophthalmoscopy*
7. instrument for viewing microscopic objects   *microscope*
8. visual examination of the ear   *otoscopy*

An **endo+scope** is an illuminated instrument for the visualization of the interior of a body cavity or organ (Figure 4-6). Although the endoscope is generally introduced through a natural opening (e.g., mouth, rectum), it may also be inserted through an incision, such as into the chest cavity through an incision in the chest wall. The visual inspection of the body by means of an endoscope is **endoscopy**.

> endo- = inside
> -scope = instrument for viewing

A **catheter** is a hollow flexible tube that can be inserted into a cavity of the body to withdraw or instill fluids, perform tests, or visualize a vessel or cavity. The introduction of a catheter is **catheterization**, and to introduce a catheter is to **catheterize** (Figure 4-7). The Latin term **cannula** is also used to mean a hollow flexible tube that is inserted into vessels or cavities.

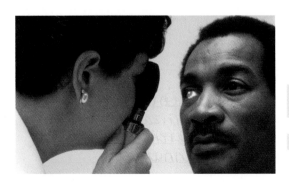

> ophthalm/o = eye
> -scopy = visual examination

Figure 4-5 Ophthalmoscopy. Proper technique for ophthalmoscopic visualization of the interior of the eye.

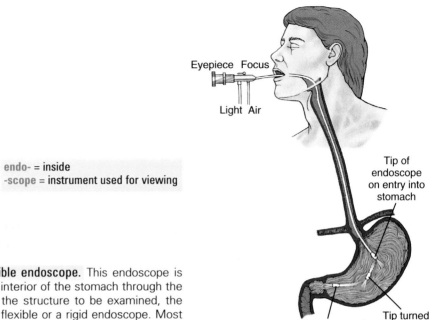

endo- = inside
-scope = instrument used for viewing

Figure 4-6 Example of flexible endoscope. This endoscope is being used to examine the interior of the stomach through the esophagus. Depending on the structure to be examined, the physician chooses either a flexible or a rigid endoscope. Most of the interior stomach can be examined, including the antrum, located in the lower part of the stomach.

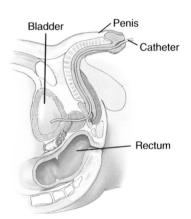

Figure 4-7 Urinary catheter inserted into the male bladder. The most common route of catheterization is insertion of the catheter through the external opening of the urethra into the urethra and into the bladder. This procedure is done to drain or remove fluid from the bladder, or to introduce fluids for various tests or treatments.

WRITE IT!
EXERCISE 5

Write terms for these meanings.
1. visual inspection of the body using an endoscope   *endoscopy*
2. the process of inserting a catheter into the body   *catheterization*
3. to introduce a catheter into the body   *catheterize*
4. a hollow flexible tube; catheter   *cannula*

Diagnostic Radiology

Radiology is the branch of medicine concerned with x-rays, radioactive substances, and the diagnosis and treatment of disease by using any of the various sources of radiant energy. Several of these procedures are noninvasive, whereas an **invasive procedure** requires entry of a body cavity (e.g., **catheterization**) or interruption of normal body function (e.g., surgical incision).

Diagnostic radiology is used to establish or confirm a diagnosis. Digital radiography uses a computer to store and manipulate radiographic data. For example, in **computed radiography**, the image data are digitized and immediately displayed on a monitor or recorded on film.

> radi/o = radiant energy
> -graphy = process of recording

Learn the word parts pertaining to radiology and their meanings.

Word Parts: Radiology

Combining Form	Meaning
ech/o, son/o	sound
electr/o	electricity
fluor/o	emitting or reflecting light
radi/o*	radiant energy
tom/o	to cut

Prefix	
ultra-	excessive

Use the electronic flashcards on the Evolve site or make your own set of flashcards using the above list. Select the word parts just presented, and study them until you know their meaning. Do this each time a set of word parts is presented.

Sometimes means radius, a bone of the forearm.

FIND IT!
EXERCISE 6

Find the combining forms used in these terms, and write the combining form and its meaning.

	Combining Form	Meaning
1. echogram	ech/o	sound
2. fluoroscope	fluor/o	emitting/reflecting light
3. radiography	radi/o	radiant energy
4. tomogram	tom/o	to cut
5. ultrasonography	son/o	sound

Radio+graphy was the predominant means of diagnostic imaging for many years, with x-rays providing film images of internal structures. An x-ray image is a **radio+graph**; however, the suffix -graph refers to an instrument used for recording. The radiograph is made by projecting x-rays through organs or structures of the body onto a photographic film. X-rays that pass through the patient expose the radiographic film or digital image receptor to create the image. X-radiation passes through different substances in the body to varying degrees. Where penetration is greater, the image is black or darker; where the x-rays are absorbed by the subject, the image is white or

 QUICK TIP
Similar usage is found in "photograph," the picture obtained in photography.

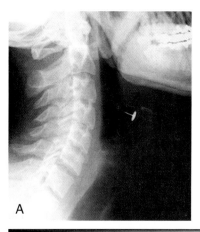

A

Figure 4-8 Penetration of x-radiation by various substances in an x-ray image. **A,** Radiograph of an aspirated thumbtack. The lodged tack appears white because it absorbs most of the x-rays and prevents them from reaching the film or image receptor. Note also the different appearances of air, soft tissue, bone, and teeth. **B,** Schematic representation of how substances appear on an x-ray image, depending on the amount of x-radiation the substance absorbs.

| Air =
black | Fat =
dark gray | Muscle/tissue =
light gray | Bone =
very light
or white | Metal =
white |

B

QUICK TIP

One *o* in radi/o + opaque is omitted to facilitate pronunciation.

light gray. Thus, air appears black, fat appears dark gray, muscle tissue appears light gray, and bone appears very light or white. Heavy substances, such as lead or steel, appear white because they absorb the rays and prevent them from reaching the image receptor (Figure 4-8).

Substances that do not permit the passage of x-rays are described as **radiopaque**. **Radiolucent** describes substances that readily permit the passage of x-rays.

Additional diagnostic imaging modalities include the following:
• Computed tomography (CT)
• Magnetic resonance imaging (MRI)
• Sono+graphy, also called **echo+graphy**, ultra+sono+graphy, and ultra+sound
• Contrast imaging
• Nuclear imaging (placing radioactive materials into body organs for the purpose of imaging)

QUICK TIP

CT is also called a "CAT" scan (*A* for "axial").

Computed tomography uses ionizing radiation to produce a detailed image of a cross section of tissue, similar to what one would see if the body or body part were actually cut into sections. The procedure, however, is painless and noninvasive. Figure 4-9 shows a CT (or CAT) scanner and a **tomogram**, the record produced.

Magnetic resonance imaging creates images of internal structures based on the magnetic properties of chemical elements within the body and uses a powerful magnetic field and radiowave pulses rather than ionizing radiation such as x-rays. MRI produces superior soft tissue resolution for distinguishing adjacent structures (Figure 4-10). Patients must remain motionless for a time and may experience anxiety because of being somewhat enclosed inside the scanner. Open MRI scanners have eliminated much of the anxiety and can accommodate larger patients.

ultra- = beyond
son/o = sound
-graphy = process
   of recording

Also called **ultrasonography**, diagnostic ultrasound, and other names, **sonography** is the process of imaging deep structures of the body by sending and receiving high-frequency sound waves that are reflected back as echoes from tissue interfaces.

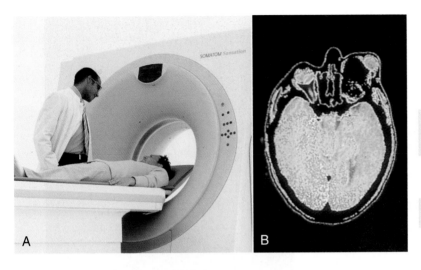

-graphy = process of recording
-ic = pertaining to
tom/o = to cut

Figure 4-9 Computed tomography (CT) of the brain. A, Positioning of patient for CT. B, CT image of the brain.

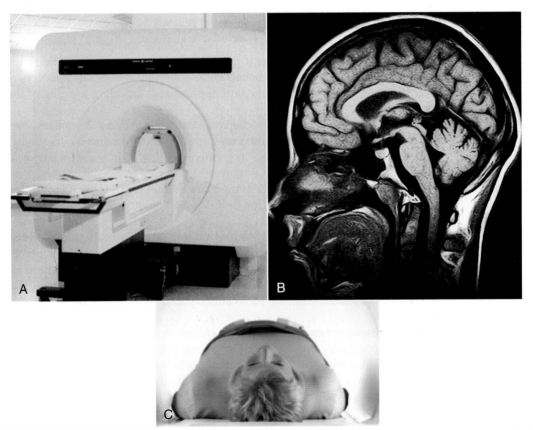

Figure 4-10 Magnetic resonance imaging (MRI). A, Clinical setting for MRI. B, MR image of the head. C, Open MRI scanner.

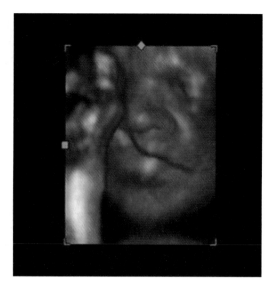

-gram = process of recording
son/o = sound
ultra- = beyond

Figure 4-11 Three-dimensional sonogram of fetus. This three-dimensional ultrasound image shows a normal fetal face of late pregnancy. Sonograms provide important information to the obstetrician and pictures for the parents as the fetus develops.

Conventional sonography provides two-dimensional images, but the more recent scanners are capable of showing a three-dimensional perspective. The record produced is called a **sonogram** or an **echogram**. Sonography is very safe and does not use ionizing radiation. It has many medical applications, including imaging of the fetus (Figure 4-11).

Contrast imaging is the use of radiopaque materials to make internal organs visible on x-ray images. A contrast medium may be swallowed, introduced into a body cavity, or injected into a vessel, resulting in greater visibility of internal organs or cavities outlined by the contrast material (Figure 4-12).

fluor/o = emitting or
reflecting light
-scopy = visual
examination

Fluoroscopy is the visual examination of an internal organ using a **fluoroscope**. This technique offers continuous imaging of the motion of internal structures and immediate serial images.

Nuclear scans involve administering radio+pharmaceuticals to a patient orally, into the vein, or by having the patient breathe the material in vapor form. **Pharmaceuticals** are medicinal drugs, and radiopharmaceuticals are those that are radioactive. Computerized scanners called gamma cameras detect the radioactivity emitted by the patient and map its location to form an image of the organ or system (Figure 4-13).

Positron emission tomography (PET) combines tomography and radioactive substances to produce enhanced images of selected body structures, especially the heart, blood vessels, and the brain. The radioactive materials used in PET are very short-lived, so the patient is exposed to extremely small amounts of radiation.

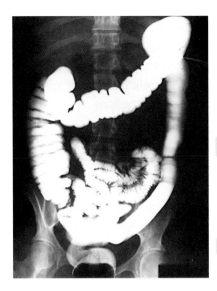

radi/o = radiant energy

Figure 4-12 Contrast imaging. In this example of a barium enema, radiopaque barium sulfate is used to make the large intestine clearly visible.

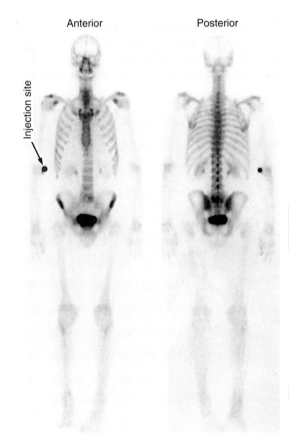

Anterior   Posterior

Injection site

-al = pertaining to
pharmaceut/i = drugs or medicine
radi/o = radiant energy

Figure 4-13 Nuclear medicine. Administration of a radio-pharmaceutical allows its accumulation in a specific organ or structure, providing information about function and, to some degree, structure.

MATCH IT!

EXERCISE 7

Match the descriptions in the left column with the imaging modalities in the right column.

__E__ **1.** Imaging of internal structures by measuring and recording sound waves

__D__ **2.** Placing radioactive materials into body organs and using computerized scanners

__A__ **3.** Producing detailed images of cross sections of tissue as though cuts had been made

__B__ **4.** Using radiopaque materials to make internal organs or vessels visible

__C__ **5.** Visualizing internal structures based on the magnetic properties of chemical elements

A. computed tomography
B. contrast imaging
C. magnetic resonance imaging
D. nuclear medicine
E. sonography

Radiation and Other Therapeutic Interventions

radi/o = radiant
energy
-therapy =
treatment

X-rays and radioactive materials are helpful in diagnosing disease and are also used in **radio+therapy**, the treatment of tumors using radiation to destroy cancer cells. The radiation may be applied by directing a beam of radiation toward the tumor with a machine that delivers radiation doses many times higher in intensity than those used for diagnosis. Alternately, the radiation may be introduced through the bloodstream or may be surgically implanted. Radiation therapy is also called **radiation oncology** (Figure 4-14).

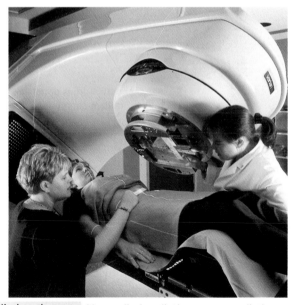

Figure 4-14 Radiation therapy. Also called radiotherapy or radiation oncology, radiation therapy treats neoplastic disease by using powerful x-rays or gamma rays to prevent the malignant cells from increasing in number.

Radiotherapy can produce undesirable side effects because of incidental destruction of normal body tissues. Most of the side effects disappear with time and include nausea and vomiting, hair loss, ulceration or dryness of mucous membranes, and suppression of bone marrow activity.

Therapeutic means "pertaining to therapy." Learn the word parts for treatment and their meanings.

Word Parts: Treatment

Combining Form	Meaning
algesi/o	sensitivity to pain
chem/o	chemical
pharmac/o, pharmaceut/i	drugs or medicine
plast/o	repair
therapeut/o	treatment
tox/o	poison

Suffix	
-therapy	treatment

FIND IT!

EXERCISE 8

Find the combining forms used in these terms, and write the combining form and its meaning.

	Combining Form	Meaning
1. algesic	alge si/o	sensitivity to pain
2. chemotherapy	chem/o	chemical
3. pharmaceutical	pharmaceut/i	drugs/medicine
4. therapeutic	therapeut/o	treatment
5. toxic	tox/o	poison

PROGRAMMED LEARNING

Remember to cover the answers (left column) with folded paper or the bookmark. Write an answer in each blank, and then check your answer before proceeding to the next frame.

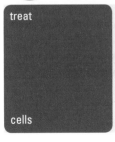

treat

1. Therapeutic radiology uses radiation to _____ cancer. Radiation therapy, also called radiation oncology, is the treatment of cancer using ionizing radiation, such as x-rays.

2. In addition to radiation, several approaches are used to treat cancer, including surgery to remove the cancer and **chemo+therapy**, treatment of disease by chemical agents. The combining form chem/o means chemical. **Cyto+tox+ic** agents are used in cancer treatment to kill cancer _____.

cells

new

3. A neoplasm is a _____ growth of tissue (a tumor) that is either benign or malignant. Anti+neo+plast+ics are medications that are used to treat neoplasms. Malignant tumors are called carcinomas. Many malignant tumors are curable if detected and treated at an early stage. Invasive carcinoma is a malignant tumor that infiltrates and destroys surrounding tissues and may continue spreading. Remission, whether spontaneous or the result of therapy, is the disappearance of the characteristics of a malignant tissue.

4. **Pharmaco+therapy** is the treatment of diseases with drugs or medicine. The combining form therapeut/o means treatment. Write an adjective that means pertaining to treatment by combining therapeut/o and -ic:

therapeutic

_____. A second meaning of this term is curative.

5. An **an+alges+ic** is a drug that relieves pain. The term results from combining an- + algesi/o + -ic. Notice that one *i* is omitted to facilitate pronunciation. The

pain

combining form algesi/o means sensitivity to _____.
    An analgesic such as aspirin is a type of pharmaceutical. The term *pharmaceutical* refers to pharmacy or drugs, but it also means a medicinal drug. Some drugs require a physician's prescription and others, such as aspirin, are over-the-counter (OTC) drugs, in other words, not requiring a prescription.

6. **Narcotic** means pertaining to a substance that produces insensibility or

stupor

_____. The term also means a narcotic drug. Narcotic analgesics alter perception of pain, induce a feeling of euphoria, and may induce sleep. Repeated use of narcotics may result in physical and psychologic dependence. In large amounts, as in an overdose (OD), narcotics can depress respiration.

7. **Anti+microbials** are drugs that destroy or inhibit the growth of microbes (microorganisms). **Anti+bio+tics** are antimicrobial agents that are derived from cultures of a microorganism or produced semisynthetically and used to treat infections. Penicillin is a well-known antibiotic. Literal translation of

against

antimicrobials indicates that they are used _____ microbes.

8. Both heat and cold are used to treat disease, especially to relieve pain and speed healing. Treating with heat is **thermo+therapy,** which can be helpful in relaxing muscles and promoting blood circulation. It may be administered as dry heat (e.g., heat lamps, electrical pads) or moist heat (e.g., warm compresses, warm water soaks). Write the term that means treatment of

thermotherapy

disease with heat: _____.

cryotherapy

9. Use thermotherapy as a model to write a term that means treatment using cold temperatures: _____. Cold compresses, such as an ice pack, are used to reduce pain and swelling, especially after surgery. You learned in Chapter 3 that destruction of tissue by the application of subfreezing temperature to destroy tissue is cryosurgery.

BUILD IT!   EXERCISE 9

Combine the words parts to write terms.

1. an- + algesi/o + -ic   _____
2. anti- + ne/o + plast/o + -ic   _Antineoplastic_
3. chem/o + -therapy   _chemotherapy_
4. cry/o + -therapy   _cryofort_ _cryotherapy_
5. cyt/o + tox/o + -ic   _cytotoxic_
6. pharmac/o + -therapy   _pharmacotherapy_
7. radi/o + -therapy   _radiotherapy_
8. therm/o + -therapy   _thermotherapy_

⚠ Be Careful with These!

palpation (part of physical exam) versus *palpitation* (heart flutter)

Opposites
acute versus *chronic*
radiopaque versus *radiolucent*
signs (objective) versus *symptoms* (subjective)

SELF-TEST   Work the following exercises to test your understanding of the material in Chapter 4. It is best to do all the exercises before checking your answers against the answers in Appendix VIII.

A. MATCH IT!   *Choose A or B from the right column to classify the descriptions as a sign or a symptom.*

_B_ **1.** The patient says he has a sore throat.   **A.** sign
_A_ **2.** The patient has a fever.   **B.** symptom
_A_ **3.** The patient's blood pressure is elevated.
_A_ **4.** The patient has an abnormal laboratory result.
_B_ **5.** The patient says she has a headache.

Match the terms in the left column with their descriptions in the right column.

_____ **6.** auscultation   **A.** feeling internal body parts with the hands on the external surface
_____ **7.** inspection   **B.** tapping the patient's body with the fingertips or fist
_____ **8.** palpation   **C.** using a stethoscope to listen for sounds within the body
_____ **9.** percussion   **D.** using the eyes to observe the patient

B. WRITE IT!   *List three vital signs. (Remember: Blood pressure is not strictly a vital sign.)*

1. _____
2. _____
3. _____

SELF-TEST   (cont'd)

C.   CIRCLE IT!   *Circle the one correct answer (a, b, c, or d) for each question.*

1. Which term means the "probable outcome of a disease"?
(a) diagnosis   (b) prognosis   (c) sign   (d) symptom
2. Which diagnostic procedure produces a detailed image of a cross section of tissue, similar to what one would see if the organ were actually cut into sections?
(a) computed tomography   (b) contrast imaging   (c) electrocardiography   (d) nuclear medicine imaging
3. What is the term for the rhythmic expansion of an artery as the heart beats?
(a) blood pressure   (b) pulse   (c) respiration   (d) systolic pressure
4. Which diagnostic procedure creates images based on the magnetic properties of chemical elements within the body?
(a) computed tomography   (b) magnetic resonance imaging   (c) nuclear scanning
(d) positron emission tomography
5. Which of the following is the same as radiation therapy?
(a) diagnostic radiology   (b) fluoroscopy   (c) positron tomography   (d) radiation oncology

D. FINDING THE CLUE!   *Use a clue to write terms for the descriptions. Solve Question 1; each ending letter becomes the clue for the first letter of the next answer.*

1. opposite of chronic _____Acute_____
2. sonogram _____
3. opposite of benign _____malignant_____
4. pertaining to therapy _____therapeutic_____
5. destructive or damaging to cells _____
6. term that often precedes tomography _____computed_____
7. identification of disease by signs, symptoms, and history _____diagnosis_____
8. instrument often used in auscultation _____stethoscope_____
9. heart tracing _____
10. term that often precedes resonance _____

E. WRITE IT!   *Write a term for each definition.*

1. drug that produces insensibility or stupor _____
2. drug that relieves pain _____
3. objective evidence of an illness _____
4. pertaining to therapy _____
5. treatment of disease by chemical agents _____
6. having severe symptoms and lasting a short time _____
7. permitting the passage of x-rays _____
8. not allowing passage of x-rays _____
9. showing little change or slow progression _____
10. act of tapping the body in physical diagnosis _____

SELF-TEST (cont'd)

F. SPELL IT! *Circle all incorrectly spelled terms, and write their correct spelling.*

1. floroscopy   _____

2. neoplazm   _____

3. ~~simptom~~   symptom

4. ~~stethoskope~~   stethoscope

5. thermometer   _____

Use Appendix VIII to check your answers, paying particular attention to spelling.

Q&E List

Use the Companion CD or audio CDs to review the terms presented in Chapter 4. Look closely at the spelling of each term as it is pronounced.

acute (**ə-kūt´**)
analgesic (**an´´əl-je´zik**)
antibiotic (**an´´te-, an´´ti-bi-ot´ik**)
antimicrobial (**an´´te-, an´´ti-mi-kro´be-əl**)
auscultation (**aws´´kəl-ta´shən**)
blood pressure (**blud presh´ər**)
cannula (**kan´u-lə**)
catheter (**kath´ə-tər**)
catheterization (**kath´´ə-tur-ĭ-za´shən**)
catheterize (**kath´ə-ter-īz**)
chemotherapy (**ke´´mo-ther´ə-pe**)
chronic (**kron´ik**)
computed radiography (**kom-pu´tid ra´´de-og´rə-fe**)
computed tomography (**kom-pu´tid to-mog´rə-fe**)
cryotherapy (**kri´´o-ther´ə-pe**)
cytotoxic (**si´to-tok´´sik**)
diagnosis (**di´´əg-no´sis**)
diastolic pressure (**di´´ə-stol´ik presh´ər**)
echogram (**ek´o-gram**)
echography (**ə-kog´rə-fe**)
endoscope (**en´do-skōp**)
endoscopy (**en-dos´kə-pe**)
fluoroscope (**floor´o-skōp**)
fluoroscopy (**floŏ-ros´kə-pe**)
inspection (**in-spek´shən**)
invasive procedure (**in-va´siv pro-se´jər**)
magnetic resonance imaging (**mag-net´ik rez´o-nəns im´ə-jing**)

narcotic (**nahr-kot´ik**)
palpation (**pal-pa´shən**)
percussion (**pər-kŭ´shən**)
pharmaceutical (**fahr´´mə-soo´tĭ-kəl**)
pharmacotherapy (**fahr´´mə-ko-ther´ə-pe**)
positron emission tomography (**poz´ĭ-tron e-mish´ən to-mog´rə-fe**)
prognosis (**prog-no´sis**)
pulse (**puls**)
radiation oncology (**ra´´de-a´shən ong-kol´ə-je**)
radiograph (**ra´de-o-graf´´**)
radiography (**ra´´de-og´rə-fe**)
radiologic (**ra´´de-o-loj´ik**)
radiolucent (**ra´´de-o-loo´sənt**)
radiopaque (**ra´´de-o-pāk´**)
radiotherapy (**ra´´de-o-ther´ə-pe**)
respiration (**res´´pĭ-ra´shən**)
sign (**sīn**)
sonogram (**son´o-gram**)
sonography (**sə-nog´rə-fe**)
stethoscope (**steth´o-skōp**)
symptom (**simp´təm**)
systolic pressure (**sis-tol´ik presh´ər**)
therapeutic (**ther´´ə-pu´tik**)
thermotherapy (**thur´´mo-ther´ə-pe**)
tomogram (**to´mo-gram**)
tympanic thermometer (**tim-pan´ik thər-mom´ə-tər**)
ultrasonography (**ul´´trə-sə-nog´rə-fe**)

 Don't forget the games on the Companion CD and http://evolve.elsevier.com/Leonard/quick/ for additional review, including questions on Spanish terms.

Enhancing Spanish Communication

English	Spanish (pronunciation)
acute	agudo **(ah-GOO-do)**
antibiotic	antibiótico **(an-te-be-O-te-co)**
blood pressure	presión sanguínea **(pray-se-ON san-GEE-nay-ah)**
chronic	crónico **(CRO-ne-co)**
diagnosis	diagnóstico **(de-ag-NOS-te-co)**
laboratory	laboratorio **(lah-bo-rah-TO-re-o)**
physical examination	examen físico **(ek-SAH-men FEE-se-co)**
radiograph	radiografía **(rah-de-o-grah-FEE-ah)**
radiology	radiología **(rah-de-o-lo-HEE-ah)**
symptom	síntoma **(SEEN-to-mah)**
temperature	temperatura **(tem-pay-rah-TOO-rah)**
therapy	terapia **(ter-ah-PEE-ah)**
thermometer	termómetro **(ter-MO-may-tro)**
treatment	tratamiento **(trah-tah-me-EN-to)**
x-ray image	radiografía **(rah-de-o-grah-FEE-ah)**

CHAPTER 5

The Body as a Whole

CONTENTS

Organization of the Body
   Reference Planes
   Body Cavities
   Body Regions
Body Fluids
   Blood

Body Defenses and Immunity
   Pathogens
   Bioterrorism
Self-Test
Q&E List
Enhancing Spanish Communication

OBJECTIVES

After completing Chapter 5, you will be able to:

1. Recognize the relationship of cells, tissues, and organs, and list the major body systems.
2. List four types of tissue, and recognize terms for abnormal tissue development.
3. Recognize the directional terms and planes of the body, match them with their descriptions, and write their combining forms.
4. Identify the body cavities, the body regions, and the four abdominal quadrants.
5. Recognize the terms for diagnostic procedures and disorders presented in Chapter 5.
6. Recognize the meanings of Chapter 5 word parts and use them to build and analyze medical terms.
7. Write terms pertaining to body fluids and blood and their disorders, as well as associated terms.
8. Write terms about body defenses, immunity, and bioterrorism when given their definitions, or match them with their meanings.
9. Spell medical terms correctly.

Organization of the Body

All parts of the human body, from atoms to visible structures, work together as a functioning whole (Figure 5-1). Starting with the simplest and proceeding to the most complex, the six levels of organization in the body can be represented as follows:

Chemicals → Cells → Tissues → Organs → Body Systems → Organism

WRITE IT!

EXERCISE 1

Which is simpler? Decide which of the two choices is simpler, then write the name of the simpler organizational level of the body in the blank (Question 1 is done as an example).

1. cell versus organ   *Cell* _____
2. organ versus tissue   _____
3. organ versus body system   _____
4. body system versus organism   _____
5. chemical versus tissue   _____

Check all your answers to the exercises in Chapter 5 with Appendix VIII, Answers to Exercises.

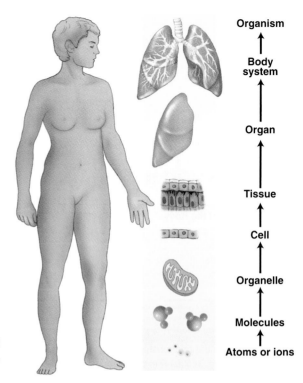

Figure 5-1 Organization scheme of the body. All of its parts, from tiny atoms to visible structures, work together to make a functioning whole.

somat/o = body

The cell is the fundamental unit of life. Nerve cells, muscle cells, and blood cells are examples of different types of somatic, or body, cells. Somat+ic cells account for all the body's cells except the reproductive cells—the sperm and ova. Groups of cells that perform the same basic activity are called *tissues*.

The four main types of tissue and their functions are epithelial (covering), connective (supporting and protecting), muscular (contracting), and nervous (conducting impulses) tissues. Label the four types of tissues in Figure 5-2.

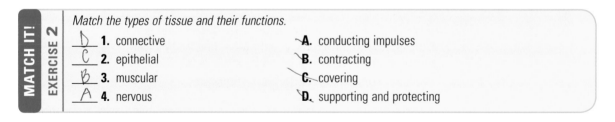

MATCH IT!
EXERCISE 2

Match the types of tissue and their functions.

D **1.** connective

C **2.** epithelial

B **3.** muscular

A **4.** nervous

A. conducting impulses

B. contracting

C. covering

D. supporting and protecting

-plasia = formation
dys- = bad
a- = without
hypo- = below
  normal
hyper- = above
  normal

Two or more tissue types that work together to perform one or more functions and form a more complex structure make up *organs*. The skin, stomach, and ear are examples of organs.

Terms used to describe abnormal changes in tissue or organ formation ususally contain the suffix -plasia. **Dys+plasia** is any abnormal development of tissues, and is recognized by cells that differ in size, shape, and appearance. **A+plasia** is the lack of development of an organ or tissue. **Hypo+plasia** is less severe than aplasia. **Hyper+plasia** means an abnormal increase in the number of normal cells in tissue. Hyperplasia

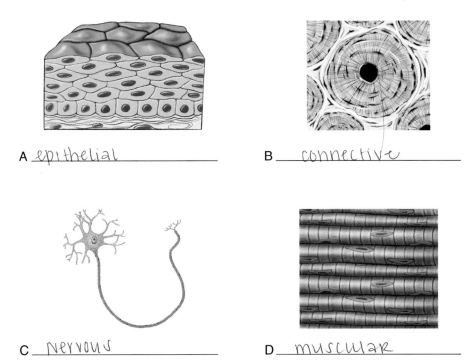

A _epithelial_   B _connective_

C _Nervous_   D _muscular_

Figure 5-2 Major types of tissue. Label the types of tissue: **A,** epithelial tissue of the type that comprises several cellular layers; **B,** connective tissue of elastic fibers; **C,** nervous tissue; **D,** muscle tissue of the striated type.

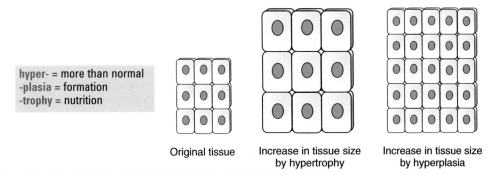

hyper- = more than normal
-plasia = formation
-trophy = nutrition

Original tissue   Increase in tissue size by hypertrophy   Increase in tissue size by hyperplasia

Figure 5-3 Comparison of hypertrophy and hyperplasia. A representation of tissue enlargement by hypertrophy and hyperplasia.

contrasts with another term, **hyper+trophy**, which means an increase in the size of an organ caused by an increase in the *size* of the cells rather than the number of cells (Figure 5-3). A change in the structure and orientation of cells, characterized by a loss of differentiation and reversal to a more primitive form, is characteristic of malignancy. This change in cell structure is **ana+plasia**.

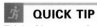

home/o =
sameness
-stasis = **controlling**

QUICK TIP

Think of homeostasis
as equilibrium.

A *body system* consists of several organs that work together to accomplish a set of functions. Body systems are covered in Chapters 6 through 14 of this book. Some systems are combined in the same chapter; for example, the skeletal and muscular systems are presented in Chapter 6. Table 5-1 lists the major body systems and their functions.

The most complex level in the organizational scheme is the *organism,* the human body. **Homeo+stasis** refers to the constant internal environment that is naturally maintained by the body.

During development, cells become specialized or differentiated. Undifferentiated cells that have the ability to divide without limit and give rise to specialized cells are called *stem cells.* Stem cells are used in bone marrow transplants and can be used in research for organ or tissue regeneration.

Table 5-1 Major Body Systems

Body System (Chapter)	Major Functions
Muscular system (6)	Makes movement possible
Skeletal system (6)	Provides protection, form, and shape for the body; stores minerals and forms some blood cells
Cardiovascular system (7)	Delivers oxygen, nutrients, and vital substances throughout the body; transports cellular waste products to the lungs and kidneys for excretion
Lymphatic system (7)	Helps maintain the internal fluid environment; produces some types of blood cells; regulates immunity
Respiratory system (8)	Brings oxygen into the body and removes carbon dioxide and some water waste
Digestive system (9)	Provides the body with water, nutrients, and minerals; removes solid wastes
Urinary system (10)	Filters blood to remove wastes of cellular metabolism; maintains the electrolyte and fluid balance
Reproductive system (11)	Facilitates procreation (producing offspring)
Integumentary system (12)	Provides external covering for protection; regulates the body temperature and water content
Nervous system (13)	Coordinates the reception of stimuli; transmits messages to stimulate movement
Endocrine system (14)	Secretes hormones and helps regulate body activities

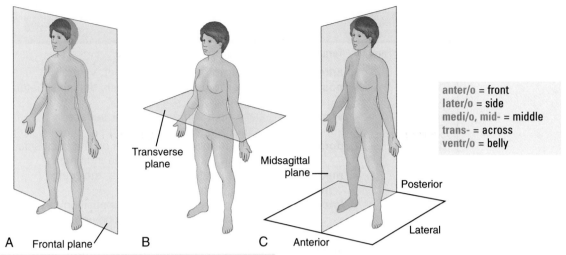

anter/o = front
later/o = side
medi/o, mid- = middle
trans- = across
ventr/o = belly

Figure 5-4 Anatomic position with reference systems. The erect anterior view with palms forward is used as the point of reference in anatomic nomenclature. **A,** Frontal plane; **B,** transverse plane; **C,** midsagittal plane, also showing the posterior, lateral, and anterior aspects.

Reference Planes

Anatomists use directional terms and planes to describe the position and direction of various body structures or parts. Locations and positions are described relative to the body in the anatomic position, that is, the position that a person is in while standing erect with the arms at the sides and the palms forward (Figure 5-4). The three reference planes are as follows:

- Frontal plane
- Transverse plane
- Sagittal plane

The three planes are imaginary flat surfaces. A **frontal plane**, or coronal plane, divides the body into front and back portions. A **transverse plane** divides the body into upper and lower portions; it may be drawn at any level. A **sagittal plane** divides the body into right and left sides, and a **midsagittal plane** divides the body into two equal halves.

trans- = across

Unless otherwise stated, descriptions of location and position assume that the body is in the **anatomic** position. Three important aspects are shown in Figure 5-4 and are used to describe locations:

- Anterior (front)
- Posterior (behind)
- Lateral (side)

Commit to memory these three aspects and additional terms that relate to directions in the body. These directional terms, their combining forms, and their meanings are presented in the following table.

Directional Terms

Combining Form	Term	Meaning
anter/o	**anterior**	nearer to or toward the front; ventral
poster/o	**posterior**	nearer to or toward the back; dorsal; situated behind
ventr/o	**ventral**	belly side; same as anterior surface in humans
dors/o	**dorsal**	directed toward or situated on the back side; same as posterior surface in humans
medi/o	**medial, median**	middle or nearer the middle; the prefix mid- also means middle
later/o	**lateral**	toward the side; denoting a position farther from the midline of the body or from a structure
super/o	**superior**	uppermost or above
infer/o	**inferior**	lowermost or below
proxim/o	**proximal**	nearer the origin or point of attachment
dist/o	**distal**	far or distant from the origin or point of attachment
cephal/o	**cephalad**	toward the head
caud/o	**caudad**	toward the tail or in an inferior direction in humans

Use the electronic flashcards on the Evolve site or make your own set of flashcards using the above list. Select the word parts just presented, and study them until you know their meaning. Do this each time a set of word parts is presented.

WRITE IT!

EXERCISE 3

Write the meanings of the combining forms, and then provide the corresponding anatomic term. (Question 1 is done as an example).

Combining Form	Meaning	Anatomic Term
1. anter/o	*front*	*anterior*
2. caud/o	tail/inferior	caudad
3. cephal/o	Head	cephalad
4. dist/o	Far/distant	distal
5. dors/o	back side	dorsal
6. infer/o	lowermost/below	inferior
7. later/o	side	lateral
8. medi/o	middle	medial, median
9. poster/o	back	posterior
10. proxim/o	nearer the origin	proximal
11. super/o	uppermost/above	superior
12. ventr/o	belly side	ventral

WRITE IT!

EXERCISE 4

Using terms from the list you just studied, write terms that mean the opposite of these terms.

1. anterior   *posterior*
2. inferior   *superior*
3. proximal   *distal*
4. ventral (in humans)   ~~posterior~~ *dorsal*

FIND IT IN NEW TERMS!

EXERCISE 5

Write the combining forms and their meanings for these new terms (Question 1 is done as an example). A short definition is provided for each term.

Term/Meaning		Combining Forms
1. **anteromedian** *anter/o, front*		*medi/o, middle*
located in front and toward the middle		
2. **posteroexternal** *poster/o, back*		*external (L. externus)*
situated toward the back and outer side		
3. **posteromedian** *poster/o, back*		*medi/o, middle*
situated in the middle of the back		
4. **dorsolateral** *dors/o, back side*		*later/o, side*
pertaining to the back and the side		
5. **posterolateral** *poster/o, back*		*later/o, side*
pertaining to a position behind and to the side		
6. **anterolateral** *anter/o, front*		*later/o, side*
pertaining to the front and one side		
7. **mediolateral** *medi/o, middle*		*later/o, side*
pertaining to the middle and one side		
8. **anterosuperior** *anter/o, front*		*super/o, above*
indicates a position in front and above		
9. **posterosuperior** *poster/o, back*		*super/o, above*
indicates a position behind and above		
10. **inferomedian** *infer/o, below*		*medi/o, middle*
situated in the middle of the underside		

PROGRAMMED LEARNING

Remember to cover the answers (left column) with folded paper or the bookmark. Write an answer in each blank, and then check your answer before proceeding to the next frame.

anterior	1. The body is facing forward in the anatomic position. Anterior means toward the front; therefore the anatomic position refers to the _____ aspect or front of the body.
back	2. **Postero+internal** means situated toward the _____ and the inner side.

front

back

back

ventral

anterior

posterior

median

tail

near

nearer

far (distant), distal

distant

telecardiogram

down

3. In radiology, directional terms are used to specify the direction of the x-ray beam from its source to its exit surface before striking the image receptor. In an **antero+posterior** projection, the x-ray beam strikes the anterior aspect of the body first. In other words, the beam passes from the _____ of the body to the back.

4. **Postero+anterior** means from the posterior to the anterior surface—in other words, from _____ to front. (Figure 5-5 shows three radiographic positions.)

5. Dorsal also means directed toward or situated on the back side. **Dorso+ventral** pertains to the _____ and belly surfaces. Dorsoventral sometimes means passing from the back to the belly surface. For example, the path of a bullet resulting from a shot in the back could be described as dorsoventral.

6. The term for belly side is _____.

7. In humans, the ventral surface is the same as the _____ aspect of the body.

8. Similarly, the dorsal surface in humans is the same as the _____ aspect of the body.

9. Two terms that mean middle are medial and _____.

10. Caudad means toward the tail. **Caud+al** means pertaining to the _____, or to a tail-like structure. Sometimes caudal is also used to mean inferior in position.

11. Proximal describes the position of structures that are nearer their origin or point of attachment. The combining form proxim/o is used in words that refer to proximal, or _____.

12. The proximal end of the thigh bone joins with the hip bone. This means that the proximal end of the thigh bone is _____ the hip bone than is the other end of the thigh bone.

13. Distal is the opposite of proximal. Distal means far or distant. It also means away from the origin or point of attachment. The lower end of the thigh bone is _____ to the hip bone.

14. Distal is derived from the same word root as *distant*, which should help you to remember the term. The combining form tel/e also means distant. A **tele+cardio+gram**, for example, is a tracing of the electrical impulses of the heart recorded by a machine _____ from the patient.

15. Telecardiograms can be sent by telephone. With a _____, the cardiologist and the patient may be in different cities.

16. Physicians rely on additional positions for examination or surgery. **Prone** and **supine** are terms used to describe the position of a person who is lying face (head) down and lying on the back, respectively (Figure 5-6). If a person is prone, is the face turned up or down? _____

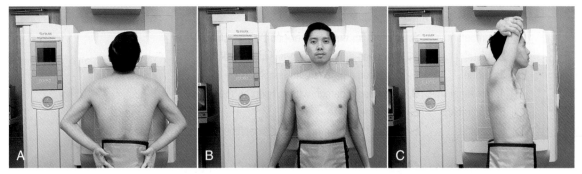

Posteroanterior projection   Anteroposterior projection   Left lateral projection

Figure 5-5 **Patient positioning for a chest x-ray. A,** In a posteroanterior (PA) projection, the anterior aspect of the chest is closest to the image receptor. **B,** In an anteroposterior (AP) projection, the posterior aspect of the chest is closest to the image receptor. **C,** In a left lateral chest projection, the left side of the patient is placed against the image receptor.

-al = pertaining to
anter/o = anterior
  (front)
later/o = side
poster/o = posterior

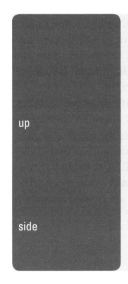

17. Pronation and supination are generally used to indicate positioning of the hands and feet, but their complete meaning includes the act of lying prone or face downward and the assumption of a supine position. **Pronation** of the arm is the rotation of the forearm so that the palm faces downward. **Supination** is the rotation of a joint that allows the hand or foot to turn upward. Supination of the elbow and wrist joints allows the palm to turn

up

    _____.

    Compare pronation and supination of the wrist in Figure 5-6, C. (*Helpful hint:* Think of <u>sup</u>ination as "palm up so I can hold a cup of <u>soup</u>." Pronation is the opposite: palm down.)

18. **Recumbent** means lying down. The patient assumes the lateral recumbent position by lying on the side because *lateral* means pertaining to the

side

    _____.

    Ambulant describes a person who is able to walk. It is also correct to say that the person is *ambulatory.*

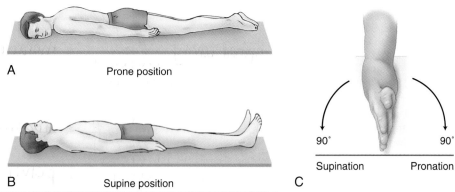

A   Prone position

B   Supine position   C

Figure 5-6 **Comparison of pronation and supination. A,** Prone, lying facedown. **B,** Supine, lying on the back. **C,** Supination and pronation of the elbow and wrist joints, which permit the palm of the hand to turn up (supination) or down (pronation).

MATCH IT!
EXERCISE 6

Match the terms with the descriptions.

  C **1.** ambulant   **A.** away from the origin or point of attachment
  A **2.** distal   **B.** describes a person who is lying facedown
  B **3.** prone   **C.** describes a person who is able to walk
  F **4.** proximal   **D.** describes a person who is lying on the back
  E **5.** recumbent   **E.** lying down
  D **6.** supine   **F.** nearer the origin or point of attachment

Body Cavities

The body has two major cavities, which are spaces within the body that contain internal organs. The two principal body cavities are the *dorsal cavity,* located near the posterior part of the body, and the *ventral cavity,* located near the anterior part (Figure 5-7).

The dorsal cavity is divided into the **cranial** and **spinal** cavities. The cranial cavity contains the brain, and the spinal cavity contains the spinal cord and the beginnings of the spinal nerves. The other principal body cavity is the ventral cavity. Large organs contained in the ventral cavity are called **viscera**. The ventral cavity is subdivided into the **thoracic** cavity and the **abdominopelvic** (abdominal and pelvic) cavity. The muscular **diaphragm** divides the thoracic and abdominopelvic cavities. The diaphragm is a dome-shaped partition that functions in respiration (see Figure 8-1, p. 192).

thorac/o = chest

The abdominopelvic cavity can be thought of as a single cavity or as two cavities, the abdominal and pelvic cavities, although no wall separates them. A membrane called the **periton+eum** lines the abdominopelvic cavity and enfolds the internal organs. The peritoneum, as with all serous membranes, secretes a lubricating fluid that allows the organs to glide against one another or against the cavity wall. A sticking together of two structures that are normally separated is called an **adhesion**. Abdominal adhesions are usually caused by inflammation or trauma (injury) and are treated surgically if they cause intestinal obstruction or excessive discomfort.

periton/o = peritoneum
-eum = membrane

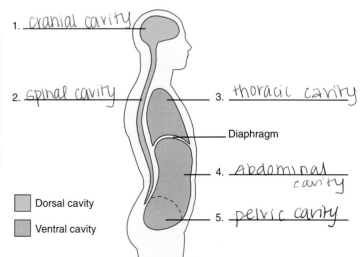

abdomin/o = abdomen
crani/o = skull
dors/o = back
pelv/i = pelvis
spin/o = spine
thorac/o = chest
ventr/o = belly

1. cranial cavity
2. spinal cavity
3. thoracic cavity
   Diaphragm
4. Abdominal cavity
5. pelvic cavity

Dorsal cavity
Ventral cavity

Figure 5-7 The dorsal and ventral cavities. Label the numbered structures as you read. The dorsal cavity is divided into the cranial cavity *(1)* and spinal cavity *(2)*. The ventral cavity is divided into the thoracic cavity *(3)* and the abdominopelvic cavity, which is subdivided into the abdominal cavity *(4)* and the pelvic cavity *(5)*.

MATCH IT! **EXERCISE 7**

Choose A or B from the right column to identify the body cavities in the left column as a dorsal or a ventral cavity.

_A B_ **1.** abdominopelvic cavity
_A_ **2.** cranial cavity
_A_ **3.** spinal cavity
_B_ **4.** thoracic cavity

A. dorsal cavity
B. ventral cavity

Body Regions

The major regions of the body are the following:

- Head
- Neck
- Torso
- Extremities

> **QUICK TIP**
> Torso is also called the trunk.

The head contains the brain and special sense organs such as the mouth, the nose, the eyes, and the ears. Senses that we possess include sight, hearing, smell, taste, touch, and pressure. The neck connects the head with the **torso**, which includes the chest, abdomen, and pelvis. The extremities are the four limbs (arms and legs). The arms, wrists, hands, and fingers make up the upper extremities. The thighs, knees, legs, ankles, feet, and toes make up the lower extremities.

WRITE IT! **EXERCISE 8**

List the four major regions of the body.

1. _Head_
2. _Neck_
3. _Torso_
4. _extremities_

Combining Forms for Select Body Regions or Structures

Combining Form	Meaning
abdomin/o	abdomen
acr/o	extremities (arms and legs)
blephar/o	eyelid
cyst/o	cyst, bladder, or sac
dactyl/o	digit (toes, fingers, or both)
lapar/o	abdominal wall
omphal/o	umbilicus (navel)
onych/o	nail
pelv/i	pelvis
periton/o	peritoneum
som/a, somat/o	body
thorac/o	chest (thorax)

Use the electronic flashcards on the Evolve site, or make your own set of flashcards using the Combining Forms list. Select the word parts just presented, and study them until you know their meaning.

Commit the combining forms in the following table to memory.

WRITE IT!

EXERCISE 9

Write combining forms for these meanings.

1. abdominal wall   _Lapar/o_
2. body   _som/a, somat/o_
3. digit   _dactyl/o_
4. extremities   _acr/o_
5. eyelid   _blephar/o_
6. nail   _onych/o_
7. chest   _thorac/o_
8. umbilicus   _omphal/o_

The chest is also called the **thorax**. The chest and pelvis are the upper part and lower part of the torso, respectively. The **abdomen** is the portion of the body trunk that is located between the chest and the pelvis. The division of the abdomen into quadrants is the convenient method of using imaginary lines to divide the abdomen into regions. **Abdominal quadrants** are often used to describe the location of pain or body structures. The four abdominal quadrants are the right upper quadrant (RUQ), left upper quadrant (LUQ), right lower quadrant (RLQ), and left lower quadrant (LLQ) (Figure 5-8).

abdomin/o =
    abdomen
-centesis = surgical
    puncture

Abdominothoracic is an adjective that pertains to the abdomen and the thorax. **Abdomino+centesis**, usually called abdominal **paracentesis**, is a surgical procedure that is performed to remove excess fluids from the abdominal cavity or to inject a therapeutic agent (Figure 5-9). Abnormal accumulation of fluid in the peritoneal cavity is called **ascites** (Figure 5-10). **Periton+itis** can result if infectious microorganisms gain access by way of surgical incisions or by the rupture or perforation of viscera or associated structures (as in rupture of the appendix). Microorganisms can also spread to the peritoneum from the bloodstream or lymphatic vessels.

periton/o =
    peritoneum
-itis = inflammation

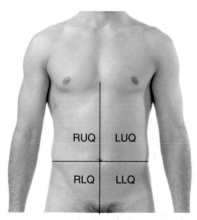

abdomin/o = abdomen
quad- = four

Figure 5-8 Abdominal quadrants. The four quadrants in this anatomic division of the abdomen are determined by drawing a vertical and horizontal line through the umbilicus. RUQ, LUQ, RLQ, and LLQ are abbreviations for right upper quadrant, left upper quadrant, right lower quadrant, and left lower quadrant, respectively.

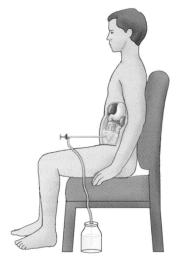

abdomin/o = abdomen
-centesis = surgical puncture
para- = beside

Figure 5-9 Abdominal paracentesis. In this surgical puncturing of the abdomen, fluid is withdrawn for diagnosis or to remove excess fluid.

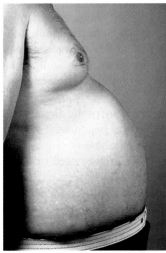

abdomin/o = abdomen
-al, -eal = pertaining to
periton/o = peritoneum

Figure 5-10 Ascites. This abnormal accumulation of a fluid in the peritoneal cavity is treated with dietary therapy and drugs. Abdominal paracentesis may be performed to relieve the pressure of the accumulated fluid.

Thoracic means pertaining to the chest. Thoracic surgery is another way of saying "chest surgery." Surgical puncture of the chest wall for aspiration of fluids could be called **thoracocentesis**, but **thoracentesis** is the more common term.

> thorac/o = thorax or chest

Incision of the abdominal wall is called **laparotomy. Laparoscopy** is examination of the interior of the abdomen by means of a **laparoscope**, an instrument that is inserted into the peritoneal cavity to inspect it.

> lapar/o = abdominal wall
> -tomy = incision

The **pelvis** is the lower portion of the body trunk. The word pelvis can refer to any basin-like structure, so you will also see it in other terms (e.g., the renal pelvis, a funnel-shaped structure within the kidney). **Pelvic** means pertaining to a pelvis, usually the bony pelvis, as is the case here. A "cephalopelvic disproportion" is a situation in which the head of the fetus is too large for the pelvis of the mother. In such cases, vaginal delivery is difficult or impossible. **Cephalo+pelvic** refers to the head of the fetus and the maternal pelvis.

> cephal/o = head
> pelv/i = pelvis

Omphalos is Greek for the umbilicus, or navel. Many new terms can be formed using omphal/o with various suffixes that you have already learned. **Omphal+ic** means

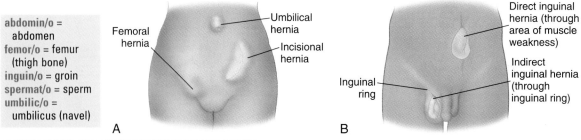

abdomin/o =
abdomen
femor/o = femur
(thigh bone)
inguin/o = groin
spermat/o = sperm
umbilic/o =
umbilicus (navel)

Figure 5-11 Common types of abdominal hernias. A, *Umbilical* hernias result from a weakness in the abdominal wall around the umbilicus. An *incisional* hernia is herniation through inadequately healed surgery. In a *femoral* hernia, a loop of intestine descends through the femoral canal into the groin (femoral means pertaining to the thigh). **B,** *Inguinal* hernias are of two types. A *direct* hernia occurs through an area of weakness in the abdominal wall. In an *indirect* hernia, a loop of intestine descends through the inguinal canal, an opening in the abdominal wall for passage of the spermatic cord in males, and a ligament of the uterus in females.

concerning the **umbilicus. Umbilical** also means pertaining to the umbilicus. An inflamed condition of the navel is **omphalitis.** Rupture of the navel is **omphalorrhexis,** and umbilical hemorrhage is **omphalorrhagia.** Congenital herniation of the navel is an **omphalo+cele.** A *hernia* is protrusion of an organ through an abnormal opening in the wall of the cavity that surrounds it. Types of abdominal hernias include umbilical, **femoral,** incisional, and **inguinal** (Figure 5-11).

cephal/o = head
-metry =
measurement

Cephalad means toward the head. **Cephalo+metry** is measurement of the dimensions of the head. **Cephalgia** and **cephalodynia** mean pain in the head or headache.

Blepharal means pertaining to the eyelid; **blepharoplegia** is paralysis of one or both eyelids. Terms for twitching of, surgical incision of, and plastic surgery performed on the eyelid are **blepharospasm, blepharotomy,** and **blepharoplasty,** respectively.

acr/o = extremities
hypo- = below
normal
therm/o =
temperature
-y = condition
-megaly = enlarged

Acral means pertaining to the extremities of the body (arms and legs). **Acro+dermat+itis** is dermatitis of the extremities. In **acro+cyan+osis,** cyanosis of the extremities, the arms and legs appear bluish. Abnormal coldness of the extremities is **acrohypothermy. Acromegaly** is a disorder in which there is abnormal enlargement of the body extremities, including the nose, jaws, fingers, and toes, caused by hypersecretion of growth hormone after maturity.

WRITE IT!

EXERCISE 10

Write terms for these descriptions.

1. cyanosis of the extremities   *acrocyanosis*
2. examination of the interior of the abdomen   *laparoscopy*
3. inflammation of the peritoneum   *peritonitis*
4. measurement of the head   *cephalometry*
5. pertaining to the abdomen and the chest   *abdominothoracic*
6. pertaining to the arms and legs   *acral*
7. plastic surgery of the eyelid   *blepharoplasty*
8. rupture of the umbilicus   *omphalorrhexis*
9. shortened term for thoracocentesis   *thoracentesis*
10. surgical incision of the chest wall   *thoracotomy*

A finger or toe is a digit. The combining form dactyl/o is often used in words that pertain to the fingers and toes. **Dactylo+graphy** is the study of fingerprints. **Dactylospasm** means cramping of a finger or toe. Inflammation of the bones of the fingers and toes is **dactylitis**.

Chiro+pody means pertaining to the hands and feet. It is also the art or profession of a **chiropodist**, a specialist who treats corns, bunions, and other afflictions of the hands and feet. Cramping of the hand, such as writer's cramp, is **chirospasm**. Plastic surgery of the hand is **chiroplasty**.

The combining form onych/o refers to the nails. An **onycho+phag+ist** habitually bites the nails. **Onychopathy** is any disease of the nails, and **onycho+myc+osis** means a disease of the nails caused by a fungus. Surgical removal of the nail is **onychectomy**, which also means declawing of an animal.

onych/o = nails
phag/o = eat
-ist = one who

FIND IT IN NEW TERMS! **EXERCISE 11**

Write the combining form and suffix and their meanings for these new terms. A short definition is provided for each term.

Term/Meaning	Combining Form	Suffix
1. blepharitis — inflammation of eyelid	blephar/o ~ eyelid	-itis ~ inflammation
2. blepharedema — swelling of eyelid, as from blepharitis and crying	blephar/o - eyelid	-edema - swelling
3. blepharoptosis — prolapse (drooping) of the upper eyelid	blephar/o - eyelid	-ptosis - prolapse (drooping)
4. onychomalacia — softening of nails	onych/o - nails	-malacia - softening
5. thoracodynia — pain in thorax, as distinguished from chest pain caused by angina pectoris, a heart condition	thorac/o - chest	-dynia - pain
6. thoracotomy — surgical incision of the chest wall	thorac/o - chest	-tomy - surgical incision
7. thoracoplasty — chest wall surgery in which portions of the ribs are removed to collapse areas of the lung	thorac/o - chest	-plasty - surgical repair
8. thoracoscopy — diagnostic examination of chest cavity	thorac/o - chest	-scopy - visual examination

Body Fluids

Fluids constitute more than 60% of an adult's weight under normal conditions (Figure 5-12). These fluids are vital in the transport of nutrients to all cells and removal of wastes from the body. Fluid balance is maintained through intake and output of water.

Water leaves the body by way of urine, feces, sweat, tears, and other fluid discharges (e.g., pus, sputum, mucus). Blood and lymph, two of the body's main fluids, are circulated through two separate but interconnected networks.

Water is the most important component of body fluids. These fluids are not distributed evenly throughout the body, and they move back and forth between compartments that are separated by cell membranes. Body fluids are found either within the

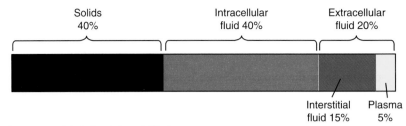

Figure 5-12 The body's fluid compartments. Fluid makes up 60% of the adult's body weight, and most is intracellular fluid. Two types of extracellular fluid are interstitial fluid and plasma. Plasma is the fluid part of the blood.

extra- = outside
inter- = between
intra- = within

cells (**intra+cellular**) or outside the cells (**extra+cellular**). Approximately one fourth of the extracellular fluid is plasma, the fluid part of the blood. Another type of extracellular fluid, called **interstitial** fluid, fills the spaces between most of the cells of the body. Accumulation of fluid in the interstitial compartment results in a condition called **edema**. Several word parts that relate to body fluids are presented next. Commit the word parts to memory.

Select Word Parts That Pertain to Body Fluids

Combining Form/Word Part	Meaning
crin/o, -crine	secrete
dacry/o, lacrim/o	tear, tearing, crying
-emia	condition of the blood
hem/o, hemat/o	blood
hidr/o	sweat or perspiration
hydr/o	water
lymph/o	lymph (sometimes refers to the lymphatics)
muc/o	mucus
-poiesis	production
-poietin	substance that causes production
py/o	pus
sial/o	saliva (sometimes refers to salivary glands)
ur/o	urine (sometimes refers to the urinary tract)

MATCH IT!

EXERCISE 12

Match the word parts with their meanings.

- E **1.** crin/o
- G **2.** dacry/o
- A **3.** hidr/o
- H **4.** hydr/o
- B **5.** -poiesis
- F **6.** -poietin
- C **7.** py/o
- D **8.** sial/o

- **A.** perspiration
- **B.** production
- **C.** pus
- **D.** saliva
- **E.** secrete
- **F.** substance that causes production
- **G.** tear
- **H.** water

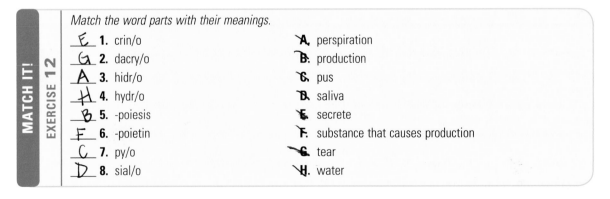

PROGRAMMED LEARNING

Remember to cover the answers (left column) with folded paper or the bookmark. Write an answer in each blank, and then check your answer before proceeding to the next frame.

crying	1. The combining forms dacry/o and lacrim/o mean tear, as in crying. The **lacrimal** gland produces fluid that keeps the eye moist. Tears are lacrimal fluid. If more lacrimal fluid is produced than can be removed, the person is _____ or "tearing."
tears	2. **Lacrimation** refers to crying, or the discharge of _____.
inflammation	3. Ophthalmitis may lead to excessive lacrimation. **Ophthalm+itis** refers to _____ of the eye.
stone	4. **Calculi** (stones or concretions) sometimes form in the lacrimal passages. A **dacryo+lith** is a lacrimal _____ or calculus. Dacryoliths are also called "tear stones."
stones	5. **Dacryo+lith+iasis** is the presence of lacrimal _____.
dacryocyst	6. The **dacryo+cyst** is the tear sac. The dacryocyst collects lacrimal fluid. Another name for the tear sac is _____.
inflammation	7. **Dacryo+cyst+itis** is _____ of the tear sac.
dacryolith	8. Write the word that means tear stone: _____.
sialolith	9. Stones can also occur in a salivary gland or duct. The combining form sial/o is used to form words that pertain to a **salivary** gland or to the fluid of these glands, called **saliva.** Use dacryo+lith as a model to write a word that means a salivary calculus: _____.
salivary	10. **Sialo+graphy** is x-ray imaging of the ducts of the _____ glands. Sialography sometimes demonstrates the presence of calculi in the salivary ducts.
inside	11. In addition to salivary glands, the body contains many other types of glands. On the basis of the presence or absence of ducts, glands are classified as exocrine or endocrine glands. You previously learned that endo- means _____. The prefix exo- in this case means outside.
exocrine	12. The combining form crin/o and the suffix -crine mean secrete. **Exo+crine** glands have ducts that carry their secretions to an epithelial surface, sometimes to the outside (e.g., sweat glands secrete perspiration onto the skin surface). Salivary glands also have ducts. Are salivary glands exocrine or endocrine glands? _____
endocrine	13. **Endo+crine** glands are ductless and secrete their hormones into the bloodstream. There are many ductless glands, including the sex glands, the **thyroid,** and the **adrenal** glands. Ductless glands are classified as _____ glands.

14. Sweat glands are also called **sudoriferous** glands, because the Latin word *sudor* means sweat. The combining form for sweat that you will use, however, is hidr/o. **Hidr+osis** means the formation and excretion of _____. A second meaning of hidrosis is excessive sweating, but **diaphoresis** is the term that is usually used to mean excessive sweating.

> sweat

15. Remembering that aden/o means gland, **hidr+aden+itis** is inflammation of a _____ gland. (Notice that when hidr/o is joined with aden/o, the *o* is dropped from hidr/o to make it easier to pronounce.)

> sweat

16. Now write a word that means tumor of a sweat gland: _____.

> **hidradenoma**

17. The combining form hydr/o means water. Do not confuse hydr/o and hidr/o. Remembering that a water hydrant is spelled with a y might help. **Hydro+therapy** refers to treatment using _____.

> water

18. As you learned earlier, "hydrophobia" is an obsolete term for rabies, a viral disease transmitted by the bite of an infected animal. The disease was given the name hydrophobia after it was observed that rabid animals avoid water. It was later learned that they avoid water because the muscles of the throat are paralyzed and they cannot swallow. Translated literally, hydro+phobia means an abnormal fear of _____.

> water

19. The combining form ur/o means urine. Translated literally, **an+uria** means without _____. Production of less than 100 mL of urine in 24 hours constitutes anuria.

> urine

20. Using poly- and -uria, write a word that means excessive urination: _____.

> **polyuria**

21. **Hemat+uria** is _____ in the urine.

> blood

22. **Lymph** is another type of body fluid. It is a transparent fluid found in **lymphatic** vessels. The lymphatic system (also called the lymphatics) collects tissue fluids from all parts of the body and returns the fluids to the blood circulation. Lymph/o usually refers to the lymphatics but sometimes refers to its fluid, _____.

> lymph

23. The combining form muc/o means **mucus. Mucoid** means resembling _____.

> mucus

24. **Mucous** means pertaining to mucus. Notice the slight difference in the spelling of mucous and mucus. Mucous also means secreting, producing, containing, or covered with mucus. The adjective that means pertaining to mucus is _____.

> mucous

25. Membranes that line passages and cavities that communicate with the air are called mucous membranes. A mucous membrane is also called a **mucosa.** Mucous membranes usually contain mucus-secreting cells. Passages and cavities that communicate with the air are lined with _____ membranes.

> mucous

26. **Muco+lytic** agents, including those used to treat certain diseases (e.g., **bronchial asthma**), break up or destroy _____.

> mucus

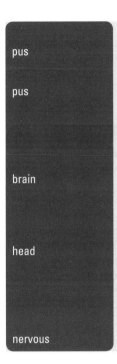

pus

pus

brain

head

nervous

27. Pus is a type of body fluid that is the liquid product of inflammation. The combining form py/o means pus. **Py+uria** is _____ in the urine.

28. **Pyo+genic** microorganisms are those that produce _____. A localized collection of pus in a cavity surrounded by healthy tissue is called an **abscess** (Figure 5-13).

29. Fluid that flows through and protects the brain and spinal column is **cerebrospinal** fluid. Dividing cerebrospinal into its component parts, cerebr/o means _____ and spinal means pertaining to the spine.

30. **Hydrocephalus** is a condition characterized by an abnormal accumulation of cerebrospinal fluid (CSF). The combining forms hydr/o and cephal/o mean water and _____, respectively.

31. When hydrocephalus occurs in an infant, the head enlarges at an abnormal rate because the soft bones of the skull push apart (Figure 5-14). If hydrocephalus occurs later in life, the bones of the skull forming the skull have fused, so symptoms are primarily neurologic. **Neuro+logic** means pertaining to the _____ system.

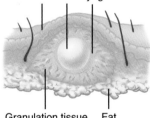

Skin Pus Pyogenic membrane

Granulation tissue   Fat

-genic = produced by
py/o = pus

Figure 5-13 **An abscess.** The pus is contained within a thin, pyogenic membrane surrounded by harder granulation tissue, the tissue's response to the infection.

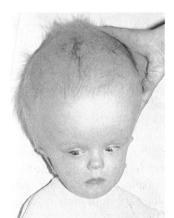

cephal/o = head
hydr/o = water

Figure 5-14 Four-month-old child with hydrocephalus. Hydrocephalus is usually caused by obstruction of the flow of cerebrospinal fluid. If hydrocephalus occurs in an infant, the soft bones of the skull push apart as the head increases in size.

Blood

Blood circulates through the heart and blood vessels, carrying oxygen, nutrients, vitamins, antibodies, and other needed substances. It carries away carbon dioxide and other wastes.

Study the following word parts.

Select Word Parts Pertaining to Blood

Combining Form	Meaning	Suffix	Meaning
coagul/o	coagulation	-cyte	cell
cyt/o	cell	-osis	generally, "increased"
erythr/o	red		or "abnormal"
hem/a, hemat/o	blood		when describing
leuk/o	white		cellular components
thromb/o	clot (thrombus)	-penia	deficiency
		-poiesis	production

WRITE IT! **EXERCISE 13**

Write the combining form for these meanings.

1. cell   _cyt/o_
2. clot   _thromb/o_
3. coagulation   _coagul/o_
4. red   _erythr/o_
5. white   _leuk/o_

MATCH IT! **EXERCISE 14**

Match the meanings with the word parts.

_B_ 1. blood   A. -cyte
_A_ 2. cell   B. hemat/o
_D_ 3. deficiency   C. -osis
_C_ 4. increased or abnormal   D. -penia
_E_ 5. production   E. -poiesis

Approximately half of the blood is composed of formed elements (cells or cell fragments), and the remainder is a straw-colored fluid, **plasma** (Figure 5-15). The cells are packed at the bottom of the tube when treated blood is spun in a **centrifuge**.

Three formed elements are found in the blood:

- Erythrocytes (red blood cells)
- Leukocytes (white blood cells)
- Blood platelets (also called thrombocytes)

Hemato+logy is the study of blood and the blood-forming tissues. The blood-forming tissues are bone marrow and lymphoid tissue (spleen, tonsils, and lymph nodes). Hemat/o means blood, but in the word hematology, the definition includes the blood-forming tissues.

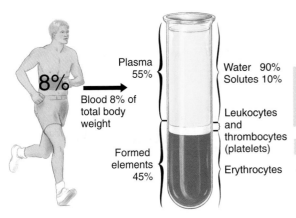

Plasma 55%

8%

Blood 8% of total body weight

Formed elements 45%

Water 90%
Solutes 10%

Leukocytes and thrombocytes (platelets)

Erythrocytes

-cyte = cell
erythr/o = red
leuk/o = white
thromb/o = clot

Figure 5-15 Composition of the blood. The cells and cell fragments are heavier than the liquid matrix, the plasma. When treated blood is spun in a centrifuge, the heavier elements (erythrocytes, leukocytes, and blood platelets) are packed into the bottom of the tube.

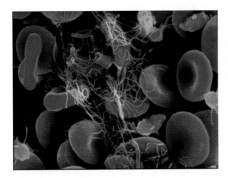

coagul/o = coagulation
fibr/o = fiber or fibrous
-graph = instrument for recording
micro- = small

Figure 5-16 Blood coagulation. This scanning electron micrograph has been colored to emphasize the different structures. Red blood cells *(red)* are entangled with the fibrin *(yellow)*. Note the thin center and the thick edges that give red blood cells a concave appearance. The platelets *(blue)*, which initiate clotting, are also visible.

WRITE IT! EXERCISE 15

Write terms for the formed elements of the blood.
1. blood platelets   *thrombocytes*
2. red blood cells   *Erythrocytes*
3. white blood cells   *Leukocytes*

A **hematoma** is a localized collection of blood, usually clotted, in an organ, tissue, or space, resulting from a break in the wall of a blood vessel. Hematomas can occur almost anywhere in the body and are usually not serious. Bruises are familiar forms of hematomas. Hematomas that occur inside the skull, however, are dangerous. The word hematoma is derived from the former meaning of tumor, a swelling, so named because there is a raised area wherever a hematoma occurs.

hemat/o = blood
-oma = tumor

Hemolysis is the destruction of red blood cells with the liberation of hemoglobin.

Hemodialysis is the process of diffusing blood through a semipermeable membrane to remove toxic materials from the bodies of persons with impaired kidney function.

hem/o = blood
-lysis = destruction

Blood **coagulation** (blood clotting), the transforming of blood from a liquid to a solid, occurs when blood is removed from the body (Figure 5-16). **Fibrin** forms in the

Figure 5-17 Stained blood. There are normally many more erythrocytes (red blood cells) than leukocytes (white blood cells). Only one leukocyte is shown here, although there are many types, each containing a nucleus. Platelets, tiny cell fragments, are also shown.

-cyte = cell
erythr/o = red
leuk/o = white

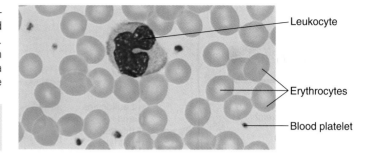

Leukocyte

Erythrocytes

Blood platelet

clot, entangling trapped cells. A substance that delays or prevents blood from clotting is an **anticoagulant**. Blood can be treated with an anticoagulant as soon as it is removed from the body, which prevents coagulation. In a blood transfusion, blood from the donor is transferred into a blood vessel of the recipient. Some blood transfusions require the use of whole blood, whereas in other types of transfusions, only part of the blood is needed. The white cells, red cells, plasma, and blood platelets are blood fractions that can be used in a transfusion. A transfusion reaction is any adverse effect that occurs after a transfusion. There are many types of reactions, ranging from acute reactions, which are life threatening, to relatively benign allergic reactions.

thromb/o = clot
-osis = condition

Some patients tend to form clots within blood vessels. **Thrombosis**, formation of internal blood clots, is a serious condition that can cause death. Special anticoagulant therapy is indicated for such persons to prevent internal clot formation.

Blood can be stained so that erythrocytes, leukocytes, and platelets can easily be recognized. Circulating erythrocytes in normal blood do not contain a nucleus, unlike leukocytes. There are several types of leukocytes, and all still have a nucleus in circulating blood (Figure 5-17).

A red blood cell (RBC) count, often called a red cell count, is enumeration of the number of erythrocytes. A white blood cell (WBC) count, often shortened to white cell count, is the enumeration of the leukocytes. A differential WBC count is an examination and enumeration of the distribution of the various types of leukocytes in a stained blood smear. This laboratory test provides information related to infections and various diseases. All three of these tests are included in a complete blood count (CBC).

thromb/o = blood
   clot
-cyte = cell
-penia = deficiency

Blood **platelets** are small structures in the blood that are important for blood clotting. Blood platelets are also called **thrombo+cytes**, but they are not really cells, only cell fragments. A reduction in the number of blood platelets is called **thrombocytopenia** or **thrombopenia**. This results in a prolonged clotting time.

an- = without
-emia = blood

Erythrocytes contain **hemoglobin** (hem/o, blood + globin, a type of protein). Hemoglobin is a red, iron-containing pigment that transports oxygen to the tissues and waste carbon dioxide to the lungs, where it is exchanged for fresh oxygen. **An+emia** is a condition in which the number of red blood cells or the concentration of hemoglobin (or both) is decreased. **Pallor** (paleness) and tachycardia are some typical signs of mild anemia, whereas more serious problems, such as difficulty breathing, shortness of breath (SOB), headache, fainting, and even congestive heart failure, can occur in severe anemia.

🔔 **QUICK TIP**

Anemia is a broad classification of disease. Compare with erythropenia, a decrease in erythrocytes.

The major function of **leukocytes** is body defense, helping to combat infection. Many leukocytes are highly **phago+cytic. Phagocytes** are cells that can ingest and destroy particulate substances such as bacteria, protozoa, cells, and cell debris. **Leukopenia**, or **leukocytopenia**, is an abnormal decrease in the total number of white blood cells. **Leukocytosis** is an abnormal increase in the total number of white blood cells. Leukocytosis can be transitory, but it is often associated with a bacterial infection.

phag/o = eat
cyt/o = cell
leuk/o = white
-penia = deficiency
-emia = blood

Leukemia is a progressive, malignant disease of the blood-forming organs. It is characterized by a marked increase in the number of leukocytes and by the presence of immature forms of leukocytes in the blood and bone marrow. Leukemias are classified according to the type of leukocyte in greatest number and according to the severity of the disease (acute or chronic).

> **QUICK TIP**
> Leukemia is a disease. Leukocytosis is descriptive of the leukocytes only.

Table 5-2 summarizes terms associated with changes in the numbers of different blood cells.

Hemato+poiesis is the formation and development of blood cells. Hematopoiesis generally takes place in the bone marrow, but some types of white blood cells are produced in lymphoid tissue. **Erythro+poietin** (-poietin, substance that causes production), a hormone produced mainly in the kidneys and released into the bloodstream, causes the production of red blood cells. By studying their word parts, you obtain only a partial insight into the meanings of **erythropoiesis** and erythropoietin. Various proteins are produced by the body to stimulate the production of the different types of white blood cells.

hemat/o = blood
-poiesis = production

MATCH IT! EXERCISE 16

Match the descriptions with the cell types in the right column (a choice may be used more than once).

B **1.** red blood cell
C **2.** white blood cell
B **3.** cell that is often decreased in anemia
C **4.** major cell type that is increased in leukemia
A **5.** has an important function in blood clotting

A. blood platelet
B. erythrocyte
C. leukocyte

Table 5-2   Changes in Numbers of Formed Elements of Blood

Cell (Function)	Common Name	Condition/Deficiency
erythrocyte (transports oxygen)	red blood cell (RBC)	**erythrocytosis** (erythr/o, red + cyt/o, cell + -osis, condition) **erythrocytopenia**, **erythropenia** (erythr/o, red + cyt/o, cell + penia, deficiency)
leukocyte (body defense)	white blood cell (WBC)	leukocytosis (leuk/o, white + cyt/o, cell + -osis, condition) leukopenia, leukocytopenia (leuk/o, white + cyt/o, cell + -penia, deficiency)
thrombocyte (blood clotting)	platelet (blood platelet)	**thrombocytosis** (thromb/o, clot + cyt/o, cell + -osis, condition) thrombopenia, thrombocytopenia (thromb/o, clot + cyt/o, cell + -penia, deficiency)

Write a term in each blank to complete these sentences.

1. The fluid portion of blood is called __plasma__.
2. A term for a localized collection of blood in an organ, tissue, or space is __Hematoma__.
3. Destruction of erythrocytes with the liberation of hemoglobin is __Hemolysis__.
4. The process of diffusing blood through a semipermeable membrane to remove toxic materials is called __Hemodialysis__.
5. Another term for clotting of blood when it is removed from the body is __coagulation__.
6. A substance that prevents blood from clotting when it is removed from the body is called a(n) __Anticoagulant__.
7. The term for formation of internal blood clots is __thrombosis__.
8. A shortened term for thrombocytopenia is __thrombopenia__.
9. The condition in which erythrocytes, hemoglobin, or both are decreased is __Anemia__.
10. Cells that can digest and destroy particulate matter are called __phagocytes__.
11. The formation and development of blood cells is __Hematopoiesis__.
12. An abnormal increase in the number of white blood cells is __leukocytosis__.
13. A shorter term that means the same as leukocytopenia is __leukopenia__.
14. A term that has the opposite meaning of erythrocytopenia is __Erythrocytosis__.

Body Defenses and Immunity

Susceptibility is being vulnerable to a disease or disorder. **Resistance** is the body's natural ability to counteract microorganisms or toxins. Our immune system usually protects us from pathogenic organisms. Unlike most body systems, the immune system is not contained within a single set of organs, but depends on several body systems.

The body's first line of defense is *nonspecific resistance* (directed against all pathogens). Several body systems or structures help prevent foreign substances from entering the body:

- Intact skin: no cuts or open sores.
- Tearing apparatus of the eyes: fluids contain destructive enzymes; wash out microorganisms.
- Urinary system: urine's composition and outflow aid in ridding the body of microorganisms.
- Mucous membranes: mucus traps foreign particles.
- Digestive system: acids and enzymes produced by the stomach destroy many invaders that are swallowed.
- Respiratory system: moist respiratory membranes and hairs in the nose trap some organisms that are breathed; coughing and sneezing help expel foreign matter.
- Lymphatic system: lymphatic structures trap pathogens and produce cells that are vital to immunity.

This initial defense mechanism also includes **inflammation** (a protective response of body tissue that increases circulation to an area after irritation or injury), **phagocytosis** (ingestion and destruction of microorganisms), and production of interferon and

QUICK TIP

Barriers against microbes may be mechanical, fluid, or chemical (stomach acids).

complement. **Interferon** is a cell-produced protein that protects the cells from viral infection. **Complement** is a protein that not only promotes inflammation and phagocytosis, but also causes bacterial cells to rupture.

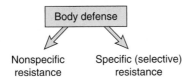

The second type of defense is *selective* or *specific resistance* (directed against particular pathogens).

The body's ability to counteract the effects of infectious organisms is **immunity**. This immune reaction, known as the antigen-antibody reaction, attacks foreign substances and destroys them. An **antigen** is any substance (e.g., bacterium, virus, toxin) that the body regards as foreign. An **antibody** is a disease-fighting protein produced by the immune system in response to the presence of a specific antigen. The body produces many types of antibodies, and each type of antibody destroys or neutralizes a specific type of antigen that caused its production. Two types of lymphocytes, T lymphocytes (also called T cells) and B lymphocytes (B cells), are involved in specific resistance.

Both nonspecific and specific defenses occur simultaneously and work together to overcome pathogens.

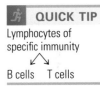

QUICK TIP

Lymphocytes of specific immunity

B cells   T cells

MATCH IT!

EXERCISE 18

Choose A or B from the right column to classify the characteristics as examples of specific or nonspecific resistance.

A **1.** Antigen-antibody reaction destroys microorganisms.

B **2.** Digestive acids destroy many swallowed microorganisms.

B **3.** Sneezing expels foreign matter.

A **4.** The immune reaction attacks foreign substances.

B **5.** Urine aids in eliminating microorganisms.

A. specific resistance

B. nonspecific resistance

Antibodies are generally acquired by having a disease or by receiving a vaccination. **Immunization** is the process by which resistance to an infectious disease is induced or augmented. *Active immunity* occurs when the individual's own body produces an immune response to a harmful antigen. *Passive immunity* results when the immune agents develop in another person or animal and then are transferred to an individual who was not previously immune. This second type of immunity is "borrowed" immunity that provides immediate protection but is effective for only a short time.

In both active and passive immunity, the recognition of specific antigens is called *specific immunity*. The terms *natural* and *artificial* refer to how the immunity is obtained (Figure 5-18).

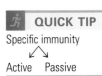

QUICK TIP

Specific immunity

Active   Passive

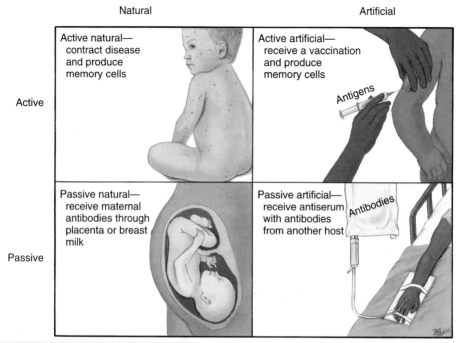

Natural   Artificial

Active natural—
contract disease
and produce
memory cells

Active artificial—
receive a vaccination
and produce
memory cells

Antigens

Active

Passive natural—
receive maternal
antibodies through
placenta or breast
milk

Passive artificial—
receive antiserum
with antibodies
from another host

Antibodies

Passive

Figure 5-18 Four types of specific immunity. Active natural immunity and passive natural immunity, as the names imply, occur through the normal activities of either an individual contracting a disease or a fetus being exposed to maternal antibodies. Both active artificial and passive artificial immunities require deliberate actions of receiving vaccinations or antibodies.

MATCH IT!
EXERCISE 19

Choose A or B to classify the events as active or passive immunity.

A **1.** having a disease
A **2.** receiving a vaccination
B **3.** receiving antibodies from a host
B **4.** receiving antibodies through the placenta

A. active immunity
B. passive immunity

A **vaccination** is the administration of antigenic material (inactivated or killed microbes or their products) to induce immunity. Vaccinations are available to immunize against many diseases, including typhoid, diphtheria, polio, measles, and mumps. Depending on its type, a vaccine is administered orally or by injection, or sprayed into the nostrils.

An **immuno+compromised** person is one whose immune response has been weakened by a disease or an **immunosuppressive** agent. Radiation and certain drugs are **immunosuppressants**.

Immunodeficiency diseases are caused by a defect in the immune system and are characterized by a susceptibility to infections and chronic diseases. Acquired immunodeficiency syndrome (AIDS) is a viral disease involving a defect in immunity that is manifested by various *opportunistic infections*. These infections are caused by normally nonpathogenic organisms in a host with decreased resistance. There is no known cure for AIDS, and the prognosis is poor. AIDS is caused by either of two types of the human immunodeficiency virus, HIV-1 or HIV-2. AIDS is transmitted by sexual intercourse or exposure to contaminated body fluid of an infected person. It was originally found in homosexual men and intravenous (IV) drug users but now occurs increasingly among heterosexual men and women and babies born of HIV-infected mothers.

Occasionally, the interaction of our defense mechanisms with an antigen results in injury. This excessive reaction to an antigen is called **hypersensitivity. Allergies** are conditions in which the body reacts with an exaggerated immune response to common, harmless substances, most of which are found in the environment.

Anaphylaxis and anaphylactic reactions are exaggerated, life-threatening hypersensitivity reactions to a previously encountered antigen. The suffix -phylaxis means protection. With a wide range in the severity of symptoms, the reactions may include generalized itching, difficulty breathing, airway obstruction, and shock. Insect stings and penicillin are two common causes of *anaphylactic shock,* a severe and sometimes fatal systemic hypersensitivity reaction.

Pathogens

Pathogens are any disease-producing agent or microorganism. Viruses and bacteria are responsible for a large number of infections, but bacteria are easier to study and grow in the laboratory. A special staining technique serves as a primary means of identifying and classifying bacteria into three major types: **cocci, bacilli,** or **spirilla** (Figure 5-19).

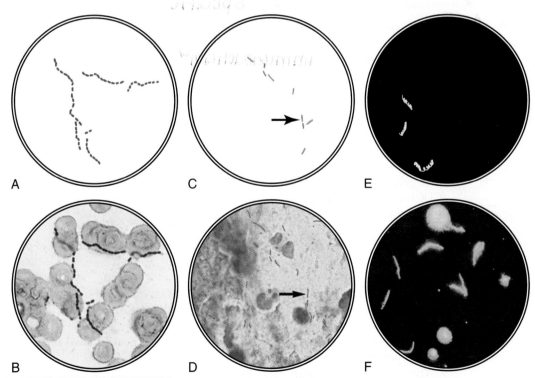

Figure 5-19 Bacteria in body fluids. A, Schematic drawing of gram-positive cocci, which appear as tiny purple spheres. The cocci are in chains in this example. **B,** Gram-positive cocci in a Gram stain of a direct smear. Note the small size of the bacteria (which stain purple) compared with the much larger cells. **C,** Schematic of gram-negative bacilli, which appear as tiny pinkish rods. **D,** Gram-negative bacilli *(arrow)* in the presence of numerous leukocytes in a Gram stain of a direct smear. **E,** Schematic of spirochetes, which appear as long, tightly coiled spirals**. F,** Spirochetes in a special preparation from material collected from a chancre, a skin lesion that occurs in syphilis.

Types of pathogenic microorganisms include bacteria, fungi, protozoa, and viruses. Our immune system is not always able to prevent *infection*, the invasion of the body by pathogenic microorganisms that cause disease.

The body's defense mechanisms, particularly the phagocytes, are important in impeding the spread of cancer and other diseases. You learned that **benign** means "favorable for recovery" and "not having a tendency to spread." **Malignant** means tending to grow worse, to spread, and possibly become life threatening. Cancer cells are malignant, exhibiting the properties of invasion and **metastasis** (spreading from one part of the body to another part). Cancer cells **metastasize** (spread to sites away from where they originate) by several means, including the bloodstream, lymphatic system, and direct extension to neighboring tissue. The immune system acts against cancer cells to block or impede their spread and invasion of sites distant from their source.

WRITE IT!   EXERCISE 20

Write words in the blanks to complete these sentences.

1. A foreign substance that induces production of antibodies is called a(n) _antigen_.
2. Lack of resistance is being _susceptible_ to a disease.
3. Phagocytosis of pathogens is part of the body's _nonspecific_ defense mechanism.
4. Antibody-mediated immunity is part of the body's _specific_ defense mechanism.
5. _Active_ immunity occurs when an individual's body produces an immune response to a harmful antigen.
6. AIDS is an abbreviation for acquired _immunodeficiency_ syndrome.

Bioterrorism

Weapons of mass destruction (WMD) have been a concern for many years but have come to the forefront as acts of terrorism have increased. Health care providers must be trained to recognize and deal with these emergencies. The Federal Emergency Management Agency (FEMA) and the Centers for Disease Control and Prevention (CDC) use the following categories to define weapons of mass destruction:

B Biological
N Nuclear
I Incendiary (incendiaries, flammable substances used to ignite fires, or explosives)
C Chemical
E Explosive

QUICK TIP

Use "Be Nice" to remember the WMD categories.

bi/o = life

Bio+terrorism is the use of pathogenic biological agents to cause terror in a population. High-priority agents include microorganisms that pose a risk to national security largely for the following reasons:

1. They can be easily disseminated (distributed over a general area) or transmitted from person to person.
2. They cause high mortality rates and a major public health impact.
3. They can cause public panic and social disruption.
4. They require special action for public health preparedness.

WRITE IT! EXERCISE 21

Write words in the blanks to complete these sentences.

1. WMD is an abbreviation for __weapons__ of mass destruction.
2. CDC is an abbreviation for Centers for __Disease__ Control and Prevention.
3. The use of pathogenic biological agents to cause terror in a population is called __bioterrorism__.
4. A term that means scattered or distributed over a general area is __disseminated__.

⛔ Be Careful with These!

Opposites

anter/o versus *poster/o*
ventr/o versus *dors/o*
proxim/o versus *dist/o* or *tel/e*
medial versus *lateral*
prone versus *supine* (pronation vs. supination)

Know the Difference!

anaplasia, aplasia, dysplasia, hypoplasia, hyperplasia, and *hypertrophy*
dacry/o (tears) versus *dactyl/o* (digits)

SELF-TEST   Work the following exercises to test your understanding of the material in Chapter 5. Complete all the exercises before checking your answers against those in Appendix VIII.

A. MATCH IT!   *Match the directional aspects of the body with the meanings in the right column.*

____ **1.** anterior
____ **2.** caudad
____ **3.** cephalad
____ **4.** distal
____ **5.** dorsal
____ **6.** inferior
____ **7.** lateral
____ **8.** medial
____ **9.** proximal
____ **10.** superior

A. above
B. below
C. far
D. middle
E. nearer the origin
F. toward the back
G. toward the front
H. toward the head
I. toward the side
J. toward the tail

Continued

SELF-TEST (cont'd)

B. WRITE IT!   *Write a word in each blank to complete these sentences.*

1. The fundamental unit of life is the _____.
2. Similar cells acting together to perform a function is called a(n) _____.
3. Tissue types working together to perform a function is called a(n) _____.
4. Abnormal development of tissues or organs is called _____.
5. An abnormal increase in the number of normal cells in tissue is called _____.
6. Blepharal means pertaining to the _____.
7. Acral means pertaining to the _____.
8. Thoracotomy means surgical incision of the _____ wall.
9. Onychomalacia means softening of the _____.
10. The _____ cavity of the body is divided into the cranial and spinal cavities.
11. Dividing the abdomen into _____ uses imaginary lines to distinguish four parts.
12. Laparotomy means incision of the _____ wall.
13. Fluid that is found within the cells is called _____ fluid.
14. Lacrimation refers to the discharge of _____.
15. Blood _____ are called thrombocytes.

C. CIRCLE IT!   *Choose the one correct answer (a, b, c, or d) for each question.*

1. Which term means the opposite of distal?
   (a) proximal   (b) inferior   (c) superior   (d) ventral
2. What membrane lines the abdominopelvic cavity and enfolds the internal organs?
   (a) lymph   (b) pericardium   (c) peritoneum   (d) visceral
3. Which term means inflammation of the navel?
   (a) dactylitis   (b) dermatitis   (c) omphalitis   (d) sialitis
4. Which term means the presence of lacrimal stones?
   (a) allergic rhinitis   (b) dacryocystitis   (c) dacryolithiasis   (d) sialitis
5. Which term means a sticking together of two structures that are normally separated?
   (a) abdominocentesis   (b) adhesion   (c) laparogastrotomy   (d) mucosa
6. Which glands are ductless and therefore secrete their hormones into the bloodstream?
   (a) endocrine   (b) exocrine   (c) salivary   (d) sudoriferous
7. Which term means formation and excretion of sweat?
   (a) adrenal   (b) ascites   (c) hidradenoma   (d) hidrosis
8. Which term means belly side?
   (a) lateral   (b) posterior   (c) superior   (d) ventral
9. What is the term for the fluid part of the blood?
   (a) intracellular   (b) lymph   (c) plasma   (d) thrombosis
10. Which term means pertaining to an immune response that has been weakened by disease or by an agent that suppresses the immune system?
    (a) immunocompromised   (b) malignancy   (c) resistance   (d) susceptibility

SELF-TEST   (cont'd)

D. WRITE IT!   *List the four main types of tissue.*

1. _____   3. _____

2. _____   4. _____

E. FINDING THE CLUE!   *Use a clue to write terms for these descriptions: Solve Question 1; each ending letter becomes the clue for the first letter of the next answer.*

1. bluish appearance of the extremities   _____

2. type of plane that divides the body into right and left parts   _____

3. instrument used in laparoscopy   _____

4. abnormal accumulation of fluid   _____

5. descriptive of one who is able to walk   _____

6. cardiogram that is transmitted electronically   _____

7. to spread to sites away from where cancer originated   _____

8. red blood cell   _____

9. pertaining to outside of a cell   _____

10. lying down   _____

F. WRITE IT!   *Write one word for each of these meanings.*

1. substance that induces an immune response   _____

2. substance that prevents coagulation   _____

3. formation and development of blood cells   _____

4. in front and to one side   _____

5. lack of development of an organ or tissue   _____

6. pertaining to the abdomen and thorax   _____

7. presence of a thrombus   _____

8. use of pathogenic agents to cause terror   _____

9. white blood cells   _____

10. within a cell   _____

G. SPELL IT!   *Circle all incorrectly spelled terms, and write the correct spelling.*

1. anafalaxis   _____

2. fibren   _____

3. hypertrofy   _____

4. immunosupressant   _____

5. supination   _____

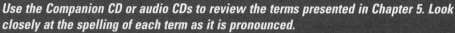

Q&E List

Use the Companion CD or audio CDs to review the terms presented in Chapter 5. Look closely at the spelling of each term as it is pronounced.

abdomen (**ab´də-mən, ab-do´mən**)
abdominal quadrant (**ab-dom´ĭ-nəl kwod´rənt**)
abdominocentesis (**ab-dom˝ĭ-no-sen-te´sis**)
abdominopelvic (**ab-dom˝ĭ-no-pel´vik**)
abdominothoracic (**ab-dom˝ĭ-no-thə-ras´ik**)
abscess (**ab´ses**)
acral (**ak´rəl**)
acrocyanosis (**ak´ro-si˝ə-no´sis**)
acrodermatitis (**ak˝ro-dur˝mə-ti´tis**)
acrohypothermy (**ak˝ro-hi´po-thur˝me**)
acromegaly (**ak˝ro-meg´ə-le**)
adhesion (**ad-he´zhən**)
adrenal (**ə-dre´nəl**)
allergy (**al´ər-je**)
ambulant (**am´bu-lənt**)
anaphylaxis (**an˝ə-fə-lak´sis**)
anaplasia (**an˝ə-pla´zhə**)
anatomic (**an˝ə-tom´ik**)
anemia (**ə-ne´me-ə**)
anterior (**an-tēr´e-ər**)
anterolateral (**an˝tər-o-lat´ər-əl**)
anteromedian (**an˝tər-o-me´de-ən**)
anteroposterior (**an˝tər-o-pos-tēr´e-ər**)
anterosuperior (**an˝tər-o-soo-pēr´e-ər**)
antibody (**an´tĭ-bod˝e**)
anticoagulant (**an˝te-, an˝ti-ko-ag´u-lənt**)
antigen (**an´tĭ-jən**)
anuria (**an-u´re-ə**)
aplasia (**ə-pla´zhə**)
ascites (**ə-si´tēz**)
bacilli (**bə-sil´i**)
benign (**bə-nīn´**)
blepharal (**blef´ə-ral**)
blepharedema (**blef˝ə-rĭ-de´mə**)
blepharitis (**blef˝ə-ri´tis**)
blepharoplasty (**blef´ə-ro-plas˝te**)
blepharoplegia (**blef˝ə-ro-ple´jə**)
blepharoptosis (**blef˝ə-rop-to´sis**)
blepharospasm (**blef´ə-ro-spaz˝əm**)
blepharotomy (**blef˝ə-rot´ə-me**)
bronchial asthma (**brong´ke-əl az´mə**)
calculi (**kal´ku-li**)
caudad (**kaw´dad**)

caudal (**kaw´dəl**)
centrifuge (**sen´tri-fūj**)
cephalad (**sef´ə-lad**)
cephalgia (**sə-fal´jə**)
cephalodynia (**sef˝ə-lo-din´e-ə**)
cephalometry (**sef˝ə-lom´ə-tre**)
cephalopelvic (**sef˝ə-lo-pel´vik**)
cerebrospinal (**ser˝ə-bro-spi´nəl**)
chiroplasty (**ki´ro-plas˝te**)
chiropodist (**ki-rop´ə-dist**)
chiropody (**ki-rop´ə-de**)
chirospasm (**ki´ro-spaz˝əm**)
coagulation (**ko-ag˝u-la´shən**)
cocci (**kok´si**)
complement (**kom´plə-mənt**)
cranial (**kra´ne-əl**)
dacryocyst (**dak´re-o-sist˝**)
dacryocystitis (**dak˝re-o-sis-ti´tis**)
dacryolith (**dak´re-o-lith˝**)
dacryolithiasis (**dak˝re-o-lĭ-thi´ə-sis**)
dactylitis (**dak˝tə-li´tis**)
dactylography (**dak˝tə-log´rə-fe**)
dactylospasm (**dak´tə-lo-spaz˝əm**)
diaphoresis (**di˝ə-fə-re´sis**)
diaphragm (**di´ə-fram**)
distal (**dis´təl**)
dorsal (**dor´səl**)
dorsolateral (**dor˝so-lat´ər-əl**)
dorsoventral (**dor˝so-ven´trəl**)
dysplasia (**dis-pla´zhə**)
edema (**ə-de´mə**)
endocrine (**en´do-krīn, en´do-krin**)
erythrocyte (**ə-rith´ro-sīt**)
erythrocytopenia (**ə-rith˝ro-si˝to-pe´ne-ə**)
erythrocytosis (**ə-rith˝ro-si-to´sis**)
erythropenia (**ə-rith˝ro-pe´ne-ə**)
erythropoiesis (**ə-rith˝ro-poi-e´sis**)
erythropoietin (**ə-rith˝ro-poi´ə-tin**)
exocrine (**ek´so-krin**)
extracellular (**eks˝trə-sel´u-lər**)
femoral (**fem´or-əl**)
fibrin (**fi´brin**)
frontal plane (**frun´təl plān**)

hematology (he´´mə-tol´ə-je)

hematoma (he´´mə-to´mə)

hematopoiesis (he´´mə-, hem´´ə-to-poi-e´sis)

hematuria (he´´mə-tu´re-ə, hem´´ə-tu´re-ə)

hemodialysis (he´´mo-di-al´ə-sis)

hemoglobin (he´mo-glo´´bin)

hemolysis (he-mol´ə-sis)

hidradenitis (hi´´drad-ə-ni´tis)

hidradenoma (hi-drad´´ə-no´mə)

hidrosis (hi-dro´sis)

homeostasis (ho´´me-o-sta´sis)

hydrocephalus (hi´´dro-sef´ə-ləs)

hydrotherapy (hi´´dro-ther´ə-pe)

hyperplasia (hi´´pər-pla´zhə)

hypersensitivity (hi´´pər-sen´´si-tiv´i-te)

hypertrophy (hi-pur´trə-fe)

hypoplasia (hi´´po-pla´zhə)

immunity (ĭ-mu´nĭ-te)

immunization (im´´u-nĭ-za´shən)

immunocompromised (im´´u-no-kom´prə-mīzd)

immunodeficiency (im´´u-no-də-fish´ən-se)

immunosuppressant (im´´u-no-sə-pres´ənt)

immunosuppressive (im´´u-no-sə-pres´iv)

inferior (in-fēr´e-ər)

inferomedian (in´´fər-o-me´de-ən)

inflammation (in´´flə-ma´shən)

inguinal (ing´gwĭ-nəl)

interferon (in´´tər-fēr´on)

interstitial (in´´tər-stish´əl)

intracellular (in´´trə-sel´u-lər)

lacrimal (lak´rĭ-məl)

lacrimation (lak´´rĭ-ma´shən)

laparoscope (lap´ə-ro-skōp´´)

laparoscopy (lap´´ə-ros´kə-pe)

laparotomy (lap´´ə-rot´ə-me)

lateral (lat´ər-əl)

leukemia (loo-ke´me-ə)

leukocyte (loo´ko-sīt)

leukocytopenia (loo´´ko-si´´to-pe´ne-ə)

leukocytosis (loo´´ko-si-to´sis)

leukopenia (loo´´ko-pe´ne-ə)

lymph (limf)

lymphatic (lim-fat´ik)

malignant (mə-lig´nənt)

medial (me´de-əl)

median (me´de-ən)

mediolateral (me´´de-o-lat´ər-əl)

metastasis (mə-tas´tə-sis)

metastasize (mə-tas´tə-sīz)

midsagittal plane (mid-saj´ĭ-təl plān)

mucoid (mu´koid)

mucolytic (mu´´ko-lit´ik)

mucosa (mu-ko´sə)

mucous (mu´kəs)

mucus (mu´kəs)

neurologic (noor´´o-loj´ik)

omphalic (om-fal´ik)

omphalitis (om´´fə-li´tis)

omphalocele (om´fə-lo-sēl´)

omphalorrhagia (om´´fə-lo-ra´jə)

omphalorrhexis (om´´fə-lo-rek´sis)

onychectomy (on´´ĭ-kek´tə-me)

onychomalacia (on´´ĭ-ko-mə-la´shə)

onychomycosis (on´´ĭ-ko-mi-ko´sis)

onychopathy (on´´ĭ-kop´ə-the)

onychophagist (on´´ĭ-kof´ə-jist)

ophthalmitis (of´´thəl-mi´tis)

pallor (pal´ər)

paracentesis (par´´ə-sən-te´sis)

pelvic (pel´vik)

pelvis (pel´vis)

peritoneum (per´´ĭ-to-ne´əm)

peritonitis (per´´ĭ-to-ni´tis)

phagocyte (fa´go-sīt)

phagocytic (fa´´go-sit´ik)

phagocytosis (fa´´go-si-to´sis)

plasma (plaz´mə)

platelets (plāt´ləts)

polyuria (pol´´e-u´re-ə)

posterior (pos-tēr´e-ər)

posteroanterior (pos´´tər-o-an-tēr´e-ər)

posteroexternal (pos´´tər-o-ek-ster´nəl)

posterointernal (pos´´tər-o-in-tur´nəl)

posterolateral (pos´´tər-o-lat´ər-əl)

posteromedian (pos´´ter-o-me´de-ən)

posterosuperior (pos´´tər-o-soo-pēr´e-ər)

pronation (pro-na´shən)

prone (prōn)

proximal (prok´sĭ-məl)

pyogenic (pi´´o-jen´ik)

pyuria (pi-u´re-ə)

recumbent (re-kum´bənt)

continued

resistance (**re-zis´təns**)
sagittal plane (**saj´ĭ-təl plān**)
saliva (**sə-li´və**)
salivary (**sal´ĭ-var-e**)
sialography (**si´´ə-log´rə-fe**)
sialolith (**si-al´o-lith**)
spinal (**spi´nəl**)
spirilla (**spi-ril´ə**)
sudoriferous (**soo´´do-rif´ər-əs**)
superior (**soo-pēr´e-ər**)
supination (**soo´´pĭ-na´shən**)
supine (**soo´pīn**)
susceptibility (**sə-sep´´tĭ-bil´ĭ-te**)
telecardiogram (**tel´´ə-kahr´de-o-gram**)
thoracentesis (**thor´ə-sen-te´sis**)
thoracic (**thə-ras´ik**)
thoracocentesis (**thor´´ə-ko-sən-te´sis**)
thoracodynia (**thor´´ə-ko-din´e-ə**)

thoracoplasty (**thor´ə-ko-plas´´te**)
thoracoscopy (**thor´´ə-kəs´kə-pe**)
thoracotomy (**thor´´ə-kot´ə-me**)
thorax (**thor´aks**)
thrombocyte (**throm´bo-sīt**)
thrombocytopenia (**throm´´bo-si´´to-pe´ne-ə**)
thrombocytosis (**throm´´bo-si-to´sis**)
thrombopenia (**throm´´bo-pe´ne-ə**)
thrombosis (**throm-bo´sis**)
thyroid (**thi´roid**)
torso (**tor´so**)
transverse plane (**trans-vərs´ plān**)
umbilical (**əm-bil´ĭ-kəl**)
umbilicus (**əm-bil´ĭ-kəs**)
vaccination (**vak´´sĭ-na´shən**)
ventral (**ven´trəl**)
viscera (**vis´ər-ə**)

 Don't forget the games on the Companion CD and http://evolve.elsevier.com/Leonard/quick/ for additional review, including questions on Spanish medical terms.

Enhancing Spanish Communication

English	Spanish (pronunciation)
abdomen	abdomen (**ab-DOH-men**), vientre (**ve-EN-tray**)
anemia	anemia (**ah-NAH-me-ah**)
ankle	tobillo (**to-BEEL-lyo**)
arm	brazo (**BRAH-so**)
armpit	sobaco (**so-BAH-co**), axila (**ac-SEE-lah**)
back	espalda (**es-PAHL-dah**)
belly	barriga (**bar-REE-gah**)
cheek	mejilla (**may-HEEL-lyah**)
chest	pecho (**PAY-cho**)
collarbone	clavícula (**clah-VEE-coo-lah**)
cry, to cry	llorar (**lyo-RAR**)
diaphragm	diafragma (**de-ah-FRAHG-mah**)
elbow	codo (**CO-do**)
extremities	extremidades (**ex-tray-me-DAHD-es**)
eyeball	globo del ojo (**GLO-bo del O-ho**)
eyebrow	ceja (**SAY-hah**)
eyelash	pestaña (**pes-TAH-nyah**)
finger	dedo (**DAY-do**)

English	Spanish (pronunciation)
fingerprint	impresión digital (**im-pray-se-ON de-he-TAHL**)
foot (pl., feet)	pie, pies (**PE-ay, PE-ays**)
forearm	antebrazo (**an-tay-BRAH-so**)
hair	pelo (**PAY-lo**)
headache	dolor de cabeza (**do-LOR day cah-BAY-sa**)
heel	talón (**tah-LON**)
hip	cadera (**cah-DAY-rah**)
jaw	mandíbula (**man-DEE-boo-lah**)
knee	rodilla (**ro-DEEL-lyah**)
kneecap	rótula (**RO-too-lah**)
leg	pierna (**pe-ERR-nah**)
lip	labio (**LAH-be-o**)
lung	pulmón (**pool-MON**)
lymph	linfa (**LEEN-fah**)
mouth	boca (**BO-cah**)
mucus	moco (**MO-co**)
nails	uñas (**OO-nyahs**)
navel	ombligo (**om-BLEE-go**)
neck	cuello (**coo-EL-lyo**)
palm	palma (**PAHL-mah**)
perspiration	sudor (**soo-DOR**)
rib	costilla (**cos-TEEL-lyah**)
skeleton	esqueleto (**es-kay-LAY-to**)
skull	cráneo (**CRAH-nay-o**)
sole	planta (**PLAHN-tah**)
spine	espinazo (**es-pe-NAH-so**)
sweat	sudor (**soo-DOR**)
tears	lágrimas (**LAH-gre-mahs**)
temple	sien (**se-AYN**)
thigh	muslo (**MOOS-lo**)
thumb	pulgar (**pool-GAR**)
toe	dedo del pie (**DAY-do del pe-AY**)
tongue	lengua (**LEN-goo-ah**)
trauma	herida (**ay-REE-dah**)
urine	orina (**o-REE-nah**)
wrist	muñeca (**moo-NYAY-cah**)

CHAPTER 6

Musculoskeletal System

CONTENTS

Function First
Structures of the Musculoskeletal System
    Major Bones of the Body
    Cartilage
    Articulations and Associated Structures
    Muscles and Associated Structures
Diseases, Disorders, and Diagnostic Terms
    Stress and Trauma Injuries
    Infections

Tumors and Malignancies
Metabolic Disturbances
Congenital Defects
Arthritis and Connective Tissue Diseases
Surgical and Therapeutic Interventions
Self-Test
Q&E List
Enhancing Spanish Communication

OBJECTIVES

After completing Chapter 6, you will be able to:

1. Recognize or write the functions of the musculoskeletal system.
2. Recognize or write the meanings of Chapter 6 word parts and use them to build and analyze medical terms.
3. Write terms for selected structures of the musculoskeletal system, or match terms with their descriptions.
4. Write the names of the diagnostic terms and pathologies related to the musculoskeletal system when given their descriptions, or match terms with their meanings.
5. Match surgical and therapeutic interventions for the musculoskeletal system, or write the names of the interventions when given their descriptions.
6. Spell terms for the musculoskeletal system correctly.

Function First

The musculoskeletal system provides protection, support, and movement for the body. Bones store mineral salts and are important in **hematopoiesis.** Muscles move an organ or part of the body by contracting and relaxing. Because of the close association of the body's skeleton and muscles, the two systems are often referred to as one, the musculoskeletal system. Muscles are also closely related to the nervous system because nerve impulses stimulate the muscles to contract.

    In addition to support and movement, the bones function in the formation of blood cells, storage of fat in the bone marrow, and storage and release of minerals, especially calcium.

hemat/o = blood
-poiesis = production

muscul/o = muscle

Write words associated with functions of the musculoskeletal system; the first letter is provided. (Question 1 is done as an example.)

1. protection
2. s upport
3. m ovement
4. f ormation   of blood cells
5. bone marrow storage of f at
6. storage and release of m inerals

Use Appendix VIII to check the answers to all the exercises in Chapter 6.

Structures of the Musculoskeletal System

Musculoskeletal means pertaining to the muscles and the skeleton. The musculoskeletal system includes all of the muscles, bones, joints and related structures. The muscular system includes all types of muscle, including the ones you're most familiar with. The skeletal system consists of the bones and cartilage of the body, which collectively provide the supporting framework for the muscles and organs as well as places for the attachment of tendons, ligaments, and muscles. A good example of this is the knee, the joint that connects the thigh bone with the lower leg (Figure 6-1).

orth/o = straight
ped/o = child
-ic = pertaining to

Orthopedics is the branch of medicine involved in the prevention and correction of deformities or diseases of the musculoskeletal system, especially those of the bones, muscles, joints, ligaments, and tendons. Ortho+ped+ics was so named because the **orthopedist** originally aligned children's bones and corrected deformities. Today, however, an orthopedist specializes in disorders of the bones and associated structures in people of all ages.

Calcium in bone is radiopaque; thus, bones can block x-rays so that they do not reach the image receptor. Bones are represented by light areas on radiographic images. Metal objects, such as metal fixation devices that are used to stabilize a joint, are also radiopaque (see Figure 4-8, p. 86).

-ar = pertaining to
articul/o = joint

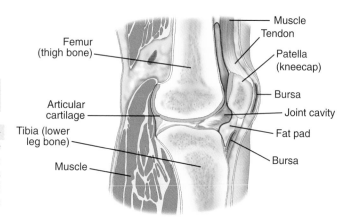

Figure 6-1 Bone with associated muscle, cartilage, and a tendon. This lateral view of the knee joint shows attachment of the thigh bone with one of the two lower leg bones. Cartilage covers the ends of the opposing bones. The fat pad and bursa provide protective cushions, and muscles make it possible to bend the knee.

Femur (thigh bone)
Articular cartilage
Tibia (lower leg bone)
Muscle
Muscle
Tendon
Patella (kneecap)
Bursa
Joint cavity
Fat pad
Bursa

Major Bones of the Body

The adult human skeleton usually consists of 206 named bones (Figure 6-2). The skull, spinal column, breastbone, and ribs are a major division of the skeleton, and together these bones form the vertical axis of the body (bone-colored in Figure 6-2). Write the name of the bones on the illustration as you read the legend.

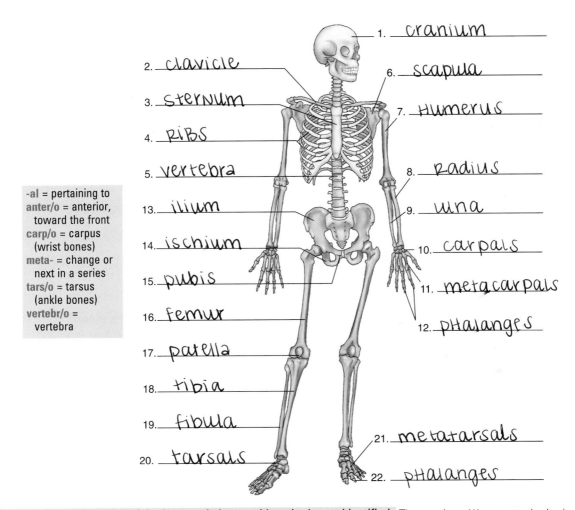

1. *cranium*

2. *clavicle*

3. *sternum*

4. *ribs*

5. *vertebra*

6. *scapula*

7. *humerus*

8. *radius*

9. *ulna*

10. *carpals*

11. *metacarpals*

12. *phalanges*

13. *ilium*

14. *ischium*

15. *pubis*

16. *femur*

17. *patella*

18. *tibia*

19. *fibula*

20. *tarsals*

21. *metatarsals*

22. *phalanges*

-al = pertaining to
anter/o = anterior, toward the front
carp/o = carpus (wrist bones)
meta- = change or next in a series
tars/o = tarsus (ankle bones)
vertebr/o = vertebra

Figure 6-2 Anterior view of the human skeleton, with major bones identified. The cranium *(1)* protects the brain and forms the framework of the face. The clavicle *(2)* is attached to the upper end of the sternum *(3)*. Also associated with the sternum are the ribs *(4)*, which support the chest wall and protect the lungs and heart. The vertebrae protect the spinal cord. A vertebra *(5)* is part of the vertebral or spinal column. The scapula *(6)* is a large triangular bone that joins the upper end of the longest bone of the arm, the humerus *(7)*. The bones of the forearm are the radius *(8)* and the ulna *(9)*. The wrist is composed of eight carpal bones, or carpals *(10)*. The bones of the palm are the metacarpals *(11)*, and the bones of the fingers are the phalanges *(12)*. The bones of the pelvis are the ilium *(13)*, the ischium *(14)*, and the pubis *(15)*. The femur *(16)* is the upper leg bone. The kneecap, or patella *(17)*, overlaps the bottom end of the femur and protects the knee joint, where the femur and tibia *(18)* meet. The smaller bone of the lower leg is the fibula *(19)*. The ankle is composed of seven tarsal bones, or tarsals *(20)*. The bones located between the ankle and toes are the metatarsals *(21)*. As with the bones of the fingers, bones of the toes are called phalanges *(22)*.

The table below lists the combining forms for the major bones, as well as their common names (when appropriate). Commit this information to memory.

Major Bones of the Body		
Bone	**Combining Form**	**Common Name**
Bones That Form the Vertical Axis of the Body		
clavicle	clavicul/o	collarbone
cranium	crani/o	skull
costa	cost/o	rib
scapula	scapul/o	shoulder blade
sternum	stern/o	breastbone
spine	rachi/o, spin/o	backbone
vertebrae, in general	spondyl/o, vertebr/o	spinal bones
cervical vertebrae	cervic/o	
thoracic vertebrae	thorac/o	
lumbar vertebrae	lumb/o	spinal bones
sacrum (sacral vertebrae)	sacr/o	
coccyx (coccygeal vertebrae)	coccyg/o*	
Bones of the Upper Extremities		
humerus	humer/o	upper arm bone
radius	radi/o	bones of the forearm
ulna	uln/o	
carpals	carp/o	wrist bones
metacarpals	metacarp/o	bones of the hand
phalanges	phalang/o	bones of the fingers
Bones of the Pelvis	pelv/i	
ilium	ili/o	
ischium	ischi/o	pelvic bones
pubis	pub/o	
Bones of the Lower Extremities		
femur	femor/o	thigh bone
patella	patell/o	kneecap
fibula	fibul/o	bones of the lower leg
tibia	tibi/o	
tarsals	tars/o†	ankle bones
calcaneus	calcane/o	heel bone
metatarsals	metatars/o	bones of the feet
phalanges	phalang/o	bones of the toes

Use the electronic flashcards on the Evolve site or make your own set of flashcards using the above list. Select the word parts just presented, and study them until you know their meanings. Do this each time a set of word parts is presented.

*coccyg/o *refers to the tailbone, which represents fused coccygeal bones.*
†tars/o *refers to the ankle (the tarsus) or to the ankle bones; tars/o also means the edge of the eyelid, because a second meaning of tarsus is "a curved plate of dense white fibrous tissue forming the supporting structure of the eyelid."*

EXERCISE 2

Match the names of bones in the left column with their common names in the right column (a choice may be used more than once).

_____ **1.** carpals
_____ **2.** clavicle
_____ **3.** cranium
_____ **4.** femur
_____ **5.** ilium
_____ **6.** ischium
_____ **7.** patella
_____ **8.** phalanges
_____ **9.** pubis
_____ **10.** scapula
_____ **11.** sternum
_____ **12.** tarsals

A. ankle bones
B. bones of the fingers or toes
C. breastbone
D. collarbone
E. pelvic bone
F. kneecap
G. shoulder blade
H. skull
I. thigh bone
J. wrist bones

EXERCISE 3

Match the names of bones in the left column with their common names in the right column (a choice may be used more than once).

_____ **1.** fibula
_____ **2.** humerus
_____ **3.** radius
_____ **4.** tarsal
_____ **5.** ulna
_____ **6.** vertebra

A. ankle bone
B. bone of the forearm
C. bone of the lower leg
D. spinal bone
E. upper arm bone

PROGRAMMED LEARNING

Remember to cover the answers (left column) with folded paper or the bookmark. Write an answer in each blank, and then check your answer before proceeding to the next frame.

skull	**1.** The common name for cranium is _____. Cranium usually refers to the skull, but a second meaning of cranium is the specific portion of the skull that encloses and protects the brain. The skull is composed of **cranial** bones and **facial** bones (Figure 6-3).
spine	**2.** The vertebral or spinal column, commonly called the backbone, is attached at the base of the skull. It encloses the spinal cord, supports the head, and serves as a place of attachment for the ribs and muscles of the back. Spin/o, rach/i, and rachi/o mean spine. **Rachio+dynia** and **rachi+algia** both mean painful _____. Inflammation of a vertebra is spondylitis.
between	**3.** **Inter+vertebral** means _____ two adjoining vertebrae. Cushions of cartilage between adjoining vertebrae are called intervertebral disks. These layers of cartilage absorb shock.

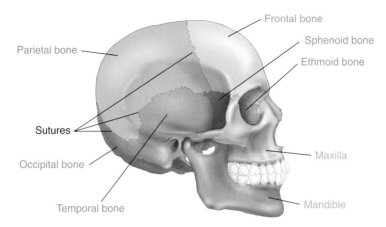

Frontal bone

Sphenoid bone

Ethmoid bone

Parietal bone

Sutures

Occipital bone

Temporal bone

Maxilla

Mandible

Figure 6-3 **The skull, the bony structure of the head.** The skull consists of the cranium and the skeleton of the face. Sutures are immovable fibrous joints between many of the cranial bones. Labels for the cranial bones (parietal, occipital, temporal, frontal, sphenoid, and ethmoid) are shown in blue, whereas labels for the facial bones are shown in orange (only the maxilla and mandible are labeled).

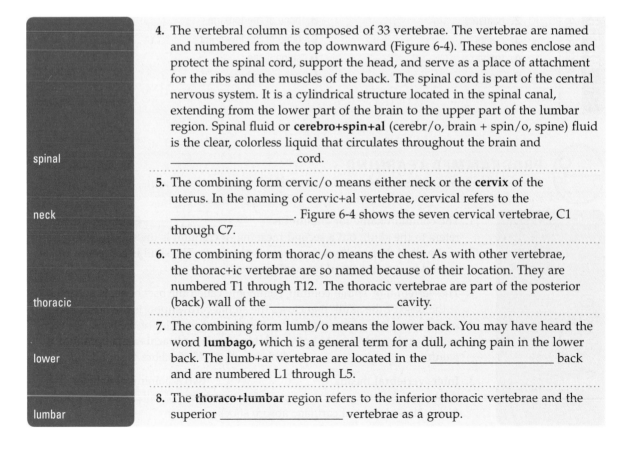

spinal

neck

thoracic

lower

lumbar

4. The vertebral column is composed of 33 vertebrae. The vertebrae are named and numbered from the top downward (Figure 6-4). These bones enclose and protect the spinal cord, support the head, and serve as a place of attachment for the ribs and the muscles of the back. The spinal cord is part of the central nervous system. It is a cylindrical structure located in the spinal canal, extending from the lower part of the brain to the upper part of the lumbar region. Spinal fluid or **cerebro+spin+al** (cerebr/o, brain + spin/o, spine) fluid is the clear, colorless liquid that circulates throughout the brain and _____ cord.

5. The combining form cervic/o means either neck or the **cervix** of the uterus. In the naming of cervic+al vertebrae, cervical refers to the _____. Figure 6-4 shows the seven cervical vertebrae, C1 through C7.

6. The combining form thorac/o means the chest. As with other vertebrae, the thorac+ic vertebrae are so named because of their location. They are numbered T1 through T12. The thoracic vertebrae are part of the posterior (back) wall of the _____ cavity.

7. The combining form lumb/o means the lower back. You may have heard the word **lumbago,** which is a general term for a dull, aching pain in the lower back. The lumb+ar vertebrae are located in the _____ back and are numbered L1 through L5.

8. The **thoraco+lumbar** region refers to the inferior thoracic vertebrae and the superior _____ vertebrae as a group.

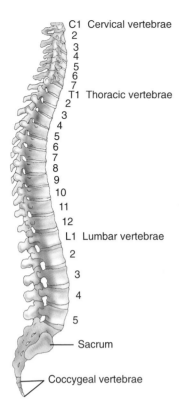

C1 Cervical vertebrae
2
3
4
5
6
7
T1 Thoracic vertebrae
2
3
4
5
6
7
8
9
10
11
12
L1 Lumbar vertebrae
2
3
4
5
Sacrum
Coccygeal vertebrae

cervic/o = neck
coccyg/o = coccyx
lumb/o = lumbar
sacr/o = sacrum
thorac/o = thorax (chest)
vertebr/o = vertebrae

Figure 6-4 The vertebral column, showing the five types of vertebrae. The vertebrae are numbered from the top downward. There are seven cervical vertebrae (C1 to C7) in the neck region, 12 thoracic vertebrae (T1 to T12) behind the chest cavity, five lumbar vertebrae (L1 to L5) supporting the lower back, five sacral vertebrae fused into one bone called the sacrum, and four coccygeal vertebrae fused into one bone called the coccyx.

9. The combining form sacr/o refers to the sacrum, the triangular bone below the lumbar vertebrae. Five **sacr+al** vertebrae are present at birth, but in the adult, they are fused to form one bone. The sacrum is the result of fusion of five _____ bones.

sacral

10. The coccyx is also the result of the fusion of vertebrae. The combining form coccyg/o means coccyx, or tail bone. This is located at the base of the spinal column and represents four fused **coccyg+eal** bones (-eal means pertaining to). The coccyx is the result of fusion of four _____ bones.

coccygeal

ribs

11. **Cost+al** refers to the costae, or _____. There are 12 pairs of ribs, each one joined to a vertebra posteriorly (at the back). The first seven pairs, called "true ribs," attach directly to the sternum. The other five pairs, referred to as "false ribs," do not attach directly to the sternum (Figure 6-5).

ribs

12. **Inter+costal** means between the _____. Intercostal muscles lie between the ribs and draw adjacent ribs together to increase the volume of the chest when breathing.

below (under)

13. **Sub+costal** means _____ a rib or the ribs.

sternum

14. **Sterno+costal** pertains to the _____ and the ribs.

vertebra

15. **Vertebro+costal** pertains to a rib and a _____.

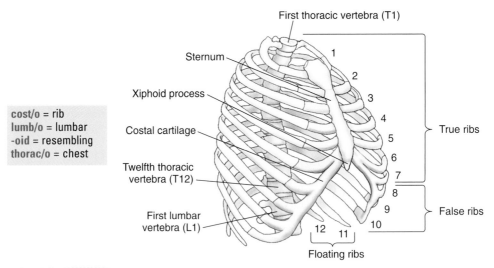

cost/o = rib
lumb/o = lumbar
-oid = resembling
thorac/o = chest

Figure 6-5 The rib cage. The ribs exist in pairs, 12 on each side of the chest, and are numbered from 1 to 12, beginning with the top rib. The upper seven pairs are joined directly with the sternum by a narrow strip of cartilage and are called "true ribs." The remaining five pairs are referred to as "false ribs" because they do not attach directly to the sternum. The last two pairs of false ribs, the "floating ribs," are attached only on the posterior aspect.

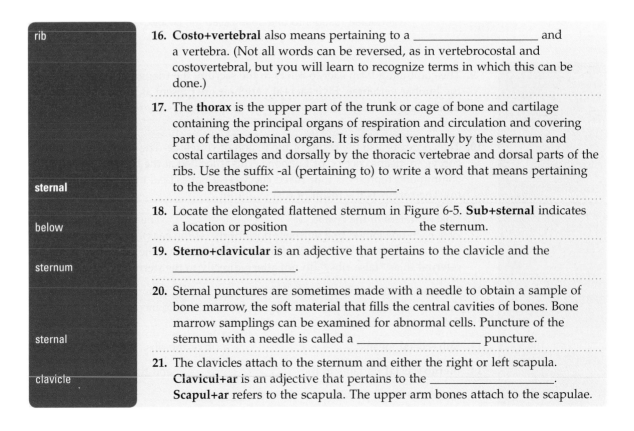

rib

16. **Costo+vertebral** also means pertaining to a _____ and a vertebra. (Not all words can be reversed, as in vertebrocostal and costovertebral, but you will learn to recognize terms in which this can be done.)

17. The **thorax** is the upper part of the trunk or cage of bone and cartilage containing the principal organs of respiration and circulation and covering part of the abdominal organs. It is formed ventrally by the sternum and costal cartilages and dorsally by the thoracic vertebrae and dorsal parts of the ribs. Use the suffix -al (pertaining to) to write a word that means pertaining to the breastbone: _____.

sternal

18. Locate the elongated flattened sternum in Figure 6-5. **Sub+sternal** indicates a location or position _____ the sternum.

below

19. **Sterno+clavicular** is an adjective that pertains to the clavicle and the _____.

sternum

20. Sternal punctures are sometimes made with a needle to obtain a sample of bone marrow, the soft material that fills the central cavities of bones. Bone marrow samplings can be examined for abnormal cells. Puncture of the sternum with a needle is called a _____ puncture.

sternal

21. The clavicles attach to the sternum and either the right or left scapula. **Clavicul+ar** is an adjective that pertains to the _____. **Scapul+ar** refers to the scapula. The upper arm bones attach to the scapulae.

clavicle

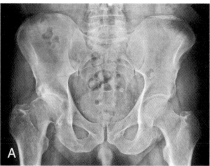

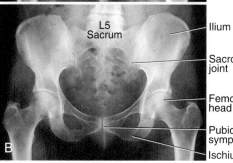

L5
Sacrum

Ilium

Sacroiliac
joint

Femoral
head

Pubic
symphysis

Ischium

---

femor/o = femur
-graph = instrument for recording
ili/o = ilium
pelv/i = pelvis
pub/o = pubis
radi/o = radiant energy
sacr/o = sacrum

Figure 6-6 Radiographs comparing male and female pelvis, anterior views. **A,** Male pelvis. Bones of the male are generally larger and heavier. The pelvic outlet, the space surrounded by the lower pelvic bones, is heart shaped. **B,** Female pelvis. The pelvic outlet is larger and more oval than that of the male. The size and shape of the female pelvis varies and is important in childbirth. L5 is the fifth lumbar vertebra. The pubic symphysis is the joint where the two pubic bones are joined.

---

pelvis

22. The lower vertebrae make up part of the pelvis, the basin-like structure formed by the sacrum, the coccyx, and the pelvic girdle (pelvic bones). The combining form pelv/i means pelvis. **Pelv+ic** means pertaining to the _____.

pubis

23. Two hip bones help form the pelvis. Each hip bone consists of three separate bones (ilium, ischium, pubis) in the newborn, but eventually the three bones fuse to form one bone. By covering the right or left half of Figure 6-6, you are observing a hip bone. Locate the ilium, the ischium, and the _____, which fuse to make up the hip bone.

ischium

24. **Ili+ac** refers to the ilium, and **ischi+al** means pertaining to the _____.

pubis

25. **Pub+ic** means pertaining to the _____.

ilium

26. **Ilio+pubic** refers to the _____ and the pubis.

ischiopubic

27. Use iliopubic as a model to write a word that means pertaining to the ischium and the pubis: _____.

ischiococcygeal

28. Use ischiopubic as a model to write a new term that means pertaining to the ischium and the coccyx: _____.

humerus

29. Technically, the arm is the portion of the upper limb of the body between the shoulder and the elbow. The bone of the upper arm is the humerus. Bones of the forearm are the ulna and the radius. The upper extremity is composed of the arm, forearm, and hand. Practice using the word parts you have learned for the bones of the arm and hand. **Humero+scapular** refers to the _____ and the scapula.

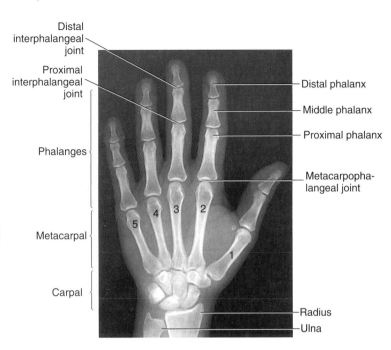

carp/o = carpus (wrist bones)
dist/o = far or distant from the origin
    or point of attachment
inter- = between
meta- = change *or* next in a series
phalang/o = phalanges
proxim/o = nearer the origin or point
    of attachment

Figure 6-7 Radiograph of the human hand. The ulna and radius are identified, as well as the bones of the hand. Eight small carpal bones make up the wrist. The palm contains five metacarpal bones, numbered 1 to 5. There are three phalanges in each finger except the thumb, which has two.

ulna	30. **Humero+ulnar** refers to both the humerus and the _____.
ulnar	31. From the previous frame, you should now recognize the adjective that means pertaining to the ulna. It is _____.
humerus	32. **Humer+al** means pertaining to the _____.
radial	33. Use humeral as a model to write an adjective that means pertaining to the radius: _____.
carpectomy	34. The wrist, also known as the **carpus,** consists of eight small bones called the carpals (Figure 6-7). Write a word that means excision of one or more bones of the wrist: _____.
carpal	35. Carpal tunnel syndrome is a complex of symptoms resulting from pressure on the median nerve in the **carpal tunnel** of the wrist. It causes pain, burning, or tingling in the fingers or hand. This complex of symptoms is called _____ tunnel syndrome.
next	36. The metacarpals are located between the carpals and the phalanges. The prefix meta- means change or next in a series. Meta+carpals lie _____ to the carpals.
fingers	37. The distal (far) ends of the metacarpals join with the fingers. **Carpo+phalang+eal** refers to the wrist and bones of the _____. There are two phalanges (singular, **phalanx**) in the thumb and three phalanges in each of the other four fingers. **Phalangitis** is inflammation of the bones of the fingers or toes.

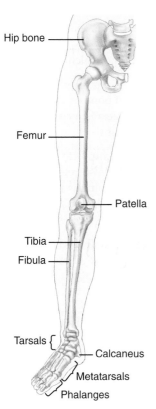

Hip bone

Femur

Patella

Tibia

Fibula

Tarsals {

Calcaneus

Metatarsals

Phalanges

meta- = change *or* next in a series
tars/o = tarsus (ankle bones)

Figure 6-8 Right lower extremity, anterior view. The lower extremity consists of the bones of the thigh, leg, foot, and the patella (kneecap). The lower leg has two bones, the tibia and fibula. The foot is composed of the ankle, instep, and five toes. The ankle has seven bones, with the calcaneus (heel bone) being the longest. The instep has five metatarsals. There are three phalanges in each of the toes, except in the great (or big) toe, which has only two.

leg

femur

femoral

kneecap

tibia

next

bone

38. Each of the lower extremities is composed of the bones of the thigh, leg, patella (kneecap), and foot (Figure 6-8). The femur is the longest and heaviest bone in the body. Femur is the name of the bone of the upper _____.

39. Ischio+femoral pertains to the ischium and the _____.

40. From the previous frame, you should recognize the adjective that means pertaining to the femur. The word is _____.

41. Patello+femoral refers to the patella, or _____, and the femur.

42. Two bones make up the lower leg. The tibia is larger than the fibula. **Tibi+algia** is pain of the _____.

43. The **tarsus**, or ankle, has seven bones. Tarsal means pertaining to the tarsus. The calcaneus is the formal name for the heel bone. The meta+tarsals lie _____ to the tarsals and also join with the bones of the toes.

44. The rigid nature of bone gives it the ability to provide shape and support for the body. However, bone also contains living cells and is richly supplied with blood vessels and nerves. The combining form oste/o means bone. **Oste+oid** means resembling _____.

calcium	**45.** The combining form calc/i means calcium. **Calcification is** the process by which organic tissue becomes hardened by deposits of _____. Calcification in soft tissue is abnormal (e.g., deposition of calcium in the walls of arteries leads to arteriosclerosis).
calcium	**46. De+calcification** is loss of _____ from bone or teeth. (The prefix de- means down, from, or reversing.) Osteomalacia is a consequence of decalcification without replacement of the lost calcium.
marrow	**47.** Bone marrow is the soft organic material that fills the central cavity of a bone. The combining form for bone marrow is myel/o, which also refers to the spinal cord. It is sometimes difficult to know which meaning is intended. When you see myel/o, you will need to decide if it means spinal cord or bone _____.
inflammation	**48. Myel+itis** means _____ of either the spinal cord or the bone marrow. **Myelo+fibr+osis** is replacement of bone marrow by fibrous tissue.
bone	**49. Osteo+myelitis** means inflammation of _____, often involving the bone marrow.
spinal	**50.** Remembering that encephal/o means brain, **myelo+encephal+itis** means inflammation of the brain and _____ cord.
	Congratulations if you knew which meaning was intended by myel/o in the last two frames! Its meaning is not always immediately apparent, but you will be able to determine which meaning is intended by the context in which the terms appear.

WRITE IT! **EXERCISE 4**

Write adjectives that describe these structures. (Question 1 is done as an example.)

1. wrist   *carpal* _____
2. skull   _____
3. femur   _____
4. humerus   _____
5. vertebra   _____
6. lower back   _____
7. pelvis   _____
8. spine   _____
9. rib   _____
10. chest   _____
11. radius   _____
12. ulna   _____

The new word parts introduced earlier in this chapter and some additional ones are presented in the following table. Be sure that you recognize their meanings.

Additional Word Parts and Their Meanings

Word Parts	Meaning
ankyl/o	stiff
arthr/o	articulation, joint
-asthenia	weakness
burs/o	bursa
calc/i	calcium
cellul/o	little cell or compartment
chondr/o	cartilage
de-	down, from, or reversing
meta-	change or next in a series
-sarcoma	malignant tumor of connective tissue
ten/o, tend/o, tendin/o	tendon

MATCH IT!

EXERCISE 5

Match the word parts in the left column with their meanings in the right column.

E 1. ankyl/o   A. cartilage
D 2. arthr/o   B. change or next in a series
F 3. -asthenia   C. down, from, or reversing
A 4. chondr/o   D. joint
C 5. de-   E. stiff
B 6. meta-   F. weakness

Cartilage

Cartilage is a specialized type of dense connective tissue that is elastic but strong and that can withstand considerable pressure or tension. Cartilage forms the major portion of the embryonic skeleton, but generally it is replaced by bone as the embryo matures. Cartilage does remain after birth, however, in the external ear, the nasal septum, the windpipe, between the vertebrae, and as a covering of bone surfaces at the places where they meet. **Chondral** means pertaining to cartilage.

FIND IT IN NEW TERMS!

EXERCISE 6

Write the combining form(s) for these new terms. A short definition is provided for each term.

Term	Combining Form(s)	Meaning
1. **subchondral**	_____	beneath the cartilage
2. **vertebrochondral**	_____	pertaining to a vertebra and its adjacent cartilage
3. **costochondral** (also **chondrocostal**)	_____	pertaining to a rib and its cartilage

Articulations and Associated Structures

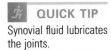

The place of union between two or more bones is called an **articulation,** or joint. Cartilage or other tissue covers the articular surfaces of bones. Joints that have cavities between articulating bones are called **synovial** joints. This type of joint is freely movable and contains synovial fluid. The elbow, knee, ankle, shoulder, and hip joints are examples of synovial joints.

Movement tends to create friction between a bone and adjacent structures. **Bursae** are sacs of fluid located in areas of friction, especially in the joints (see Figure 6-1). Four common types of joint motion are extension, flexion, rotation, and circumduction. Looking at Figure 6-9, you can see that **extension** straightens a limb and the opposite movement, **flexion,** bends a limb. **Rotation** is the movement of a bone around its own axis, and a circular movement of a limb at the far end is **circumduction.**

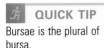

Ligaments are strong bands of fibrous connective tissue that connect bones or cartilage and serve to support and strengthen joints. Ligamentous means related to or resembling a ligament.

Muscles and Associated Structures

Muscle is composed of cells or fibers that contract and allow movement of an organ or part of the body. There are three main types of muscle tissue: *cardiac* (heart) muscle; *smooth* (**visceral** or **involuntary**) muscle found in the internal organs; and *skeletal* muscle, which is under conscious or voluntary control (Figure 6-10). The muscular system, however, usually refers only to skeletal muscle (Figure 6-11). The term **fascia** is used for the fibrous membrane that covers, supports, and separates muscles. **Tendons** are bands of strong fibrous tissue that attach the muscles to the bones. The combining forms ten/o and tend/o mean tendon.

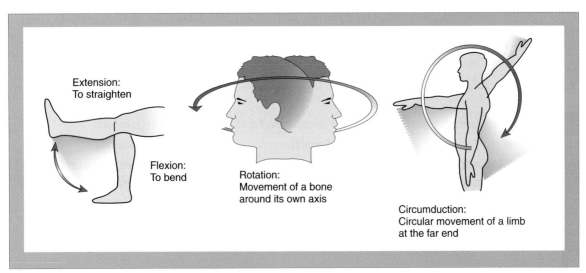

Figure 6-9 Four common types of joint motion.

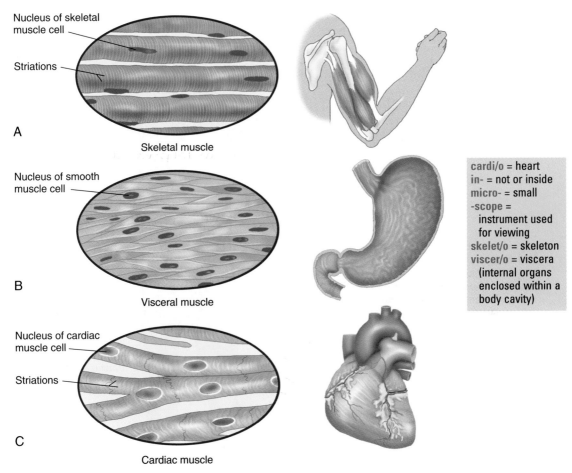

cardi/o = heart
in- = not or inside
micro- = small
-scope =
   instrument used
   for viewing
skelet/o = skeleton
viscer/o = viscera
   (internal organs
   enclosed within a
   body cavity)

Figure 6-10 Types of muscle. A, Voluntary, or skeletal, muscle is the type that is attached to bone and is controlled by the conscious part of the brain to produce movement. Under the microscope, voluntary muscle shows *striations,* alternate light and dark bands similar to those in the drawing. **B,** Visceral muscle is located in the walls of hollow internal structures, is involuntary, and lacks striations. It is also called smooth muscle. **C,** Cardiac muscle is involuntary but striated.

WRITE IT!

EXERCISE 7

Using combining forms and other word parts you have learned, write words in the blanks to complete the sentences. This exercise teaches you several new terms and is not a review.

1. **Fascial** means pertaining to ___fascia___.
2. **Myo+lysis** means ___destruction___ of muscle.
3. **Myo+pathy** means any ___disease___ of muscle.
4. **Musculo+fascial** refers to or consists of ___muscle___ and fascia.
5. **My+algia** is muscle ___pain___.

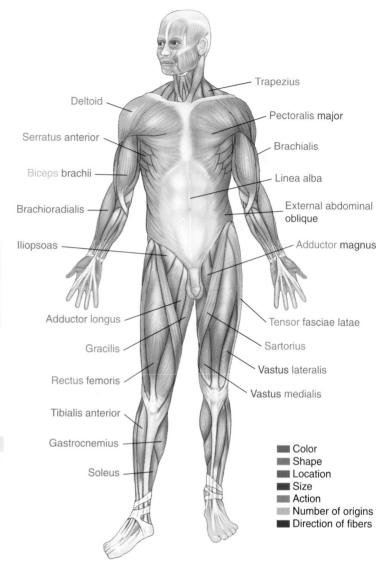

abdomin/o = abdomen
bi- = two
brachi/o = arm
pector/o = chest
radi/o = radiant energy or radius
tibi/o = tibia

Trapezius
Deltoid
Pectoralis major
Serratus anterior
Brachialis
Biceps brachii
Linea alba
Brachioradialis
External abdominal oblique
Iliopsoas
Adductor magnus
Adductor longus
Tensor fasciae latae
Gracilis
Sartorius
Rectus femoris
Vastus lateralis
Tibialis anterior
Vastus medialis
Gastrocnemius
Soleus

■ Color
■ Shape
■ Location
■ Size
■ Action
■ Number of origins
■ Direction of fibers

Figure 6-11 Major skeletal muscles of the body, anterior view. Muscle features such as size, shape, direction of fibers, location, number of attachments, origin, and action are often used in naming muscles. This is demonstrated by the use of color coding for the names. The meanings of the major word parts are identified.

Diseases, Disorders, and Diagnostic Terms

Although injury is a primary cause of problems of the musculoskeletal system, the bones, muscles, and associated tissues are subject to various pathologies, including infections, malignancies, metabolic disturbances, congenital defects, and diseases of connective tissue, such as bone, cartilage, ligaments, and tendons, which bind and support other structures. The cause of some disorders is not known, such as chronic fatigue syndrome, characterized by disabling fatigue, or **fibro+my+algia**, characterized by widespread non+articular pain of the torso, extremities, and face. In **myo+fibro+sis**, tissue is replaced by fibrous tissue, and **myasthenia gravis** is characterized by fatigue and muscle weakness resulting from a defect in the conduction of nerve impulses.

non- = not
articul/o = joint
-ar = pertaining to

Stress and Trauma Injuries

The vertebral column is composed of several bones and is, in effect, a strong, flexible rod that moves anteriorly (forward), posteriorly (backward), and laterally (from side to side). If the disks between the vertebrae become diseased, they sometimes rupture, resulting in a **herniated disk,** which can press on the spinal cord or on a spinal nerve, causing pain. Although commonly called a "slipped disk," herniated disk is a more appropriate name.

In injuries of the spine, the greatest danger is that the spinal cord may be injured by the movement of a fractured vertebra. Cord injury can cause paralysis below the point of injury. **Para+plegia** is paralysis of the lower portion of the body and of both legs. (Disease of the spinal cord, such as a tumor, can also cause paralysis.) **Quadri+plegia** or **tetra+plegia** is paralysis of the arms and legs. (In this term, quadri- refers to all four extremities, both arms and both legs.) **Paresis** is slight or incomplete paralysis. **Para+paresis** is slight or partial paralysis, and **quadriparesis** or **tetraparesis** affects all four extremities.

> para- = beside
> quadri- =
>   tetra- four
> -plegia = paralysis

A **dislocation** is the displacement of a bone from a joint (Figure 6-12). **Fracture** (fx) is the breaking of a bone, usually from sudden injury. Bones may break spontaneously, as in osteomalacia or osteomyelitis. In a *simple* fracture, the bone is broken but does not puncture the skin surface. In a *compound* fracture, the broken bone is visible through an opening in the skin. Compare simple and compound fractures (Figure 6-13).

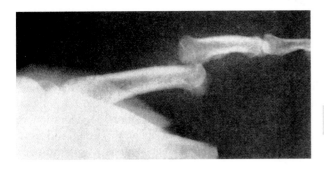

> -graph = recording instrument
> radi/o = radiant energy

Figure 6-12 Radiograph demonstrating a dislocation of the finger. Dislocations, often the result of trauma, can occur in any synovial joint but are more common in the shoulder, hip, knee, and fingers.

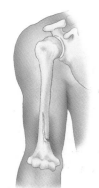 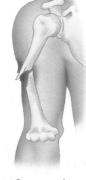

| Incomplete, simple (closed) | Complete, simple (closed) | Compound (open) |

Figure 6-13 Classification and description of the severity of fractures. Fractures are classified as complete or incomplete and are described as open (compound) or closed.

A **sprain** is injury to a joint that causes pain and disability, with the severity depending on the degree of injury to ligaments or tendons. A **strain** is excessive use of a part of the body to the extent that it is injured or trauma to a muscle caused by violent contraction or excessive forcible stretch. A **myo+cele** is a condition in which muscle protrudes through its fascial covering. This is also called a fascial hernia. **Tendin+itis** means inflammation of a tendon and is sometimes called **tendonitis.**

tendin/o = tendon
-itis = inflammation

BUILD IT!
EXERCISE 8

Combine the word parts to write terms for these descriptions.

1. replacement of normal tissue by fibrous tissue (my/o + fibr/o + -osis) __myofibrosis__

2. muscular weakness (my/o + -asthenia) __myasthenia__

3. paralysis in the lower limbs and trunk (para- + -plegia) __paraplegia__

4. paralysis of arms and legs (quadri- + -plegia) __quadriplegia__

5. fascial hernia (my/o + -cele) __myocele__

MATCH IT!
EXERCISE 9

Match the terms in the left column with their meanings in the right column.

__B__ **1.** compound fracture   **A.** bone broken, but does not protrude through skin

__D__ **2.** dislocation   **B.** bone broken, and protrudes through opening in skin

__A__ **3.** simple fracture   **C.** muscle injury caused by excessive use of body part

__C__ **4.** strain   **D.** displacement of a bone from a joint

---

Infections

cellul/o = little cell
-itis = inflammation
my/o = muscle

Cellulitis is an acute, spreading inflammation of the deep subcutaneous tissues (Figure 6-14). If the muscle is also involved, it is called **myocellulitis.**

oste/o = bone
chondr/o = cartilage

Osteitis is inflammation of a bone and may be caused by infection, degeneration, or trauma. Osteomyelitis, as mentioned earlier, is an infection of the bone and bone marrow and is caused by infectious microorganisms. **Osteochondritis** is inflammation

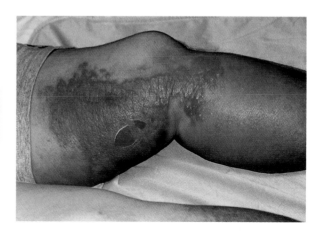

cellul/o = small cell
cutane/o = skin
-itis = inflammation
sub- = under

Figure 6-14 Cellulitis. Note the acute, diffuse (spreading) infection of the skin and subcutaneous tissue.

of bone and cartilage and tends to attack the bone-forming (ossification) centers of the skeleton.

Tumors and Malignancies

There are many types of benign tumors of the musculoskeletal system. The cause of bone tumors is largely unknown, unless cancer originates in other tissues and spreads to the bone.

Malignant bone tumors may be *primary* (originating in the bone) or *secondary* (originating in other tissue and metastasizing to the bone).

Sarcomas are cancers that arise from connective tissue, such as muscle or bone, and in general, terms using the word part -sarcoma name or describe malignant tumors (but there are rare misnomers). A **chondro+sarcoma** is composed of masses of cartilage. A **fibro+sarcoma** is a malignant tumor containing much fibrous tissue. Leukemias are chronic or acute diseases of the blood-forming tissues characterized by unrestrained growth of leukocytes and their precursors.

chondr/o = cartilage
-sarcoma = malignant tumor

Bone marrow is important in blood production and is involved in some types of leukemia. Leukemias are classified according to the predominant cell type and the severity of the disease (acute or chronic). Bone marrow studies are used to diagnose leukemia, identify tumors or other disorders of the bone marrow, and determine the extent of myelosuppression, or inhibition of the bone marrow. The posterior iliac crest is generally the preferred site for bone marrow aspiration (Figure 6-15). In adults, the anterior iliac crest or the sternum may also be used.

Multiple myeloma is a disease characterized by the presence of many tumor masses in the bone and bone marrow. It is usually progressive and generally fatal.

myel/o = bone marrow
-oma = tumor

Metabolic Disturbances

Metabolism is the sum of all the chemical processes that result in growth. Metabolic disorders result in a loss of homeostasis in the body, for example, anything that upsets the delicate balance between bone destruction and bone formation.

Osteo+porosis is a metabolic disease in which reduced bone mass leads to subsequent fractures, most often affecting postmenopausal women, sedentary individuals,

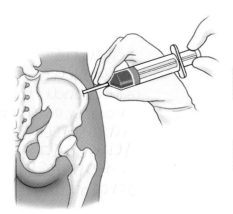

ili/o = ilium
poster/o = behind

Figure 6-15 Bone marrow aspiration from the posterior iliac crest. Cells and fluid are suctioned from the bone marrow, and results can provide important information about bone marrow function, including WBC, RBC, and platelet production.

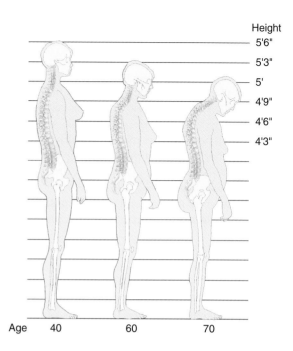

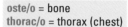

oste/o = bone
thorac/o = thorax (chest)

Figure 6-16 Osteoporotic changes in the curvature of the spine. The spine appears normal at age 40 years and shows osteoporotic changes at age 60 and 70. These changes bring about a loss of as much as 6 to 9 inches in height and the so-called dowager's hump in the upper thoracic vertebrae.

oste/o = bone
porosis = thinning
of bone

-malacia =
abnormal
softening

WORD ORIGIN

deformans (L.)
deformity or disfiguring

and patients receiving long-term steroid therapy. Osteoporosis may cause pain, especially in the lower back, and loss of height; spinal deformities are common. Figure 6-16 shows the effect of the disease on height and shape of the spine with advancing years.

Osteo+malacia is a reversible skeletal disorder characterized by a defect in the mineralization of bone. The most common cause of osteomalacia is a deficiency of vitamin D, which is necessary for proper absorption of calcium. A specific term for softening of the vertebrae is **spondylo+malacia**.

Osteitis deformans (Paget disease) is a skeletal disease of elderly persons characterized by chronic bone inflammation. This results in the thickening and softening of bones and in the bowing of the long bones.

BUILD IT!

EXERCISE 10

Combine the word parts to write terms for these descriptions.

1. acute inflammation of deep subcutaneous tissues (cellul/o + -itis)   *cellulitis*

2. infection of bone and bone marrow (oste/o + myel/o + -itis)   *osteomyelitis*

3. inflammation of bone and cartilage (oste/o + chondr/o + -itis)   *osteochondritis*

4. malignant tumor composed of cartilage (chondr/o + -sarcoma)   *chondrosarcoma*

5. malignant tumor containing fibrous tissue (fibr/o + -sarcoma)   *fibrosarcoma*

6. disease characterized by unrestrained WBC growth (leuk/o + -emia)   *leukemia*

7. abnormal loss of bone density and bone deterioration (oste/o + -porosis)   *osteoporosis*

8. abnormal mineralization and softening of bone (oste/o + -malacia)   *osteomalacia*

Congenital Defects

The skeletal system is affected by several developmental defects, including malformations of the spine. Some spinal malformations are congenital, and others can result from postural or nutritional defects or injury. **Spina bifida** is a congenital abnormality characterized by defective closure of the bones of the spine. It can be so extensive that it allows herniation of the spinal cord, or it might be evident only on radiologic examination.

Scoliosis is lateral curvature of the spine. It may be congenital but can be caused by other conditions, such as hip disease.

Exaggerated curvature of the spine from front to back gives rise to a condition called **kyphosis,** commonly known as humpback or hunchback. It can result from congenital disorders or from certain diseases, but it is also seen in osteoporosis affecting the spine, particularly in postmenopausal women with calcium deficiency. It is believed that ingestion of sufficient calcium (and estrogen therapy after menopause) can help prevent this problem. Compare scoliosis and kyphosis (Figure 6-17).

Muscular dystrophy is a group of inherited diseases characterized by weakness, atrophy (wasting) of muscle without involvement of the nervous system, and progressive disability and loss of strength.

Cranio+cele is a hernial protrusion of the brain through a defect in the skull.

The feet and hands are also subject to congenital defects, such as the presence of extra fingers or toes, or webbing between adjacent digits. Flatfoot, also known as **tarso+ptosis**, is a relatively common inherited condition characterized by the flattening out of the arch of the foot.

Arthritis and Connective Tissue Diseases

Connective tissue diseases affect tissue that supports and binds other body parts. The affected tissues include muscle, cartilage, tendons, vessels, and ligaments. **Arthr+itis** is any inflammatory condition of the joints characterized by pain, heat, swelling, redness, and limitation of movement.

Osteo+arthritis, also called degenerative joint disease (DJD), is a form of arthritis in which one or many joints undergo degenerative changes, particularly loss of articular

---

WORD ORIGIN
bifida *(L.)* divided into two (bi-) parts

WORD ORIGIN
skoliosis *(Gk)* curvature
kyphos *(Gk)* hunchback

dys- = bad
-trophy = nutrition

crani/o = skull
-cele = herniation

tars/o = ankle
-ptosis = prolapse

oste/o = bone
arthr/o = joint
-itis = inflammation

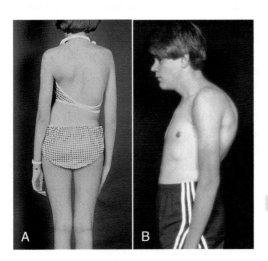

later/o = lateral or side
thorac/o = chest

Figure 6-17 Scoliosis vs. kyphosis. A, Lateral curvature of the spine, scoliosis, is a common abnormality in childhood, especially in girls. **B,** Severe kyphosis of the thoracic spine.

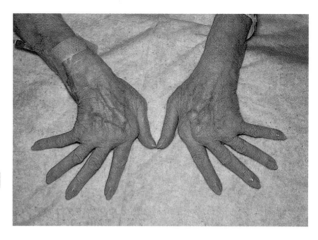

arthr/o = joint
-itis = inflammation
rheumat/o = rheumatism

Figure 6-18 Hand deformity characteristic of chronic rheumatoid arthritis. Marked deformity of the joints in the hand, causing deviation of the fingers.

cartilage. It is a chronic disease involving the bones and joints, especially joints that bear weight, which can also cause loss of spinal flexibility. Osteoarthritis is the most common type of arthritis and is often classified as a connective tissue disease. Connective tissue diseases are a group of acquired disorders that have immunologic and inflammatory changes in small blood vessels and connective tissue.

Rheumatoid arthritis (RA) is the second most common connective tissue disease. It is a chronic, systemic (pertaining to the whole body) disease that often results in joint deformities, particularly of the hands and feet (Figure 6-18). (**Rheumatism** is a general term for acute and chronic conditions characterized by inflammation, soreness, and stiffness of muscles and by pain in joints and associated structures.)

spondyl/o = vertebra
arthr/o = joint
-itis = inflammation
poly- = many

There are many other types of arthritis, including **spondylarthritis** (inflammation of a vertebra), which can be thought of as arthritis of the spine. (For easier pronunciation, the *o* is dropped from spondyl/o when it is joined with arthritis.) **Rheumatoid spondylitis** causes inflammation of cartilage between the vertebrae and can eventually cause neighboring vertebrae to fuse. Sometimes the whole spine becomes stiffened, a condition called "poker spine" or **ankylosed** spine. **Polyarthritis** is inflammation of more than one joint. Both **arthralgia** and **arthrodynia** mean painful joint. **Burs+itis** is inflammation of a bursa, but does not necessarily include joint inflammation. **Ankyl+osis** is an abnormal condition in which a joint is immobile and stiff.

burs/o = bursa
ankyl/o = stiff

Lupus erythematosus (LE) is an autoimmune disease that involves connective tissue. The disease is named for the characteristic butterfly rash that appears across the bridge of the nose in some patients (see Figure 12-9, p. 308).

Gout is a painful metabolic disease that is a form of acute arthritis. It is characterized by inflammation of the joints, especially of those in the foot or knee. It is hereditary and results from **hyper+uric+emia** and from deposits of urates in and around joints.

hyper- = excessive
uric = uric acid
-emia = inflammation

The knee, a synovial joint, is subject to many injuries, including dislocation, sprain, and fracture. The most common injury is the tearing of the cartilage, which can often be repaired during arthroscopy.

Arthro+scopy is direct visualization of the interior of a joint using a special fiberoptic **endo+scope** called an **arthro+scope**. It requires only a few small incisions (Figure 6-19). Bits of diseased or damaged cartilage can be removed during this procedure. Incision of a joint is **arthrotomy**. **Arthropathy** refers to any disease of a joint.

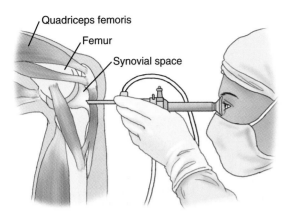

Quadriceps femoris
Femur
Synovial space

arthr/o = joint
endo- = inside
-scope = instrument used for viewing
-scopy = visual examination
synovi/o = synovium

Figure 6-19 Arthroscopy of the knee. The examination of the interior of a joint is performed by inserting a specially designed endoscope through a small incision. This procedure also permits biopsy of cartilage or damaged synovial membrane, diagnosis of conditions not obvious on radiographic images, and, in some cases, removal of loose bodies in the joint space.

WRITE IT!
EXERCISE 11

Write the correct term in the blanks to complete each sentence.

1. A congenital abnormality characterized by defective closure of the spine is spina ___bifida___.
2. Lateral curvature of the spine is ___scoliosis___.
3. A group of inherited diseases characterized by weakness, wasting of muscle, and progressive disability is muscular ___dystrophy___.
4. An inflammatory condition of the joints characterized by pain and limitation of movement is ___arthritis___.
5. Degenerative joint disease is also called ___osteoarthritis___.
6. A chronic, systemic type of arthritis is called ___rheumatoid___ arthritis.
7. Painful joint is called either arthralgia or ___arthrodynia___.
8. An autoimmune disease that involves connective tissue is lupus ___erythematosus___
9. A painful inherited form of acute arthritis that involves urate deposits in the joints is ___gout___.
10. A term for excessive uric acid in the blood is ___hyperuricemia___

BUILD IT!
EXERCISE 12

Combine these word parts to write terms for the descriptions.

1. spinal arthritis (spondyl/o + arthr/o + -itis) ___spondylarthritis___
2. inflammation of more than one joint (poly- + arthr/o + -itis) ___polyarthritis___
3. stiff joint (ankyl/o + -osis) ___ankylosis___
4. inflammation of a bursa (burs/o + -itis) ___bursitis___
5. direct visualization of the interior of a joint (arthr/o + -scopy) ___arthroscopy___

Surgical and Therapeutic Interventions

Orthopedic surgeons restore fractures to their normal positions by **reduction,** pulling the broken fragments into alignment. Management usually involves immobilization with a splint, bandage, cast, or traction. A cast immobilizes a broken bone until it heals.

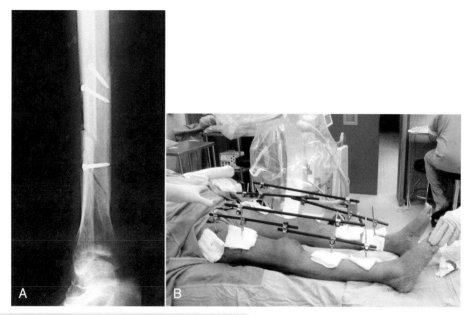

Figure 6-20 Internal vs. external fixation of fractures. A, Lateral view of a lower leg break after reduction and internal fixation using screws. **B,** External fixation of a fracture, using pins that are attached to a compression device. The pins are removed when the fracture is healed.

Traction is the use of a pulling force to a part of the body to produce alignment and rest while decreasing muscle spasm and correcting or preventing deformity.

A fracture is usually restored to its normal position by manipulation without surgery. This is called *closed* reduction. If a fracture must be exposed by surgery before the broken ends can be aligned, it is an *open* reduction. The fracture shown in Figure 6-20, *A,* was corrected by surgery that included *internal fixation* to stabilize the alignment. Internal fixation uses pins, rods, plates, screws, or other materials to immobilize the fracture. After healing, the fixation devices may be removed or left in place. *External fixation* is used in both open and closed reductions. This method uses metal pins attached to a compression device outside the skin surface (Figure 6-20, *B*).

After a bone is broken, the body begins the healing process to repair the injury. Electrical bone stimulation, bone grafting, and ultrasound treatment may be used when healing is slow or does not occur.

Persons with osteoporosis are predisposed to fractures. Calcium therapy, vitamin D, and **anti-osteoporotics** are used to treat osteoporosis. Estrogen therapy, begun soon after the start of menopause, may help in the prevention and treatment of osteoporosis. Vertebral fractures can sometimes be repaired by **vertebro+plasty**. In this procedure, a cement-like substance is injected into the body of a fractured vertebra to stabilize and strengthen it and immediately remove pain.

Excision of a bone (or a portion of it) is **oste+ectomy;** this is usually written **ostectomy.** Excision of a rib is **cost+ectomy**. **Crani+ectomy** is excision of a segment of the skull; **cranio+tomy** is incision through the skull. Plastic surgery to repair the skull is **cranio+plasty**. Excision of cartilage is **chondr+ectomy.**

QUICK TIP

One *e* is often dropped. Ostectomy versus osteectomy.

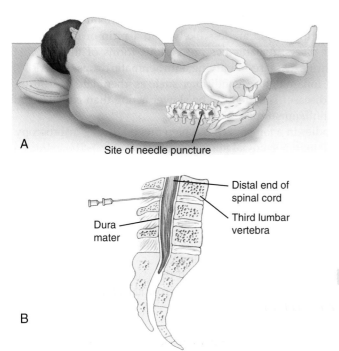

A
Site of needle puncture

B

Distal end of
spinal cord

Third lumbar
vertebra

Dura
mater

-al, -ic = pertaining to
an- = no or without
cerebr/o = brain
esthesi/o = feeling
spin/o = spine

Figure 6-21 Lumbar puncture. The needle is
inserted into the space between the third and
fourth lumbar vertebrae. A specimen of cerebrospinal fluid may be collected for examination. A
lumbar puncture is also necessary for injection of
a spinal anesthetic.

Tendons may become damaged when a person sustains a deep wound and may
require surgical repair or **tendo+plasty. Myo+plasty** is surgical repair of muscle.
Teno+myo+plasty is surgical repair of tendon and muscle.

Muscle relaxants are prescribed to relieve muscle spasms, such as the spasms
that accompany a herniated disk. If bed rest and other treatments do not alleviate
the problem, a **laminectomy** may be indicated. This is surgical removal of the bony
posterior arch of a vertebra to permit surgical access to the disk so that the herniated material can be removed. Complete excision of an intervertebral disk is a
disk+ectomy.

Spinal anesthesia is loss of feeling produced by an anesthetic injected into the spinal
canal. Spinal puncture (also called spinal tap or lumbar puncture) is puncture of the
spinal cavity with a needle, either to extract the spinal fluid for diagnostic purposes
or to introduce agents into the spinal canal for anesthesia or radiographic studies
(Figure 6-21).

Numerous surgeries are performed to straighten the toes, remove bunions (abnormal enlargement of the joint at the base of the great toe), and correct various deformities of the feet. A **bunion+ectomy** is excision of a bunion. Surgical repair to straighten
the alignment of the toes is usually done at the same time.

Many drugs are available to treat different forms of arthritis and other connective
tissue diseases. **Antiinflammatories** are generally used to reduce inflammation and pain,
especially drugs classified as nonsteroidal antiinflammatory drugs (NSAIDs). Two
examples are aspirin and ibuprofen. Physical therapy is an important part of arthritis
treatment as well as restoring function after injury or surgery.

Cyclooxygenase-2 (COX-2) inhibitors (e.g., Celebrex) are also frequently used to reduce the inflammation of arthritis and are less likely than aspirin or ibuprofen to cause stomach distress and ulcers. **Antiarthritics** are various forms of therapy that relieve the symptoms of arthritis. Disease-modifying antirheumatic drugs (DMARDs) may change the course of inflammatory conditions such as rheumatoid arthritis, slowing progression of the disease. They tend to be slower acting than NSAIDs and may be prescribed with antiinflammatories.

Torn cartilage or loose bodies in a joint space can be removed during arthroscopy. Excessive fluid can accumulate in a synovial joint after injury and must be extracted with a needle; this procedure is called **arthro+centesis.**

-centesis = surgical puncture

When other measures are inadequate to provide pain control for degenerative joint disease, surgery may be indicated, often total joint replacement. Replacement of hips, knees, elbows, wrists, shoulders, and finger or toe joints is common. Total knee replacement is the surgical insertion of a hinged device to relieve pain and restore motion to a knee that is severely affected by arthritis or injury. Any surgical reconstruction or replacement of a joint is called **arthro+plasty.**

myel/o = bone marrow
suppress = to inhibit

Cancer treatment often induces **myelosuppression.** If the patient's bone marrow is destroyed with radiation and chemotherapy, bone marrow transplants are used to stimulate the production of normal blood.

MATCH IT! EXERCISE 13

Match the surgical terms in the left column with their meanings in the right column.

_____ **1.** closed reduction   **A.** excision of a bone

_____ **2.** internal fixation   **B.** surgically exposing and aligning a broken bone

_____ **3.** open reduction   **C.** pulling a broken bone into alignment without surgery

_____ **4.** ostectomy   **D.** surgery using pins or other materials to immobilize a broken bone

---

WRITE IT! EXERCISE 14

Write terms for these meanings.

1. excision of a disk   _____

2. inhibiting bone marrow activity   _____

3. medications that reduce inflammation _____

4. surgical puncture of a synovial joint _____

5. surgical repair of muscle   _____

 Be Careful with These!

ankyl/o (stiff) does not mean ankle! *tars/o* means ankle.
metatars/o (bones of the foot) versus *metacarp/o* (bones of the hand)
paresis (incomplete paralysis) versus *paralysis*
Remember that *radi/o* can mean a bone of the forearm, not just radiation.

SELF-TEST   Work the following exercises to test your understanding of the material in Chapter 6. Complete all the exercises before using Appendix VIII to check your answers.

A. MATCH IT!   *Match the names of bones in the left column with their common names in the right column (a choice may be used more than once).*

____ **1.** carpals	**A.** ankle bones
____ **2.** clavicle	**B.** bone of the forearm
____ **3.** cranium	**C.** bone of the lower leg
____ **4.** femur	**D.** bones of the fingers or toes
____ **5.** fibula	**E.** breastbone
____ **6.** humerus	**F.** collarbone
____ **7.** ilium	**G.** pelvic bone
____ **8.** ischium	**H.** kneecap
____ **9.** patella	**I.** shoulder blade
____ **10.** phalanges	**J.** skull
____ **11.** pubis	**K.** spinal bone
____ **12.** radius	**L.** thigh bone
____ **13.** scapula	**M.** upper arm bone
____ **14.** sternum	**N.** wrist bones
____ **15.** tarsals	
____ **16.** ulna	
____ **17.** vertebra	

B. MATCH IT!   *Match the connective tissues with their descriptions (each choice is used once).*

____ **1.** bone	**A.** connects bones or cartilages
____ **2.** bursa	**B.** fluid-filled sac that helps reduce friction
____ **3.** cartilage	**C.** fluid-secreting tissue lining the joint
____ **4.** joint	**D.** place of union between two or more bones
____ **5.** ligament	**E.** provides protection and support for a joint
____ **6.** synovial membrane	**F.** strong, fibrous tissue that attaches muscles to bones
____ **7.** tendon	**G.** the most rigid connective tissue

C. WRITE IT!   *Write answers in the blanks to complete the sentences.*

1. In examining a male patient, Dr. Johnson asks him to straighten his leg. This joint motion is called

_____ .

2. A 60-year-old man undergoes a procedure in which the physician examines his right knee with an arthroscope. The name of the procedure is _____ .

3. Seventy-year-old Esther has osteoporosis and has fractured a vertebra. Dr. Bonelly injects a cement-like substance into the vertebra to stabilize and strengthen it, in a procedure known as a(n) _____ .

4. Fourteen-year-old Mary has lateral curvature of the spine. This condition is called _____ .

5. The orthopedist diagnoses an adult woman with carpal tunnel syndrome. This complex of symptoms results from pressure on the median nerve in the carpal tunnel of the _____ .

Continued

SELF-TEST   (cont'd)

D. CIRCLE IT!   *Circle the one correct response (a, b, c, or d) for each question.*

1. What does rachialgia mean?
   (a) fused spine   (b) painful spine   (c) the opposite of rachiodynia   (d) the same as spondylitis
2. What is the meaning of a myocele?
   (a) fascial hernia   (b) fibrous muscle   (c) hardened muscle   (d) painful muscle
3. Which term means inflammation of the vertebrae?
   (a) carpitis   (b) phalangitis   (c) spondylitis   (d) tarsitis
4. Which term means between the ribs?
   (a) costovertebral   (b) intercostal   (c) intracostal   (d) subcostal
5. Which term means excision of a portion of the skull?
   (a) angiectomy   (b) coccygectomy   (c) craniectomy   (d) craniotomy
6. Which term indicates a broken bone that is visible through an opening in the skin?
   (a) closed fracture   (b) complete fracture   (c) compound fracture   (d) simple fracture
7. What is the meaning of articulation?
   (a) bone   (b) cartilage   (c) fascia   (d) joint
8. Which term means rupture of an intervertebral disk?
   (a) chondrosarcoma   (b) herniated disk   (c) spondylomalacia   (d) vertebrochondritis
9. What does osteoid mean?
   (a) growth of bone   (b) inflammation of bone   (c) resembling bone   (d) softening of bone
10. Which term refers to the bones located between the toes and the bones of the ankle?
   (a) carpals   (b) metacarpals   (c) metatarsals   (d) tarsals

E. READING HEALTH CARE REPORTS   *Read the health report, and define the five underlined terms listed after the report.*

MEDICAL REPORT   **Mid-City Medical Center**

222 Medical Center Drive   **Main City, USA 63017-1000**   **Phone:** (555) 434-0000
                                                                    Fax: (555) 434-0001

DIAGNOSIS RECORD/DISCHARGE SUMMARY

Patient: Martha Watkins
Final Diagnosis: <u>Osteoarthritis</u> of the right knee
Secondary Diagnosis: <u>Rheumatoid arthritis</u>; <u>degenerative joint disease left knee</u>
Complications: Postoperative deep vein thrombosis—right lower extremity
Principal Operation/Procedure(s)/Treatment Rendered: <u>Right total knee arthroplasty</u>, posterior stabilized, cemented.
Discharge Instructions: Up ad lib with full weight bearing to <u>right lower extremity</u>. Ambulate with wheeled walker. Home health for physical and occupational therapy 3× week, and nursing visits to monitor incision and medication. Patient to change dry dressing to incision daily.
Medications: Coumadin 5 mg daily
Diet: Regular
Follow-up: Patient to make appointment with Dr. Withers for staple removal in 10 days
Date Admitted: 1/31/2006   **Date Discharged:** 2/05/2006

Dr. John Withers
(Dr. John Withers)

SELF-TEST (cont'd)

1. osteoarthritis: _____
2. rheumatoid arthritis: _____
3. degenerative joint disease left knee: _____
4. right total knee arthroplasty: _____
5. right lower extremity: _____

F. FINDING THE CLUE! *Use a clue to write terms for the descriptions. Solve Question 1; each ending letter becomes the clue for the first letter of the next answer.*

1. describing a stiffened joint _____
2. displacement of a bone from its normal position _____
3. not involving the joints _____
4. pertaining to a bone of the forearm _____
5. type of vertebra _____
6. any of a large number of arthritis-type conditions _____
7. inflammation of the bone marrow _____
8. pertaining to the breastbone _____
9. pertaining to the side _____
10. flexible band that connects bones and cartilage _____

G. WRITE IT! *Write a one-word term for each of these meanings.*

1. destruction of muscle _____
2. inflammation of the bone and cartilage _____
3. inhibition of the bone marrow _____
4. medications used to reduce inflammation _____
5. medications used to treat osteoporosis _____
6. pertaining to the collarbone _____
7. pertaining to the neck _____
8. pertaining to the upper arm bone _____
9. prolapse of the ankle _____
10. restoring a fracture to its normal position _____

H. SPELL IT! *Circle the terms that are incorrectly spelled, and write the correct spelling.*

1. ankilosis _____
2. circumduktion _____
3. femural _____
4. flexsion _____
5. laminektomy _____

Q&E List
*Use the Companion CD or audio CDs to review the terms presented in Chapter 6. Look
closely at the spelling of each term as it is pronounced.*

ankylosed (**ang´kə-lōzd**)
ankylosis (**ang´´kə-lo´sis**)
antiarthritics (**an´´te-ahr-thrit´iks**)
antiinflammatories (**an´´te-in-flam´ə-tor´´ēs**)
anti-osteoporotics (**an´´te-os´´te-o-pə-rot´iks**)
arthralgia (**ahr-thral´jə**)
arthritis (**ahr-thri´tis**)
arthrocentesis (**ahr´´thro-sen-te´sis**)
arthrodynia (**ahr´´thro-din´e-ə**)
arthropathy (**ahr-throp´ə-the**)
arthroplasty (**ahr´thro-plas´´te**)
arthroscope (**ahr´thro-skōp**)
arthroscopy (**ahr-thros´kə-pe**)
arthrotomy (**ahr-throt´ə-me**)
articulation (**ahr-tik´´u-la´shən**)
bunionectomy (**bun´´yən-ek´tə-me**)
bursa (**bər´sə**)
bursitis (**bər-si´tis**)
calcaneus (**kal-ka´ne-əs**)
calcification (**kal´´sĭ-fĭ-ka´shən**)
carpal (**kahr´pəl**)
carpal tunnel (**kahr´pəl tun´əl**)
carpectomy (**kahr-pek´tə-me**)
carpophalangeal (**kahr´´po-fə-lan´je-əl**)
carpus (**kahr´pəs**)
cartilage (**kahr´tĭ-ləj**)
cellulitis (**sel´´u-li´tis**)
cerebrospinal (**ser´´ə-bro-spi´nəl**)
cervical (**sur´vĭ-kəl**)
cervix (**sur´viks**)
chondral (**kon´drəl**)
chondrectomy (**kon-drek´tə-me**)
chondrocostal (**kon´´dro-kos´təl**)
chondrosarcoma (**kon´´dro-sahr-ko´mə**)
circumduction (**sur´´kəm-duk´shən**)
clavicle (**klav´ĭ-kəl**)
clavicular (**klə-vik´u-lər**)
coccygeal (**kok-sij´e-əl**)
coccyx (**kok´siks**)
costa (**kos´tə**)
costal (**kos´təl**)
costectomy (**kos-tek´tə-me**)

costochondral (**kos´´to-kon´drəl**)
costovertebral (**kos´´to-vur´tə-brəl**)
cranial (**kra´ne-əl**)
craniectomy (**kra´´ne-ek´tə-me**)
craniocele (**kra´ne-o-sēl´´**)
cranioplasty (**kra´ne-o-plas´´te**)
craniotomy (**kra´´ne-ot´ə-me**)
cranium (**kra´ne-əm**)
decalcification (**de-kal´´sĭ-fĭ-ka´shən**)
diskectomy (**dis-kek´tə-me**)
dislocation (**dis´´lo-ka´shən**)
endoscope (**en´do-skōp**)
extension (**ek-sten´shən**)
facial (**fa´shəl**)
fascia (**fash´e-ə**)
fascial (**fash´e-əl**)
femoral (**fem´or-əl**)
femur (**fe´mər**)
fibromyalgia (**fi´´bro-mi-al´jə**)
fibrosarcoma (**fi´´bro-sahr-ko´mə**)
fibula (**fib´u-lə**)
flexion (**flek´shən**)
fracture (**frak´chər**)
gout (**gout**)
hematopoiesis (**he´´mə-, hem´´ə-to-poi-e´sis**)
herniated disk (**hur´ne-āt´´əd disk**)
humeral (**hu´mər-əl**)
humeroscapular (**hu´´mər-o-skap´u-lər**)
humeroulnar (**hu´´mər-o-ul´nər**)
humerus (**hu´mər-əs**)
hyperuricemia (**hi´´pər-u´´rĭ-se´me-ə**)
iliac (**il´e-ak**)
iliopubic (**il´´e-o-pu´bik**)
ilium (**il´e-əm**)
intercostal (**in´´tər-kos´təl**)
intervertebral (**in´´tər-vur´tə-brəl**)
involuntary (**in-vol´ən-tar´´e**)
ischial (**is´ke-əl**)
ischiococcygeal (**is´´ke-o-kok-sij´e-əl**)
ischiofemoral (**is´´ke-o-fem´o-rəl**)
ischiopubic (**is´´ke-o-pu´bik**)
ischium (**is´ke-əm**)

kyphosis (ki-fo´sis)

laminectomy (lam´´ĭ-nek´tə-me)

leukemia (loo-ke´me-ə)

ligament (lig´ə-mənt)

lumbago (ləm-ba´go)

lumbar (lum´bər, lum´bahr)

lupus erythematosus (loo´pəs er´´ə-them´´ə-to´sis)

metacarpal (met´´ə-kahr´pəl)

metatarsal (met´´ə-tahr´səl)

multiple myeloma (mul´tĭ-pəl mi´´ə-lo´mə)

muscular dystrophy (mus´ku-lər dis´trə-fe)

musculofascial (mus´´ku-lo-fash´e-əl)

musculoskeletal (mus´´ku-lo-skel´ə-təl)

myalgia (mi-al´jə)

myasthenia gravis (mi´´əs-the´ne-ə grav´is)

myelitis (mi´´ə-li´tis)

myeloencephalitis (mi´´ə-lo-en-sef´´ə-li´tis)

myelofibrosis (mi´´ə-lo-fi-bro´sis)

myelosuppression (mi´´ə-lo-sə-presh´ən)

myocele (mi´o-sēl)

myocellulitis (mi´´o-sel´´u-li´tis)

myofibrosis (mi´´o-fi-bro´sis)

myolysis (mi-ol´ĭ-sis)

myopathy (mi-op´ə-the)

myoplasty (mi´o-plas´´te)

orthopedics (or´´tho-pe´diks)

orthopedist (or´´tho-pe´dist)

ostectomy (os-tek´tə-me)

osteectomy (os´´te-ek´tə-me)

osteitis (os´´te-i´tis)

osteitis deformans (os´´te-i´tis de-for´mans)

osteoarthritis (os´´te-o-ahr-thri´tis)

osteochondritis (os´´te-o-kon-dri´tis)

osteoid (os´te-oid)

osteomalacia (os´´te-o-mə-la´shə)

osteomyelitis (os´´te-o-mi´´ə-li´tis)

osteoporosis (os´´te-o-pə-ro´sis)

paraparesis (par´´ə-pə-re´sis)

paraplegia (par´´ə-ple´jə)

paresis (pə-re´sis)

patella (pə-tel´ə)

patellofemoral (pə-tel´´o-fem´ə-rəl)

pelvic (pel´vik)

phalanges (fə-lan´jēz)

phalangitis (fal´´ən-ji´tis)

phalanx (fa´lanks)

polyarthritis (pol´´e-ahr-thri´tis)

pubic (pu´bik)

pubis (pu´bis)

quadriparesis (kwod´´rĭ-pə-re´sis)

quadriplegia (kwod´´rĭ-ple´jə)

rachialgia (ra´´ke-al´jə)

rachiodynia (ra´´ke-o-din´e-ə)

radial (ra´de-əl)

radius (ra´de-əs)

reduction (re-duk´shən)

rheumatism (roo´mə-tiz-əm)

rheumatoid arthritis (roo´mə-toid ahr-thri´tis)

rheumatoid spondylitis (roo´mə-toid spon´´də-li´tis)

rotation (ro-ta´shən)

sacral (sa´krəl)

sacrum (sa´krəm)

sarcoma (sahr-ko´mə)

scapula (skap´u-lə)

scapular (skap´u-lər)

scoliosis (sko´´le-o´sis)

spina bifida (spi´nə bif´ĭ-də)

spine (spīn)

spondylarthritis (spon´´dəl-ahr-thri´tis)

spondylomalacia (spon´´də-lo-mə-la´shə)

sprain (sprān)

sternal (stur´nəl)

sternoclavicular (stur´´no-klə-vik´u-lər)

sternocostal (stur´´no-kos´təl)

sternum (stur´nəm)

strain (strān)

subchondral (səb-kon´drəl)

subcostal (səb-kos´təl)

substernal (səb-stər´nəl)

synovial (sĭ-no´ve-əl)

tarsal (tahr´səl)

tarsoptosis (tahr´´sop-to´sis)

tarsus (tahr´səs)

tendinitis (ten´´dĭ-ni´tis)

tendon (ten´dən)

tendonitis (ten´´də-ni´tis)

tendoplasty (ten´do-plas´´te)

tenomyoplasty (ten´´o-mi´o-plas´´te)

tetraparesis (tet´´rə-pə-re´sis)

tetraplegia (tet´´rə-ple´jə)

thoracic (thə-ras´ik)

thoracolumbar (thor´´ə-ko-lum´bər)

continued

thorax **(thor´aks)**
tibia **(tib´e-ə)**
tibialgia **(tib´´e-al´jə)**
ulna **(ul´nə)**
ulnar **(ul´nər)**

vertebra **(vur´tə-brə)**
vertebrochondral **(vur´´tə-bro-kon´drəl)**
vertebrocostal **(vur´´tə-bro-kos´təl)**
vertebroplasty **(vur´tə-bro-plas´´te)**
visceral **(vis´ər-əl)**

evolve Don't forget the games on the Companion CD and http://evolve.elsevier.com/Leonard/quick/ for additional review, including questions on Spanish medical terms.

ESPAÑOL   Enhancing Spanish Communication

English	Spanish (pronunciation)
cranium	cráneo **(CRAY-nay-o)**
fracture	fractura **(frac-TOO-rah)**
ligament	ligamento **(le-gah-MEN-to)**
phalanges	falanges **(fah-LAHN-hays)**
phosphorus	fósforo **(FOS-fo-ro)**
reduction	reducción **(ray-dooc-se-ON)**
sacrum	hueso sacro **(oo-AY-so SAH-cro)**
shoulder	hombro **(OM-bro)**
shoulder blade	espaldilla **(es-pal-DEEL-lyah)**
spinal column	columna vertebral **(co-LOOM-nah ver-tay-BRAHL)**
spine	espinazo **(es-pe-NAH-so)**
sprain, to	torcer **(tor-SERR)**
sternum	esternón **(es-ter-NON)**
stiff	tieso **(te-AY-so)**
tendon	tendón **(ten-DON)**
vertebral column	columna vertebral **(co-LOOM-nah ver-tay-BRAHL)**

CHAPTER 7

Circulatory System

CONTENTS

Function First
CARDIOVASCULAR SYSTEM
Structures of the Cardiovascular System
- Heart
- Blood Vessels

Diseases, Disorders, and Diagnostic Terms
- Heart
- Blood Vessels

Surgical and Therapeutic Interventions
- Heart
- Blood Vessels

LYMPHATIC SYSTEM
Structures of the Lymphatic System
Diseases, Disorders, and Diagnostic Terms
Surgical and Therapeutic Interventions
SELF-TEST
Q&E List
Enhancing Spanish Communication

OBJECTIVES

After completing Chapter 7, you will be able to:

1. Recognize or write the functions of the circulatory system.
2. Recognize or write the meanings of Chapter 7 word parts and use them to build and analyze medical terms.
3. Write terms for selected structures of the cardiovascular system, or match terms with their descriptions.
4. Write the names of the diagnostic terms and pathologies related to the cardiovascular system when given their descriptions, or match terms with their meanings.
5. Match surgical and therapeutic interventions for the cardiovascular system, or write the names

of the interventions when given their descriptions.
6. Write terms for selected structures of the lymphatic system, or match terms with their descriptions.
7. Write the names of the diagnostic terms and pathologies related to the lymphatic system when given their descriptions, or match terms with their meanings.
8. Match surgical and therapeutic interventions for the lymphatic system, or write the names of the interventions when given their descriptions.
9. Spell terms for the circulatory system correctly.

Function First

The **circulatory** system consists of the **cardio+vascul+ar** system (heart and blood vessels) and the **lymphatic** system (structures involved in the conveyance of the fluid **lymph**). The circulatory system cooperates with other body systems to maintain homeostasis, or equilibrium of the internal environment of the body.

Body cells must have a constant supply of food, oxygen, and other substances to function properly. Blood circulates through the heart and blood vessels, carrying

cardi/o = heart
vascul/o = vessel

home/o = sameness
-stasis = controlling

oxygen, nutrients, vitamins, antibodies, and other substances. It carries away waste and carbon dioxide.

The cardiovascular system supplies body cells with needed substances, transports waste products for disposal, maintains the acid-base balance of the body, prevents hemorrhage through blood clotting, protects against disease, and helps regulate body temperature.

WRITE IT!   EXERCISE 1

Write words that are associated with the functions of the cardiovascular system; the first letter is provided. (Question 1 is done as an example.)

The cardiovascular system carries **(1)** *oxygen* _____, (2) *n* _____, (3) *v* _____, and (4) *a* _____ to the cells. Blood carries (5) *w* _____ and (6) *c* _____ *d* _____ away from cells. This system also maintains *the* (7) *a* _____ balance, prevents (8) *h* _____ through blood clotting, and helps regulate body (9) *t* _____.

Use Appendix VIII to check the answers to all the exercises in Chapter 7.

Cardiovascular System

Structures of the Cardiovascular System

Components of the cardiovascular system include the heart and a vast network of vessels (Figure 7-1).

cardi/o, coron/o = heart
sub- = below
vascul/o = vessel

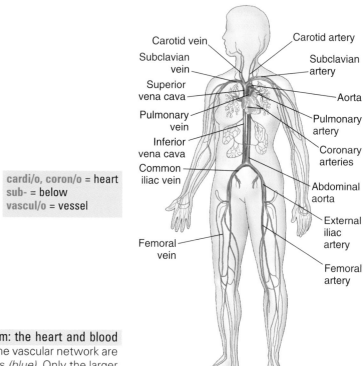

Carotid vein
Subclavian vein
Superior vena cava
Pulmonary vein
Inferior vena cava
Common iliac vein
Femoral vein

Carotid artery
Subclavian artery
Aorta
Pulmonary artery
Coronary arteries
Abdominal aorta
External iliac artery
Femoral artery

Figure 7-1 The cardiovascular system: the heart and blood vessels. Two major components of the vascular network are shown, the arteries *(red)* and the veins *(blue)*. Only the larger or more common blood vessels are labeled.

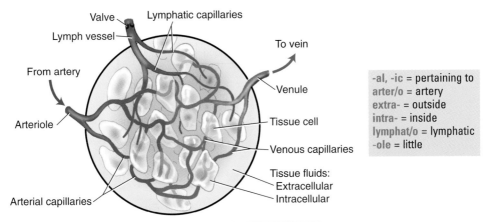

Valve
Lymph vessel
Lymphatic capillaries
From artery
To vein
Venule
Arteriole
Tissue cell
Venous capillaries
Arterial capillaries
Tissue fluids:
Extracellular
Intracellular

-al, -ic = pertaining to
arter/o = artery
extra- = outside
intra- = inside
lymphat/o = lymphatic
-ole = little

Figure 7-2 A capillary bed showing the relationship of blood vessels. Blood that is rich in oxygen is carried by the arteries, which branch many times to become arterioles. Arterioles branch to become capillaries, the site of oxygen and carbon dioxide exchange. Oxygen-poor blood is returned to the heart through the venules, which flow into the veins. The veins carry the blood to the two largest veins, the superior and inferior venae cavae, which empty into the heart. Venae cavae is plural for vena cava.

Blood that is rich in oxygen is pumped by the heart to all parts of the body. It leaves the heart by the **arteries**, which branch many times and become **arterioles**. The arterioles branch even more to become tiny vessels with one-cell-thick walls called **capillaries**.

The capillaries have the important feature of being the site where oxygen and waste carbon dioxide are exchanged. Blood leaving the capillaries returns to the heart through the **venules**, which flow into the **veins** (Figure 7-2). The veins carry blood back to the heart by way of the **venae cavae**. Before it is again pumped to the body cells, blood picks up a fresh supply of oxygen by passing through the lungs.

🏃 **QUICK TIP**
Venae cavae is the plural of vena cava.

WRITE IT!
EXERCISE 2

List the five main types of blood vessels.

1. _____
2. _____
3. _____
4. _____
5. _____

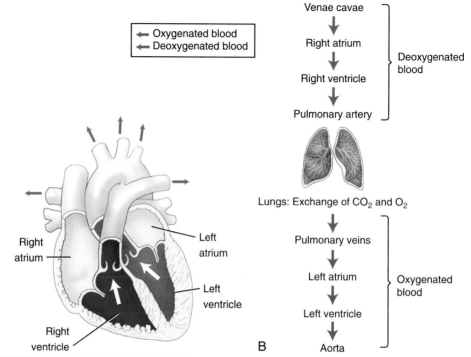

| ← Oxygenated blood |
| ← Deoxygenated blood |

Venae cavae
↓
Right atrium
↓
Right ventricle
↓
Pulmonary artery
⎫ Deoxygenated blood

Lungs: Exchange of CO_2 and O_2
↓
Pulmonary veins
↓
Left atrium
↓
Left ventricle
↓
Aorta
⎫ Oxygenated blood

Right atrium
Left atrium
Left ventricle
Right ventricle

A   B

Figure 7-3 **Circulation of blood through the heart. A,** Anterior cross section showing the heart chambers. Arrows indicate the direction of blood flow from the ventricles. **B,** Schematic representation of deoxygenated or oxygenated status of the blood as it flows through the heart.

Heart

Study Figure 7-3, *A*, and note that the heart has four chambers:
- Right **atrium**
- Left atrium
- Right **ventricle**
- Left ventricle

Deoxygenated blood, which has had much of its oxygen removed, is brought to the right atrium by the body's two largest veins, the venae cavae. The right atrium contracts and forces blood through a valve to the right ventricle. The oxygen-deficient blood is then transported to the lungs, where it absorbs oxygen. This oxygenated blood is transported back to the heart (left atrium then pumped to left ventricle) before it is pumped throughout the body (Figure 7-3, *B*).

In normal heart function, valves close and prevent backflow of blood when the heart contracts. Valves between the **atria** and ventricles are **atrio+ventricul+ar** (AV) valves: the **tricuspid** valve on the right side and the **bicuspid** or **mitral** valve on the left side. **Cuspid** refers to the small flaps that make up the atrioventricular valves (Figure 7-4). The pulmonary (or pulmonic) valve regulates the flow of blood to the lungs and the aortic valve regulates the flow of blood into the **aorta**, the artery by which blood leaves the heart to be routed throughout the body. The pulmonary and aortic valves are called **semilunar** because of their half-moon appearance when the valves are closed.

The **peri+card+ium,** a sac made up of a double membrane, encloses the heart. Notice that one *i* is dropped when cardi/o and -ium are joined (to facilitate pronunciation). The innermost layer of the pericardium is the **visceral** pericardium or **epicardium.**

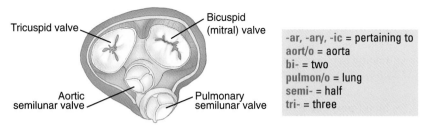

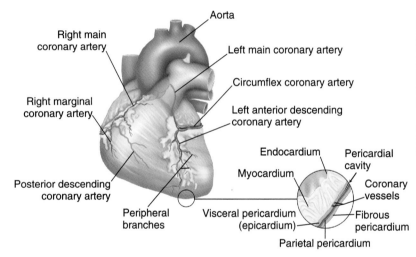

> -ar, -ary, -ic = pertaining to
> aort/o = aorta
> bi- = two
> pulmon/o = lung
> semi- = half
> tri- = three

Figure 7-4 Valves of the heart. Valves between the atria and the ventricles are the tricuspid valve on the right side of the heart and the bicuspid, or mitral, valve on the left side. Cuspid refers to the little flaps of tissue that make up the valve. Mitral indicates the mitered appearance of the bicuspid valve. The pulmonary and aortic valves are called semilunar valves because of the half-moon appearance of the valves.

> cardi/o, coron/o = heart
> endo- = inside
> fibr/o = fiber, fibrous
> my/o = muscle
> peri- = around
> viscer/o = viscera

Figure 7-5 Coronary arteries and heart tissues. The two main coronary arteries are the left coronary artery and right coronary artery. The three layers of the heart, beginning with the innermost layer, are endocardium, myocardium, and epicardium (also called the visceral pericardium).

Another membrane, the **endocardium**, forms the lining inside the heart (Figure 7-5, *inset*). The heart muscle itself is called the **myocardium**. This is the thickest tissue of the heart and is composed of muscle fibers that contract, resulting in the squeezing of blood from the heart with each heartbeat.

> endo- = inside
> my/o = muscle

Blood vessels that supply oxygen to the heart are coronary arteries (**Figure 7-5**). **Coronary** means encircling, in the manner of a crown, and refers to the way in which coronary arteries encircle the heart in a crownlike fashion.

MATCH IT!

EXERCISE 3

Match the types of heart tissue in the left column with their meanings in the right column.

_____ **1.** endocardium   **A.** muscular middle layer of the heart

_____ **2.** myocardium   **B.** lining of the heart

_____ **3.** pericardium   **C.** sac that encloses the heart

Blood Vessels

Five types of blood vessels are shown in Figure 7-2: arteries, smaller arteries called arterioles, veins, smaller veins called venules, and capillaries. The term *vascular* means pertaining to blood vessels in general. **Arterial** and **venous** mean pertaining to the arteries and veins, respectively. **Aortic** means pertaining to the aorta, the largest artery of the body.

Blood pressure is the pressure exerted by the blood on the wall of an artery. Indirect blood pressure readings generally consist of two numbers expressed as a fraction (see Figure 4-3, p. 81). A healthy young person has a blood pressure of approximately 120/80 mm Hg. The first number represents the maximum pressure on the artery. The second number is the amount of pressure that still exists when the heart is relaxed (i.e., not contracting).

Commit the meanings of the combining forms in the following table to memory.

Combining Forms: Blood Vessels

Combining Form	Meaning
angi/o, vas/o,* vascul/o	vessel
aort/o	aorta
arter/o, arteri/o	artery
arteriol/o	arteriole
ather/o	yellow fatty plaque
phleb/o, ven/o	vein
venul/o	venule

Use the electronic flashcards on the Evolve site or make your own set of flashcards using the above list. Select the word parts just presented, and study them until you know their meanings. Do this each time a set of word parts is presented.

*Sometimes means vas deferens.

MATCH IT!
EXERCISE 4

Match the combining forms in the left column with their meanings in the right column (a choice may be used more than once).

____ **1.** angi/o
____ **2.** arteri/o
____ **3.** arteriol/o
____ **4.** ather/o
____ **5.** phleb/o
____ **6.** vas/o
____ **7.** vascul/o
____ **8.** venul/o

A. arteriole
B. artery
C. vessel (in general)
D. vein
E. venule
F. yellow fatty plaque

Diseases, Disorders, and Diagnostic Terms

Heart

cardi/o = heart
my/o = muscle
-pathy = disease
-itis = inflammation

Cardiomyopathy is a general diagnostic term that designates primary disease of the heart muscle itself. An example of a cardiomyopathy is **myocarditis**, inflammation of the heart muscle. Each layer of the heart can become inflamed. **Endocarditis** is often caused by infective microorganisms that invade the endocardium, and the heart valves are frequently affected. Inflammation of the pericardium is **pericarditis**, which can be caused by infectious microorganisms, by a cancerous growth, or by other problems.

Stress tests measure the function of the heart when it is subjected to carefully controlled amounts of physiologic stress, usually using exercise but sometimes specific drugs. In a treadmill stress test, often performed when blockage of coronary arteries is suspected, an **electrocardiogram** and other measurements are taken while the patient walks on a treadmill at varying speeds and inclines. In **electrocardiography** the electrical currents of the heart muscle are recorded by an **electrocardiograph** (see Figure 3-8 p. 66).

electr/o = electrical
cardi/o = heart
-gram = a record

Cardiac catheterization is the passage of a long, flexible tube into the heart chambers through a vein in an arm or leg or the neck. Cardi+ac refers to the heart. An instrument called a **catheter** is used. This allows the collection of blood samples from different parts of the heart and determines pressure differences in various chambers (Figure 7-6). Combined with special **endo+scop+ic** equipment, cardiac catheterization allows internal parts of the heart to be viewed. An endoscopic examination uses an **endoscope**, a device consisting of a tube and an optical system that allows observation of the inside of a hollow organ or cavity.

endo- = inside
scop/o = to view
-ic = pertaining to]

Noninvasive procedures such as electrocardiography do not require entering the body or puncturing the skin and therefore are less hazardous for the patient than invasive procedures. Several noninvasive procedures are available for the diagnosis of heart disease. Conventional x-ray procedures provide information about heart size and gross abnormalities, but newer methods have contributed greatly to information about the heart.

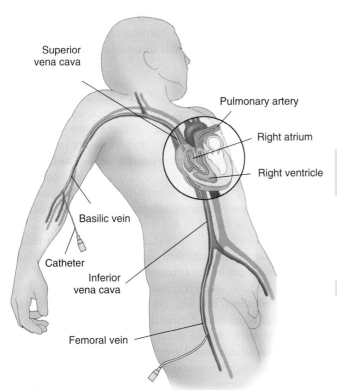

Superior vena cava

Pulmonary artery

Right atrium

Right ventricle

Basilic vein

Catheter

Inferior vena cava

Femoral vein

-ary = pertaining to
femor/o = femur (thigh bone)
pulmon/o = lung

Figure 7-6 Right-sided heart catheterization. The right side of the heart is usually examined first and may be the only side examined because examination of the left side presents more risks to the patient. The catheter is inserted into the femoral vein, a large vein in the thigh, or the basilic vein in the arm. The catheter is then advanced to the right atrium, the right ventricle, and into the pulmonary artery.

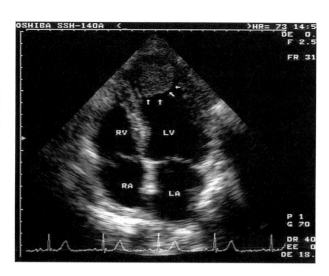

cardi/o = heart
echo- = sound
-gram = a record

Figure 7-7 Echocardiogram. The heart is viewed from the top, and the four chambers are labeled: *RV,* right ventricle; *RA,* right atrium; *LV,* left ventricle; and *LA,* left atrium. A large thrombus, a blood clot, is indicated by the arrows.

echo- = sound
-graphy = process
  of recording

Echocardiography (echo) is the term generally associated with the use of **ultrasonography** in diagnosing heart disease. The **echocardiogram** is a record of the heart obtained by directing ultrasonic waves through the chest wall (Figure 7-7). Cardiac magnetic resonance imaging (MRI) may be performed as well as computed tomography (CT).

Positron emission tomography (PET) is used in other areas of the body but is especially helpful in examining blood flow in the heart and blood vessels. In this procedure the patient is injected with a radioactive element, which becomes concentrated in the heart, and color-coded images are produced. Additional diseases and disorders that affect the heart are described in the following list.

angina pectoris severe chest pain and constriction about the heart caused by an insufficient supply of blood to the heart itself. (Angina is derived from a Latin word that means to choke. Angina is frequently used with other terms and refers to pain of that particular part. Pectoris refers to the chest and is derived from the Latin word *pectora,* meaning chest.)

arrhythmia (a-, without) irregularity or loss of rhythm of the heartbeat. Although this term is often used, **dysrhythmia** is more technically correct.

cardiomegaly (cardi/o, heart + -megaly, enlargement) enlarged size of the heart.

congenital heart defects abnormalities present in the heart at birth (congenital means existing at birth). These defects often involve the septum, a partition that divides the right and left chambers of the heart. Atrial septal defects and **ventricular** septal defects involve abnormal openings between the atria and ventricles, respectively.

congestive heart failure (CHF) condition characterized by weakness, breathlessness, and edema in lower portions of the body; the work demanded of the heart is greater than its ability to perform; also called congestive heart disease or **heart failure.**

coronary artery disease (CAD) abnormal condition that affects the heart's arteries and produces various pathologic effects, especially the reduced flow of blood to the myocardium.

coronary heart disease (CHD) heart damage resulting from insufficient oxygen caused by pathologic changes in the coronary arteries.

fibrillation severe cardiac arrhythmia in which contractions are too rapid and uncoordinated for effective blood circulation. It can sometimes be reversed by the use of a **defibrillator,** an electronic apparatus that delivers a shock to the heart, often through the placement of electrodes on the chest (de- means down, from, or reversing). **Defibrillation** may also be used to slow the heart or restore its normal rhythm.

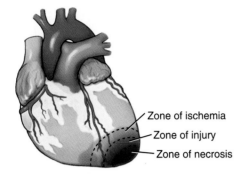

-al = pertaining to
cardi/o = heart
my/o = muscle
necr/o = dead

Zone of ischemia
Zone of injury
Zone of necrosis

Figure 7-8 Myocardial infarction. Also called a heart attack, myocardial infarction (MI) is necrosis of a portion of cardiac muscle. MI is usually caused by an obstruction in a coronary artery.

heart murmur soft blowing or rasping sound that may be heard when listening to the heart with a stethoscope; it is not necessarily pathologic.

hyperlipidemia (hyper-, excessive + -emia, blood) excessive lipids (fats) in the blood. An elevated blood level of one type of lipid, cholesterol, is associated with an increased risk of developing coronary heart disease in most individuals.

hypertension (hyper-, excessive or above normal) elevated blood pressure. Usually, if the first number is consistently above 140 or the second number is consistently above 100, the person is considered to have hypertension.

hypotension (hypo-, below normal) low blood pressure. A blood pressure of 95/60 indicates hypotension, but each person's reading must be interpreted individually.

infarction necrosis of a localized area of tissue caused by lack of blood supply to that area. Necrosis means death of tissue. It can result from **occlusion** (obstruction) or **stenosis** (narrowing) of the artery that supplies blood to that tissue. **Myocardial infarction** (MI) is the death of an area of the heart muscle that occurs as a result of oxygen deprivation; also called acute myocardial infarction (AMI).

myocardial ischemia deficiency of blood supply to the myocardium (Figure 7-8). The word ischemia refers to a temporary deficiency of blood supply to any body part.

septal defect defect in the wall separating the left and right sides of the heart. The defect is usually congenital and is either an atrial septal defect (ASD) or a ventricular septal defect (VSD).

shock serious condition in which blood flow to the heart is reduced to such an extent that body tissues do not receive enough blood. This condition can result in death. Shock may have various causes, including hemorrhage, infection, drug reaction, injury, poisoning, MI, and excessive emotional stress.

MATCH IT! EXERCISE 5

Match the following diseases, disorders, and diagnostic terms pertaining to the heart in the left column with their meanings in the right column.

_____ **1.** angina pectoris
_____ **2.** cardiomegaly
_____ **3.** cardiomyopathy
_____ **4.** congenital heart defect
_____ **5.** congestive heart failure
_____ **6.** fibrillation
_____ **7.** heart murmur
_____ **8.** myocardial infarction
_____ **9.** myocardial ischemia
_____ **10.** hypertension

A. death of an area of the heart muscle
B. abnormality present in the heart at birth
C. soft blowing or rasping heart sound
D. contractions that are too rapid and uncoordinated for effective blood circulation
E. elevated blood pressure
F. severe chest pain caused by insufficient blood supply
G. condition characterized by weakness, shortness of breath, and edema of the lower portions of the body
H. deficiency of blood supply to the heart
I. general designation for primary myocardial disease
J. enlarged heart

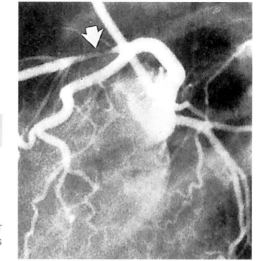

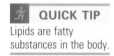

arteri/o = artery
-gram = a record

Figure 7-9 Arteriogram. Radiographic image after injection of a radiopaque contrast medium reveals blockage of an artery *(arrow)*.

Blood Vessels

Vasodilation is an increase in the diameter of a blood vessel. **Vasoconstriction** has the opposite meaning of vasodilation. The dilation and constriction of blood vessels influence blood pressure as well as distribution of blood to various parts of the body. You already know that hypertension means elevated blood pressure. The most common type has no single identifiable cause, but risk for the disorder is increased by obesity, a high blood level of cholesterol, and a family history of high blood pressure. Both **cholesterol** and **triglycerides** are **lipids**. High levels of these two lipids are associated with greater risk of hardening of the arteries. Laboratory tests for cardiovascular disorders include testing for lipids and cardiac enzymes in the blood.

Angi+omas are tumors consisting principally of blood vessels (**hemangioma**) or lymph vessels (**lymphangioma**). Such tumors are usually benign (not malignant).

Aorto+graphy is radiography of the aorta after the injection of a contrast medium to enhance the image of the aorta on an x-ray image. The record produced from this procedure is an **aortogram**.

Arterio+graphy is radiography of arteries after injection of radiopaque material into the bloodstream. The image produced is an **arteriogram** (Figure 7-9). **Angio+cardio+graphy** is radiography of the heart and great vessels after intravenous injection of a radiopaque solution. **Angiography** is a general term for radiography of vessels.

QUICK TIP

Lipids are fatty substances in the body.

---

angi/o = vessel
-oma = tumor
hem/a or hem/o = blood

PROGRAMMED LEARNING

Remember to cover the answers (left column) with folded paper or the bookmark. Write an answer in each blank, and then check your answer before proceeding to the next frame.

arteriopathy	**1.** Remembering that -pathy means disease, write a word that means any disease of the arteries: _____.
artery	**2.** **Arter+itis** is inflammation of an _____. (Notice that one *i* is omitted to make pronunciation easier.)

arteries	3. **Arterio+scler+osis** is hardening of the _____.
	4. Arteriosclerosis is a thickening and loss of elasticity of the walls of the arteries. This is a major cause of hypertension. **Athero+sclerosis**, a form of arteriosclerosis, is characterized by the formation of fatty, cholesterol-like
arteries	deposits on the walls of the _____. Ather/o means yellow fatty plaque. Atherosclerosis is a common cause of coronary artery disease.
	5. Arteries carry blood away from the heart. The aorta, the largest artery in the body, is approximately 3 cm in diameter at its origin in the left side of the heart. The aorta has many branches, and early divisions of this vessel supply the heart, head, and upper part of the body. The combining form for aorta is
aort/o	_____.
aortitis	6. Write a word that means inflammation of the aorta: _____.
	7. An **aneurysm** is a ballooning out of the wall of a vessel, usually an artery, caused by a congenital defect or weakness of the wall of the vessel. See Figure 7-10 for common sites of arterial aneurysms. Aortic aneurysms can affect any
aorta	part of which vessel? _____. A potentially dangerous effect of an aneurysm is rupture of the vessel and resulting **hemorrhage** (loss of a large amount of blood in a short time). An aortic aneurysm can be repaired by surgery.

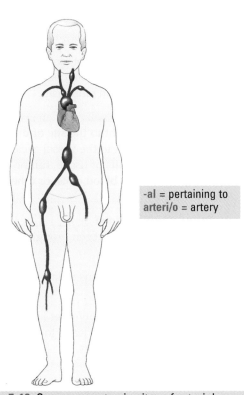

-al = pertaining to
arteri/o = artery

Figure 7-10 Common anatomic sites of arterial aneurysms.

A Hemorrhagic
stroke

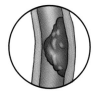
B Thrombotic
stroke

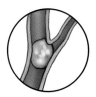
C Embolic (embolitic)
stroke

Figure 7-11 Types of stroke. A, Hemorrhagic stroke. Blood vessel bursts and allows blood to seep into brain tissue until clotting stops the seepage. **B,** Thrombotic stroke. Plaque can cause a clot to form that blocks blood flow. **C,** Embolic stroke. A blood clot or other embolus reaches an artery in the brain, lodges there, and blocks the flow of blood.

vessel	**8.** A cerebral aneurysm is a ballooning out of a blood _____ in the brain. **Cerebr+al** (cerebr/o + -al, pertaining to) refers to the cerebrum or brain. Cerebral aneurysms pose a danger of rupture and hemorrhage within the skull.
vessels	**9.** An aneurysm may rupture to produce a hemorrhagic cerebrovascular accident. In a **cerebro+vascular** accident (CVA, stroke, or stroke syndrome), blood _____ in the brain have become diseased or damaged. CVAs may also be caused by blockage of a cerebral artery by either a thrombus or an embolus (Figure 7-11).
thrombus	**10.** A **thrombus** is an internal blood clot, and a cerebral thrombus can cause a thrombotic stroke. **Thrombotic** means pertaining to a _____. Another cause of blockage is an embolism.
thrombotic	**11.** An **embolism** is the sudden blocking of an artery or lymph vessel by foreign material that has been brought to the site of blockage by the circulating blood. The foreign material brought to the vessel is called an **embolus**. Emboli (plural of embolus) can be bits of tissue, tumor cells, globules of fat, air bubbles, clumps of bacteria, blood clots, or other material. If the embolus is a blood clot, it is called a _____ embolus.
clot	**12.** A thrombotic embolus is a blood _____ that has broken loose from its place of origin and has been brought to an artery or lymph vessel by the circulating blood.
arteritis	**13.** Use -itis to write a term that means inflammation of an artery: _____.
many	**14.** **Poly+arter+itis** is a disease that involves inflammation of _____ arteries. It leads to diminished flow of blood to areas normally supplied by these arteries.

polyarteritis

15. A disease that involves inflammation of several arteries is called

_____ .

artery (arteries)

16. Arteries are used to measure the pulse rate. The **pulse** is the periodic thrust felt over the arteries; it is consistent with the heartbeat. The pulse, the rhythmic expansion of the _____, can be felt with a finger (see Figure 4-1, p. 80).

17. The normal pulse rate of an adult in a resting state is approximately 70 to 80 beats per minute. An increased pulse rate is called **tachy+cardia** (tachy-, fast + cardi/o + -ia). Use brady- to form a word that means decreased pulse

bradycardia

rate: _____ .

arterioles

18. You read earlier that arteries branch out to form what type of vessels?

_____

19. Arterioles carry blood to the smallest blood vessels, the

capillaries

_____, where exchange of oxygen and carbon dioxide occurs.

venules

20. Small vessels that collect blood from the capillaries are _____ .

21. Veins carry blood back to the heart. Write the two combining forms that mean

phleb/o

vein: ven/o and _____ .

22. Use phleb/o to write a word that means inflammation of a vein:

_____ .

phlebitis

vein

23. **Thrombo+phleb+itis** is inflammation of a _____ associated with a blood clot. Thromb/o is a combining form for thrombus, or blood clot. You should know that some specialists differentiate between the type of blood clot that occurs to prevent hemorrhage and a thrombus, a blood clot that occurs internally. Thus, it is preferable to refer to the latter as a thrombus.

vein

24. Venous **thromb+osis** is a blood clot in a _____ . This can be caused by an injury to the leg or by prolonged bed confinement, or it can be a complication of phlebitis.

25. Remember that coronary arteries supply blood to the heart. Formation of a blood clot in a coronary artery, which then leads to occlusion of the vessel, is

coronary

called _____ thrombosis. This is a common cause of myocardial infarction.

26. **Varicose** veins are swollen and knotted veins that occur most often in the legs. Sluggish blood flow, weakened walls, and incompetent valves contribute to varicose veins (Figure 7-12). A varicose vein is also called a **varicosity**.

varicose

Swollen and knotted veins are called _____ veins. **Hemorrhoids** are masses of dilated varicose veins in the **anal** canal. Hemorrhoids are often accompanied by pain, itching, and bleeding.

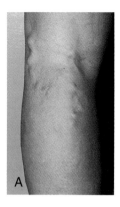

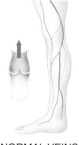
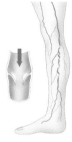

NORMAL VEINS
Functional valves aid
in flow of venous blood
back to heart

VARICOSE VEINS
Failure of valves and
pooling of blood in
superficial veins

Figure 7-12 Varicose veins. A, The appearance of superficial varicose veins in the legs, a common location. **B,** Comparison of normal veins and varicose veins. Note the large and twisted veins.

A

B

BUILD IT!
EXERCISE 6

Combine the word parts to write terms for these descriptions.

1. hardening of the arteries (arteri/o + -sclerosis)   _____

2. inflammation of the aorta (aort/o + -itis)   _____

3. pertaining to vessels of the brain (cerebr/o + vascul/o + -ar)   _____

4. inflammation of a vein associated with a blood clot
   (thromb/o + phleb/o + -itis)   _____

5. inflammation of many arteries (poly- + arter/o + -itis)   _____

MATCH IT!
EXERCISE 7

Match the definition in the left column with the appropriate term in the right column (not all selections will be used).

_____ **1.** ballooning out of the wall of a vessel

_____ **2.** condition of a blood clot in a vessel or the heart cavity

_____ **3.** increased blood pressure

_____ **4.** increased pulse rate

A. aneurysm
B. bradycardia
C. hypertension
D. hypotension
E. tachycardia
F. thrombosis

Surgical and Therapeutic Interventions

Heart

The treatment of heart disease has seen major advances, including heart transplantation, the replacement of a diseased heart with a donor organ. Open heart surgery refers to operative procedures on the heart after it has been exposed through incision of the chest wall. Atrial or ventricular septal defects usually require surgical closure of the abnormal opening.

cardi/o = heart
pulmon/o = lungs
-ary = pertaining to

Cardiopulmonary bypass is the method used to divert blood away from the heart and lungs temporarily when surgery of the heart and major vessels is performed. A heart-lung pump collects the blood, replenishes it with oxygen, and returns it to the body (Figure 7-13). **Cardiopulmonary** means pertaining to the heart and lungs.

The heart has a natural pacemaker called the **sinoatrial** (SA) node. The use of the term *pacemaker* in reference to the heart often implies an artificial cardiac pacemaker, a small battery-powered device generally used to increase the heart rate by electrically

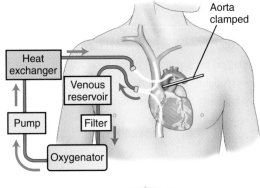

Aorta clamped

-ary, -ous = pertaining to
cardi/o = heart
pulmon/o = lungs
ven/o = vein

Figure 7-13 Cardiopulmonary bypass. Components of a cardiopulmonary bypass system used during heart surgery.

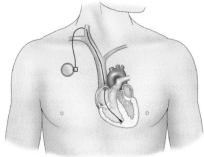

cardi/o = heart

Figure 7-14 Artificial cardiac pacemaker.

stimulating the heart muscle. Depending on the patient's need, a cardiac pacemaker may be permanent or temporary and may fire only on demand or at a constant rate (Figure 7-14). **Cardio+version**, restoring the heart's normal rhythm using electrical shock, may be used when drug therapy is ineffective in treating a cardiac dysrhythmia.

Cardiopulmonary resuscitation (CPR) is recommended as an emergency first-aid procedure to reestablish heart and lung action if breathing or heart action has stopped. It consists of closed heart massage and artificial respiration (mouth-to-mouth breathing or a mechanical means). CPR provides basic life support until it is no longer needed or until more advanced life support equipment is available.

Antiarrhythmic drugs are used to prevent, alleviate, or correct an abnormal heart rhythm. **Digoxin** is a well-known drug that is prescribed in the treatment of congestive heart failure and certain arrhythmias. Beta blockers are often given after a myocardial infarction to allow the heart to work less. The pain of angina pectoris is often relieved by rest and vasodilation of the coronary arteries with **nitroglycerin,** a coronary vasodilator.

WRITE IT! **EXERCISE 8**

Write the correct term in the blanks to complete each sentence.

1. Drugs used to correct abnormal heart rhythms are _____ drugs.

2. Operative procedures on the heart after incision of the chest wall are called

_____ heart surgeries.

3. A word that refers to the lungs and heart is _____.

4. Medications that are given after a myocardial infarction to allow the heart to work less are

_____ blockers.

5. An electrical device that can keep the heart rhythm within a desirable range is a cardiac

_____.

Match the medical terms in the left column with their meanings in the right column.

_____ **1.** cardioversion

_____ **2.** cardiopulmonary bypass

_____ **3.** cardiopulmonary resuscitation

_____ **4.** digoxin

_____ **5.** nitroglycerin

A. vasodilator often used in angina pectoris

B. drug often used in CHD and certain arrhythmias

C. method used to divert blood away from the heart and lungs during heart surgery

D. emergency first-aid procedure used to reestablish heart and lung action

E. restoring the heart's normal rhythm using electrical shock

Blood Vessels

Nonsurgical Vascular Treatments. In some cases, blood flow through vessels can be increased by using methods that do not require surgery. A blood clot is sometimes treated with a **thrombolytic** agent administered through a catheter to dissolve the clot. An oral anticoagulant, warfarin (Coumadin) or **heparin**, is prescribed in the treatment and prevention of a variety of **thrombo+embol+ic** disorders.

Vasodilators are medications that cause dilation of blood vessels. Calcium channel blockers are drugs that help diminish muscle spasms, particularly those of the coronary artery.

Antihypertensives are agents that are used to reduce high blood pressure. **Diuretics** are also used and act to reduce the blood volume through greater excretion of water by the kidneys.

Antilipidemic drugs are prescribed to lower cholesterol levels in the blood, which is generally considered to coincide with a lower incidence of coronary heart disease.

Surgical Treatments of Vascular Problems. **Angioplasty** is surgical repair of blood vessels that have become damaged by disease or injury. Balloon angioplasty uses a balloon catheter that is inflated inside an artery to flatten the plaque against the arterial wall; a stent is sometimes inserted. This procedure may be necessary in coronary artery disease (Figure 7-15). If blockage is too severe, a coronary artery bypass graft (CABG) using venous or arterial grafts may be necessary (Figure 7-16).

Other per+cutane+ous procedures to remove blockage include laser or a specially designed catheter for cutting away plaque from the lining of an artery (**atherectomy**). If a thrombus has formed, it is sometimes treated with a thrombolytic agent to dissolve the clot (**intravascular thrombolysis**, with the thrombolytic agent delivered through a catheter).

Cardiopulmonary bypass is generally required to perform **aorto+plasty**; however, the aorta can sometimes be repaired percutaneously. In the latter case, the physician threads a catheter mounted with a compressed replacement valve on a tiny balloon through an incision in a vein in the groin.

Surgical excision of a vein, or a segment of vein, is called **phleb+ectomy**. A **hemorrhoid+ectomy** is surgical excision of a hemorrhoid.

thromb/o = clot
-lytic = capable of destroying
embol/o = embolus
-ic = pertaining to

anti- = against
-emic = pertaining to blood

per- = through
cutane/o = skin
-ous = pertaining to

ather/o = yellow, fatty plaque
-ectomy = excision

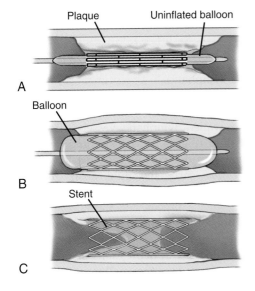

Plaque   Uninflated balloon

A

Balloon

B

Stent

C

angi/o = vessel
-plasty = surgical repair

Figure 7-15 Balloon angioplasty and placement of a coronary artery stent. A small, balloon-tipped catheter is threaded into a coronary artery and inflated to compress the plaque. A *stent,* an expandable meshlike structure, is placed over the angioplasty site to keep the coronary artery open. **A,** The stent and uninflated balloon catheter are positioned in the artery. **B,** The stent expands as the balloon is inflated. **C,** The balloon is then deflated and removed, leaving the implanted stent.

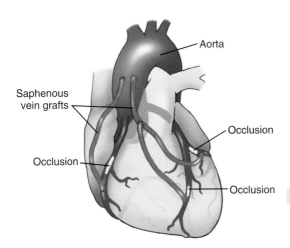

Aorta

Saphenous
vein grafts

Occlusion

Occlusion

Occlusion

Figure 7-16 Coronary artery bypass graft. Sections of blood vessels (such as the saphenous veins from the patient's leg) are grafted onto the coronary arteries to bypass the blocked coronary arteries.

WRITE IT! **EXERCISE 10**

Write a term in each blank to complete these sentences.

1. The initials of the surgery that uses venous or arterial grafts to bypass blocked coronary arteries are

_____.

2. A term for surgical repair of the aorta is _____.

3. Flattening plaque against the arterial wall with a balloon catheter is called balloon

_____.

4. Surgical excision of a vein or a segment of vein is called _____.

5. Agents used to reduce high blood pressure are called _____.

6. Agents used to lower cholesterol levels in the blood are called _____.

Lymphatic System

Structures of the Lymphatic System

The lymphatic system is also called "the lymphatics." The primary function of the lymphatic system is to collect fluid that escapes from the blood capillaries and return it to the circulation. As blood circulates, some of the fluid leaves the capillaries to bathe the tissue cells. Thin-walled lymphatic vessels, distributed throughout the body, collect the escaped fluid (Figure 7-17). This fluid, lymph, is transported by the lymphatic vessels. The system depends on muscular contraction because there is no pump, just valves that carry the fluid away from the tissue.

QUICK TIP

Lymph/o refers to either the lymphatics or the fluid *lymph*.

The lymph vessels, lymph nodes, lymph, tonsils, **thymus**, and **spleen** compose the lymphatic system (see Figure 7-17). Small knots of tissue found at intervals along the course of the lymphatic vessels are called the *lymph nodes.*

The **tonsils** are masses of lymphatic tissue located in depressions of the mucous membranes of the pharynx. We usually think of tonsils as the small masses located at the back of the throat, but these are just one type of tonsil, the **palatine tonsils**. The combining form tonsill/o generally refers to the palatine tonsil. **Pharyngeal** tonsils are commonly called **adenoids**. When the component parts of the term *adenoid* are analyzed, they are seen to mean "resembling a gland." For this reason, pharyngeal tonsil is a more appropriate name for these masses of tissue.

aden/o = gland
-oid = resembling

Commit the following combining forms and meanings to memory.

Additional Word Parts and Their Meanings

Word Part	Meaning	Word Part	Meaning
adenoid/o	adenoids	lymphat/o	lymphatics
cervic/o	neck (or the uterine cervix)	splen/o	spleen
home/o	sameness	thromb/o	thrombus, blood clot

Diseases, Disorders, and Diagnostic Terms

The lymphatic system frequently becomes involved in metastasis, the spread of cancer cells from their origin to other parts of the body. When cancer cells enter a lymphatic vessel, the cells may be trapped by the lymph nodes and begin growing there, or the cells may be carried to sites far from their origin. Lymphatic carcinoma is cancer that has spread to the lymphatics from another site. **Lymph+oma** is a general term for cancer that originates in the lymphatic system.

lymph/o = lymphatic
-oma = tumor

Lymph+ang+itis is an acute or chronic inflammation of lymphatic vessels and can be caused by various microorganisms (Figure 7-18). **Lymphangiography** is radiography of

angi/o = vessel
-itis = inflammation

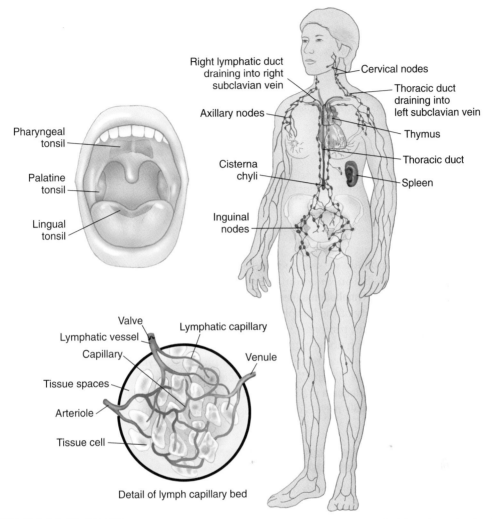

Figure 7-17 **Lymphatic system.** Only a few of the lymph nodes are shown: cervical lymph nodes in the neck, axillary lymph nodes in the armpit, and inguinal lymph nodes in the groin. The close relationship to the cardiovascular system is shown in the detailed drawing. Lymph capillaries merge to form lymphatic vessels that join other vessels to become trunks that drain large regions of the body. The right lymphatic duct receives fluid from the upper right quadrant of the body and empties into the right subclavian vein. The thoracic duct, which begins with the cisterna chyli, collects fluid from the rest of the body and empties it into the left subclavian vein. Also shown are the lymphatic organs: tonsils, thymus, and spleen.

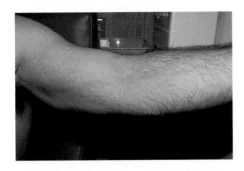

angi/o = vessel
dist/o = distant
-itis = inflammation
lymph/o = lymph or lymphatics

Figure 7-18 **Streptococcal lymphangitis.** This type of inflammatory condition of the lymph nodes is caused by streptococcal bacteria. Examination of the area distal to the affected node usually reveals the source of the infection.

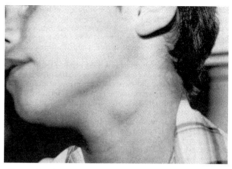

aden/o = gland
-al = pertaining to
cervic/o = neck
-itis = inflammation
lymph/o = lymph or lymphatics

Figure 7-19 Lymphadenitis. The cervical lymph node is enlarged, firm, painless, and freely movable. The node may resolve without treatment or may eventually rupture and drain.

lymph/o =
    lymphatics
-edema = swelling

-oma = swelling

splen/o = spleen
-megaly =
    enlargement

the lymphatic vessels and nodes after injection of a radiopaque substance has made them visible on x-ray film. Accumulation of lymph in tissue and the resultant swelling are called **lymphedema** (see Figure 2-11, p. 33). **Lymphangiograms** are useful for checking the integrity of the lymphatic system in lymphedema and for investigating the spread of malignant tumors.

The lymph nodes were once considered to be glands, so the word part aden/o often appears in terms related to the lymph nodes. **Lymphadenitis** is inflammation of the lymph nodes (Figure 7-19), **lymphadenopathy** refers to any disease of the lymph nodes, and **lymphadenoma** is a tumor of a lymph node. **Tonsillitis** is inflammation of the tonsils. **Spleno+megaly** means enlarged spleen and has many causes.

Surgical and Therapeutic Interventions

Infected lymph nodes or lymph vessels often respond to antibiotic therapy or resolve on their own.

Lymph nodes are frequently biopsied to determine if cancer has spread from an internal organ. **Lymph+aden+ectomy** is excision of a lymph node. Treatment of lymphoma is determined by the type of lymphoma and can include intensive radiotherapy, chemotherapy, and biologic therapies, including interferon.

A ruptured spleen often requires a **splenectomy**. Excision of the tonsils is a **tonsillectomy**. An **adenoidectomy** is performed because the adenoids are enlarged, chronically infected, or causing obstruction. Adenoids are sometimes removed at the same time as a tonsillectomy; this combined procedure is abbreviated T&A.

MATCH IT!

MATCH IT!

EXERCISE 11

Match the meanings in the left column with the medical terms in the right column (not all selections will be used).

_____ **1.** swelling caused by obstruction of a lymphatic tissue

_____ **2.** general term for cancer originating in the lymphatic system

_____ **3.** inflammation of the lymphatic vessels

_____ **4.** record produced by x-ray examination of the lymphatic vessels and nodes

_____ **5.** any disease of the lymph nodes

A. lymphadenitis
B. lymphadenoma
C. lymphadenopathy
D. lymphangiogram
E. lymphangiography
F. lymphangitis
G. lymphedema
H. lymphoma

ⓘ Be Careful with These!

arter/o and *arteri/o* (artery) versus *arteriol/o* (arteriole) versus *ather/o* (yellow fatty plaque)

ven/o (vein) versus *venul/o* (venule)

echocardiography (process using ultrasound to visualize the heart) versus *electrocardiography* (process of recording electrical impulses of the heart)

congenital heart disease (condition present from birth) versus *congestive heart failure* (condition resulting from the heart's inability to meet the body's demand)

SELF-TEST   Work the following exercises to test your understanding of the material in Chapter 7. Complete all the exercises before using Appendix VIII to check your answers.

A. LABEL IT! *Using this illustration of a capillary bed, write combining forms for the structures that are indicated. (Line 1 is done as an example.) Write two combining forms for line 2 (artery) and line 4 (vein), as indicated on the drawing.*

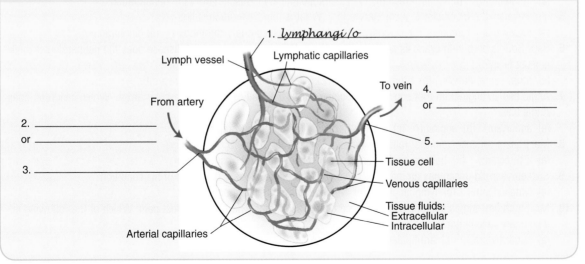

1. *lymphangi/o*

Lymph vessel

Lymphatic capillaries

From artery

To vein   4. _____
or _____

2. _____
or _____

5. _____

3. _____

Tissue cell

Venous capillaries

Tissue fluids:
Extracellular
Intracellular

Arterial capillaries

Continued

SELF-TEST   (cont'd)

B. WRITE IT!   *Write words in the blanks to complete the sentences.*

Oxygen-rich blood is pumped from the heart into the **(1)** _____ and is routed to arteries, which branch to become **(2)** _____, which branch to become capillaries. The capillaries are the site of **(3)** _____ and carbon dioxide exchange. Blood leaving the capillaries returns to the heart through the venules, which flow into the **(4)** _____. Blood returns to the heart by way of the superior and inferior venae cavae. The chamber of the heart that receives the oxygen-poor blood is the right **(5)** _____. Blood is reoxygenated by the lungs. A primary function of the **(6)** _____ system is to collect fluid that escapes from the blood capillaries and return it to the circulation.

Arteries that provide oxygen and nutrients to the heart itself are called **(7)** _____ arteries. The three layers of the heart, beginning with the innermost layer, are **(8)** _____, **(9)** _____, and **(10)** _____ (also called the visceral pericardium).

C. CIRCLE IT!   *Circle one correct response (a, b, c, or d) in each of the following multiple-choice questions.*

1. Charlie is told that he has a form of arteriosclerosis in which yellowish plaque has accumulated on the walls of the arteries. What is the name of this form of arteriosclerosis?
   (a) aortostenosis   (b) atherosclerosis   (c) cardiomyopathy   (d) coarctation
2. Which of these surgeries can be used to correct coronary occlusion?
   (a) cardioversion   (b) coronary artery bypass   (c) defibrillation   (d) lymphadenectomy
3. Kristen, a 28-year-old woman, is told she has inflammation of the lining of the heart. What is the medical term for this heart pathology?
   (a) coronary heart disease   (b) endocarditis   (c) myocarditis   (d) pericarditis
4. Jayne had ventricular fibrillation during coronary angiography. What procedure did the physician use to stop fibrillation?
   (a) atherectomy   (b) endarterectomy   (c) cardiopulmonary resuscitation   (d) defibrillation
5. Jim developed a blood clot in a coronary artery. What is Jim's condition called?
   (a) myocardial infarction   (b) coronary artery bypass   (c) coronary thrombosis   (d) fibrillation
6. Baby Seth is born with cyanosis and a heart murmur. Which congenital heart disease does the neonatologist think is most likely?
   (a) atrial septal defect   (b) atrioventricular block   (c) megalocardia   (d) pericarditis
7. Angie has an angiogram that shows a ballooning out of the wall of a cerebrovascular artery. Which condition does Angie have?
   (a) aneurysm   (b) angioma   (c) arteriosclerosis   (d) coronary thrombosis
8. Mary has a varicose vein that must be excised. What is the name of the surgery?
   (a) arterectomy   (b) balloon angioplasty   (c) phlebectomy   (d) resuscitation
9. Sixteen-year-old Jason has an inflamed cervical lymph node. What is the name of his condition?
   (a) lymphadenitis   (b) lymphangitis   (c) lymphedema   (d) lymphoma
10. Mr. Smith has angina pectoris and uses a coronary vasodilator when he has chest pain. Which of the following is a coronary vasodilator?
   (a) antiarrhythmic   (b) antilipidemic   (c) heparin   (d) nitroglycerin

SELF-TEST (cont'd)

D. READING HEALTH CARE REPORTS *Read the case study, and define the five underlined terms listed after the report.*

MEDICAL REPORT   Physician's Laboratory

222 Medical Center Drive   **Main City, USA 63017-1000**   **Phone:** (555) 434-0000
                                                                        Fax: (555) 434-0001

Pt: H. I. Wilson (male, age 60)
Sx: Mid-sternal chest pain radiating to both shoulders
Patient history: Unremarkable
Family history: Both parents deceased. Father, myocardial infarction at age 68; mother had mid-life
   hypertension and hyperlipidemia.
Physical exam: BP 160/94; apical heart rate 100 and regular; R 24. Lungs clear to auscultation.
ECG: Normal
Labs: Cardiac enzymes normal; cholesterol 250
Thallium stress test: Showed chest pain with increased cardiac activity; demonstrated need for cardiac
   catheterization.
Cardiac Cath: Coronary angiography showed blockage in three main coronary arteries.
Diagnosis: Hypercholesterolemia; CAD; angina pectoris
Plan: CABG in am

1. myocardial infarction   _____
2. hypertension   _____
3. hyperlipidemia   _____
4. cardiac catheterization   _____
5. angina pectoris   _____

E. WRITE IT *Write a one-word term for each of these meanings.*

1. abnormally low blood pressure   _____
2. agent used to reduce blood pressure   _____
3. an enlarged spleen   _____
4. any disease of the lymph nodes   _____
5. excision of the tonsils   _____
6. increased pulse rate   _____
7. fatty substances such as triglycerides _____
8. radiography of the heart and great vessels _____
9. the lining of the heart   _____
10. the smallest blood vessels   _____

Continued

SELF-TEST (cont'd)

F. SPELL IT *Circle all incorrectly spelled terms and write the correct spellings.*

1. adenoidektomy _____
2. colesterol _____
3. cardiovascular _____
4. defibrillater _____
5. infarktion _____

G. FINDING THE CLUE *Use a clue to write terms for these descriptions. Solve Question 1; each ending letter becomes the clue for the first letter of the next answer.*

1. dissolving of a blood clot _____
2. type of node that is the source of the heartbeat _____
3. inflammation of a lymph node _____
4. narrowing or stricture of a duct or canal _____
5. pertaining to a septum _____
6. a fat _____
7. pertaining to the lower blood pressure reading _____
8. pertaining to the heart _____
9. increased blood level of this increases risk of coronary heart disease _____
10. radiology of the lymph vessels using contrast medium _____

Q&E List

Use the Companion CD or audio CDs to review the terms presented in Chapter 7. Look closely at the spelling of each term as it is pronounced.

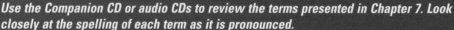

adenoidectomy (**ad˝ə-noid-ek´tə-me**)
adenoids (**ad´ə-noids**)
anal (**a´nəl**)
aneurysm (**an´u-riz˝əm**)
angina pectoris (**an-ji´nə, an´jə-nə pek´tə-ris**)
angiocardiography (**an˝je-o-kahr˝de-og´rə-fe**)
angiography (**an˝je-og´rə-fe**)
angioma (**an˝je-o´mə**)
angioplasty (**an´je-o-plas˝te**)
antiarrhythmic (**an˝te-ə-rith´mik**)
antihypertensive (**an˝te-, an˝ti-hi˝pər-ten´siv**)
antilipidemic (**an˝te-, an˝ti-lip˝ĭ-de´mik**)
aorta (**a-or´tə**)
aortic (**a-or´tik**)
aortitis (**a˝or-ti´tis**)
aortogram (**a-or´to-gram**)

aortography (**a˝or-tog´rə-fe**)
aortoplasty (**a-or´to-plas˝te**)
arrhythmia (**ə-rith´me-ə**)
arterial (**ahr-tēr´e-əl**)
arteriogram (**ahr-tēr´e-o-gram**)
arteriography (**ahr˝tēr-e-og´rə-fe**)
arteriole (**ahr-tēr´ĕ-ōl**)
arteriopathy (**ahr-tēr˝e-op´ə-the**)
arteriosclerosis (**ahr-tēr˝e-o-sklə-ro´sis**)
arteritis (**ahr˝tə-ri´tis**)
artery (**ahr´tə-re**)
atherectomy (**ath˝ər-ek´tə-me**)
atherosclerosis (**ath˝ər-o-sklə-ro´sis**)
atria (**a´tre-ə**)
atrioventricular (**a˝tre-o-ven-trik´u-lər**)
atrium (**a´tre-əm**)

bicuspid (**bi-kus′pid**)

bradycardia (**brad′′e-kahr′de-ə**)

capillaries (**kap′ĭ-lar′′ēs**)

cardiac catheterization (**kahr′de-ak
kath′′ə-tur′′ĭ-za′shən**)

cardiomegaly (**kahr′′de-o-meg′ə-le**)

cardiomyopathy (**kahr′′de-o-mi-op′ə-the**)

cardiopulmonary (**kahr′′de-o-pool′mə-nar-e**)

cardiopulmonary bypass (**kahr′′de-o-pool′mə-nar-e
bi′pas**)

cardiopulmonary resuscitation
(**kahr′′de-o-pool′mə-nar-e re-sus′′ĭ-ta′shən**)

cardiovascular (**kahr′′de-o-vas′ku-lər**)

cardioversion (**kahr′de-o-ver′′zhən**)

catheter (**kath′ə-tər**)

cerebral (**sə-re′brəl, ser′ə-brəl**)

cerebrovascular (**ser′′ə-bro-vas′ku-lər**)

cholesterol (**kə-les′tər-ol′′**)

circulatory (**sur′ku-lə-tor′′e**)

congenital heart defects (**kən-jen′ĭ-təl hahrt de′fekts**)

congestive heart failure (**kən-jes′tiv hahrt fāl′yər**)

coronary (**kor′ə-nar′′e**)

coronary artery disease (**kor′ə-nar′′e ahr′tə-re dĭ-zēz′**)

coronary heart disease (**kor′ə-nar′′e hahrt dĭ-zēz′**)

cuspid (**kus′pid**)

defibrillation (**de-fib′′rĭ-la′shən**)

defibrillator (**de-fib′′rĭ-la′tər**)

digoxin (**dĭ-jok′sin**)

diuretic (**di′′u-ret′ik**)

dysrhythmia (**dis-rith′me-ə**)

echocardiogram (**ek′′o-kahr′de-o-gram′′**)

echocardiography (**ek′′o-kahr′′de-og′rə-fe**)

electrocardiogram (**e-lek′′tro-kahr′de-o-gram′′**)

electrocardiograph (**e-lek′′tro-kahr′de-o-graf′′**)

electrocardiography (**e-lek′′tro-kahr′′de-og′rə-fe**)

embolism (**em′bə-liz-əm**)

embolus (**em′bo-ləs**)

endocarditis (**en′′do-kahr-di′tis**)

endocardium (**en′′do-kahr′de-um**)

endoscope (**en′do-skōp**)

endoscopic (**en′′do-skop′ik**)

epicardium (**ep′′ĭ-kahr′de-um**)

fibrillation (**fĭ-brĭ-la′shən**)

heart failure (**hahrt fāl′yər**)

heart murmur (**hahrt mur′mər**)

hemangioma (**he-man′′je-o′mə**)

hemorrhage (**hem′ə-rəj**)

hemorrhoidectomy (**hem′′ə-roid-ek′tə-me**)

hemorrhoids (**hem′ə-roids**)

heparin (**hep′ə-rin**)

hyperlipidemia (**hi′′pər-lip′′ĭ-de′me-ə**)

hypertension (**hi′′pər-ten′shən**)

hypotension (**hi′′po-ten′shən**)

infarction (**in-fahrk′shən**)

intravascular thrombolysis (**in′′trə-vas′kyəl-ər throm-
bol′ĭ-sis**)

lipid (**lip′id**)

lymph (**limf**)

lymphadenectomy (**lim-fad′′ə-nek′tə-me**)

lymphadenitis (**lim-fad′′ə-ni′tis**)

lymphadenoma (**lim-fad′′ə-no′mə**)

lymphadenopathy (**lim-fad′′ə-nop′ə-the**)

lymphangiogram (**lim-fan′je-o-gram′′**)

lymphangiography (**lim-fan′′je-og′rə-fe**)

lymphangioma (**lim-fan′′je-o′mə**)

lymphangitis (**lim′′fan-ji′tis**)

lymphatic (**lim-fat′ik**)

lymphedema (**lim′′fə-de′mə**)

lymphoma (**lim-fo′mə**)

mitral (**mi′trəl**)

myocardial infarction (**mi′′o kahr′de-əl in-fahrk′shən**)

myocardial ischemia (**mi′′o kahr′de-əl is-ke′me-ə**)

myocarditis (**mi′′o-kahr-di′tis**)

myocardium (**mi′′o-kahr′de-əm**)

nitroglycerin (**ni′′tro-glis′ər-in**)

occlusion (**o-kloo′zhən**)

palatine tonsil (**pal′ə-tin ton′sil**)

pericarditis (**per′′ĭ-kahr-di′tis**)

pericardium (**per′′ĭ-kahr′de-əm**)

pharyngeal (**fə-rin′je-əl**)

phlebectomy (**flə-bek′to-me**)

phlebitis (**flə-bi′tis**)

polyarteritis (**pol′′e-ahr′′tə-ri′tis**)

positron emission tomography (**poz′ĭ-tron e-mish′ən
to-mog′rə-fe**)

pulse (**puls**)

semilunar (**sem′′e-loo′nər**)

septal defect (**sep′təl de′fekt**)

shock (**shok**)

sinoatrial (**si′′no-a′tre-əl**)

continued

spleen **(splēn)**
splenectomy **(sple-nek´tə-me)**
splenomegaly **(sple´´no-meg´ə-le)**
stenosis **(stə-no´sis)**
tachycardia **(tak´´ĭ-kahr´de-ə)**
thromboembolic **(throm´´bo-em-bol´ik)**
thrombolytic **(throm´´bo-lit´ik)**
thrombophlebitis **(throm´´bo-flə-bi´tis)**
thrombosis **(throm-bo´sis)**
thrombotic **(throm-bot´ik)**
thrombus **(throm´bəs)**
thymus **(thi´məs)**
tonsil **(ton´sil)**
tonsillectomy **(ton´´sĭ-lek´tə-me)**
tonsillitis **(ton´´sĭ-li´tis)**

tricuspid **(tri-kus´pid)**
triglyceride **(tri-glis´ər-īd)**
ultrasonography **(ul´´trə-sə-nog´rə-fe)**
varicose **(var´ĭ-kōs)**
varicosity **(var´´ĭ-kos´ĭ-te)**
vasoconstriction **(vas´´o-, va´´zo-kən-strik´shən)**
vasodilation **(vas´´o-, va´´zo-di-la´shən)**
vasodilator **(vas´´o-, va´´zo-di´la-tər)**
vein **(vān)**
vena cava **(ve´nə ka´və)**
venous **(ve´nəs)**
ventricle **(ven´trĭ-kəl)**
ventricular **(ven-trik´u-lər)**
venule **(ven´ūl)**
visceral **(vis´ər-əl)**

 Don't forget the games on the Companion CD and http://evolve.elsevier.com/Leonard/quick/ for additional review, including questions on Spanish medical terms.

Enhancing Spanish Communication

English	Spanish (pronunciation)
artery	arteria **(ar-TAY-re-ah)**
capillary	capilar **(cah-pe-LAR)**
catheter	catéter **(cah-TAY-ter)**
cholesterol	colesterol **(co-les-tay-ROL)**
dizziness	vértigo **(VERR-te-go)**
high blood pressure	hipertensión, presión alta **(e-per-ten-se-ON, pray-se-ON AHL-tah)**
lymphatic	linfático **(lin-FAH-te-co)**
murmur	murmullo **(moor-MOOL-lyo)**
narrow	estrecho **(es-TRAY-cho)**
obstruction	obstrucción **(obs-trooc-se-ON)**
rhythm	ritmo **(REET-mo)**
rib	costilla **(cos-TEEL-lyah)**
same	mismo **(MEES-mo)**
sound	sonido **(so-NEE-do)**
spleen	bazo **(BAH-so)**
tonsil	tonsila **(ton-SEE-lah)**, amígdala **(ah-MEEG-dah-lah)**
varicose veins	venas varicosas **(VAY-nahs vah-re-CO-sas)**

CHAPTER 8

Respiratory System

CONTENTS

Function First
Structures of the Respiratory System
Diseases, Disorders, and Diagnostic Terms
Surgical and Therapeutic Interventions

Self-Test
Q&E List
Enhancing Spanish Communication

OBJECTIVES

After completing Chapter 8, you will be able to:

1. Recognize or write the functions of the respiratory system.
2. Recognize or write the meanings of Chapter 8 word parts and use them to build and analyze terms.
3. Write terms for selected structures of the respiratory system, or match terms with their descriptions.
4. Write the names of the diagnostic terms and pathologies related to the respiratory system when given their descriptions, or match terms with their meanings.
5. Match surgical and therapeutic interventions for the respiratory system, or write the names of the interventions when given their descriptions.
6. Spell terms for the respiratory system correctly.

Function First

Respiration is the combined activity of various processes that supply oxygen to all body cells and remove carbon dioxide. Breathing is external respiration, the absorption of oxygen from the air and the removal of carbon dioxide by the lungs. Breathing is often called pulmonary ventilation or simply ventilation. The **respiratory** system consists of a series of passages that bring outside air in contact with special structures that lie close to blood capillaries. Oxygen and carbon dioxide are exchanged at the interface between these special structures and the capillaries. This exchange of gases is part of homeo+stasis, a state of equilibrium of the internal environment of the body.

Breathing consists of the **inspiration** of air into and the **expiration** of air out of the lungs. Inspiration is also called **inhalation**, and expiration is called **exhalation**.

WORD ORIGIN
ventilare (L.)
to fan

homeostasis =
   even internal
   state

in- = in
spir/o = to breathe
ex- = out

WRITE IT!   **EXERCISE 1**

Write a term for each clue.

1. state of equilibrium of the body's internal environment _____

2. another term for inhalation _____

3. another term for exhalation _____

4. the essential gas supplied by respiration _____

Use Appendix VIII to check your answers to all the exercises in Chapter 8.

Structures of the Respiratory System

The respiratory system consists of the organs involved in the exchange of gases between an organism and the atmosphere. Figure 8-1 shows the major organs of the respiratory system. The conducting passages of this system are known as the upper respiratory tract and the lower respiratory tract. Label the numbered blanks as you read the information that accompanies the drawing.

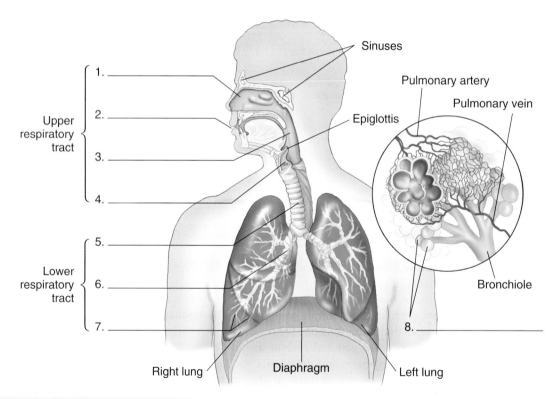

Figure 8-1 The organs of respiration. Air first enters the body through the nose and passes through the nasal cavity *(1)*, or it enters through the mouth and passes through the oral cavity *(2)*. The air reaches the pharynx *(3)* and passes to the larynx *(4)* and the trachea *(5)*. The trachea divides into a left and a right bronchus *(6)*. Each bronchus divides into smaller tubes called bronchioles *(7)*. At the end of each bronchiole are clusters of air sacs called alveoli *(8)*, where oxygen is exchanged for waste carbon dioxide. Normal quiet breathing is accomplished almost entirely by movement of the diaphragm.

The nose, nasal cavity, para+nasal sinuses (air-filled paired cavities in various bones around the nose), pharynx (throat), and larynx (voice box) comprise the upper respiratory tract (URT). The trachea, bronchi, bronchioles, alveoli (air sacs), and lungs belong to the lower respiratory tract (LRT). A lidlike structure, the epiglottis, covers the larynx during swallowing.

para- = beside
nas/o = nose
-al = pertaining to

The **diaphragm** is a muscular wall that separates the abdomen from the **thorac+ic** cavity. The diaphragm contracts and relaxes with each inspiration and expiration. **Phren+ic** means pertaining to the diaphragm, but it sometimes means pertaining to the mind (as in schizophrenic). If the meaning is unclear, use a dictionary to determine it.

thorac/o = chest

phren/o = mind *or* diaphragm
-ic = pertaining to

The chest cavity contains the lungs and many other organs. The right lung has three lobes (rounded parts), and the left lung has two lobes (study the lungs in Figure 8-1). Each lung is surrounded by a membrane called the **pleura**. The walls of the chest cavity are also lined with pleura. The space between the pleura that covers the lungs and the pleura that lines the thoracic cavity is called the **pleural** cavity.

Commit the word parts and their meanings in the table below to memory. After you have studied the list, cover the left column and check to make sure that you know the combining form(s) for each structure before working Exercise 2.

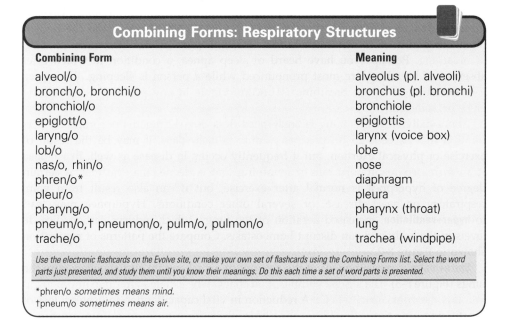

Combining Forms: Respiratory Structures

Combining Form	Meaning
alveol/o	alveolus (pl. alveoli)
bronch/o, bronchi/o	bronchus (pl. bronchi)
bronchiol/o	bronchiole
epiglott/o	epiglottis
laryng/o	larynx (voice box)
lob/o	lobe
nas/o, rhin/o	nose
phren/o*	diaphragm
pleur/o	pleura
pharyng/o	pharynx (throat)
pneum/o,† pneumon/o, pulm/o, pulmon/o	lung
trache/o	trachea (windpipe)

Use the electronic flashcards on the Evolve site, or make your own set of flashcards using the Combining Forms list. Select the word parts just presented, and study them until you know their meanings. Do this each time a set of word parts is presented.

*phren/o *sometimes means mind.*
†pneum/o *sometimes means air.*

Match the word parts in the left column with their meanings in the right column (answers will be used more than once).

_____ **1.** alveol/o		**A.** air sacs of the lungs
_____ **2.** bronch/o		**B.** branch of the trachea
_____ **3.** laryng/o		**C.** diaphragm
_____ **4.** nas/o		**D.** lung
_____ **5.** phren/o		**E.** nose
_____ **6.** pharyng/o		**F.** throat
_____ **7.** pneum/o		**G.** voice box
_____ **8.** pulm/o		**H.** windpipe
_____ **9.** rhin/o		
_____ **10.** trache/o		

Diseases, Disorders, and Diagnostic Terms

pulmon/o = lung
-logist = specialist

A **pulmonologist** is a physician who specializes in the anatomy, physiology, and pathology of the lungs.

eu = normal
dys- = bad
-pnea = breathing
orth/o = straight

Normal respiration in an adult consists of 15 to 20 breaths per minute. **Eu+pnea** means normal respiration. **Dys+pnea** is labored or difficult breathing, and the patient often complains of shortness of breath (SOB). **A+pnea** means temporary absence of breathing. Perhaps you have heard of sleep apnea, a condition in which brief absences of breathing are most pronounced while a person is sleeping. **Ortho+pnea** is a condition in which breathing is uncomfortable in any position except sitting erect or standing.

brady- = slow
tachy- = fast
hyper = more than
    normal

Abnormally slow breathing is **brady+pnea** (less than 12 breaths per minute). Respiration that exceeds 25 breaths per minute is **tachy+pnea**; it may be the result of exercise or physical exertion, but it frequently occurs in disease as well. **Hyper+pnea** is an increased respiratory rate or breathing that is deeper than normal. A certain degree of hyperpnea is normal after exercise, but it can also result from pain, respiratory or heart disease, or several other conditions. Hyperpnea may lead to **hyper+ventilation**, increased aeration of the lungs, which reduces carbon dioxide levels in the body and can disrupt homeostasis. Compare the patterns of respiration shown in Figure 8-2.

spir/o = to breathe
-metry =
    measurement

Spiro+metry is measurement of the amount of air taken into and expelled from the lungs (Figure 8-3). The largest volume of air that can be exhaled after maximum inspiration is the vital capacity (VC). A reduction in vital capacity often indicates a loss of functioning lung tissue. Inability of the lungs to perform their ventilatory function is acute respiratory failure. This leads to **hyp+ox+ia** or to **an+ox+ia**. Both terms mean a deficiency of oxygen, which can be caused by respiratory disorders but can occur under other conditions as well. Hypoxia can result from reduced oxygen concentration in the air at high altitudes or from anemia (decrease in hemoglobin or in number of erythrocytes in the blood, or both).

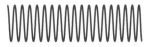

Normal (eupnea)
Regular at a rate
of 12-20 breaths per minute

Bradypnea
Slower than 12 breaths
per minute

Tachypnea
Faster than 20 breaths
per minute

Hyperpnea
Deep breathing, faster than
20 breaths per minute

brady- = slow
eu- = normal
hyper- = greater than normal
-pnea = breathing
tachy- = fast

Figure 8-2 Select patterns of respiration. Pattern of normal respiration compared with respiratory patterns seen in bradypnea, tachypnea, and hyperpnea.

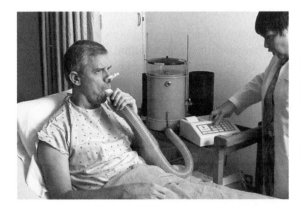

-meter = instrument used to measure
-metry = process of measuring
spir/o = to breathe (sometimes, spiral)

Figure 8-3 Spirometry. A spirometer is used to evaluate the air capacity of the lungs. It measures and records the volume of inhaled and exhaled air.

MATCH IT!

EXERCISE 3

Match the terms in the right column with their meanings in the left column.

_____ **1.** breathing air into the lungs

_____ **2.** breathing out

_____ **3.** labored or difficult breathing

_____ **4.** abnormally slow breathing

_____ **5.** acceleration in the number of breaths per minute

_____ **6.** normal respiration

A. bradypnea

B. dyspnea

C. eupnea

D. expiration

E. inspiration

F. tachypnea

Write the combining forms and their meanings for each of these new terms. A short definition is provided for each term.

Term/Meaning	Combining Form(s)	Meaning
1. **bronchial** pertaining to the bronchi	_____	_____
2. **pharyngeal** pertaining to the pharynx	_____	_____
3. **pneumatic** pertaining to respiration or air*	_____	_____
4. **pneumocardial** pertaining to the lungs and heart	_____	_____
5. **pulmonary, pulmonic** pertaining to the lungs	_____	_____

*Sometimes pertains to rarefied or compressed air, as in pneumatic tires.

PROGRAMMED LEARNING

Remember to cover the answers (left column) with folded paper or the bookmark. Write an answer in each blank, and then check your answer before proceeding to the next frame.

air

1. **Thorax** means chest. **Pneumo+thorax** refers to air or gas in the chest cavity, specifically the pleural cavity. **Hemo+thorax** means blood in the pleural cavity (Figure 8-4). **Pneumo+hemo+thorax** means the presence of _____ and blood in the pleural cavity.

lungs

2. **Pneumon+ia** or **pneumon+itis** means inflammation of the _____. There are many causes of pneumonia, but it is caused primarily by bacteria, viruses, or chemical irritants.

bronchi

3. **Broncho+pneumonia** is inflammation of the lungs and of the _____.

pneumocentesis

4. Use pneum/o to build a word that means surgical puncture of a lung: _____. (Congratulations if you remembered the suffix that means surgical puncture!) This procedure is done to remove fluid from a lung.

lungs

5. **Pulmonary edema** is **effusion** (escape) of fluid into the air spaces and tissue spaces of the _____ (**edema** is abnormal accumulation of fluid in the tissue). Although pulmonary edema can have other causes, a major cause is insufficient cardiac activity. Remember that cardi/o means heart, so cardi+ac refers to the heart.

breathing

6. Dyspnea on exertion is one of the earliest symptoms of pulmonary edema. As the condition becomes more advanced, the patient can become **ortho+pne+ic** (-pnea + -ic is shortened to -pneic), which means that _____ is difficult except when the patient is sitting erect or standing.

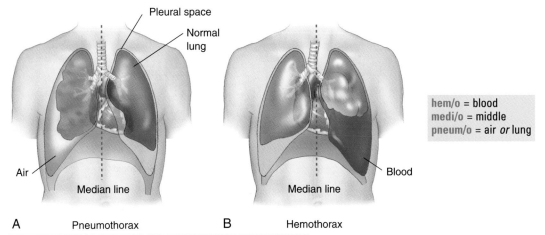

Figure 8-4 **Two abnormal conditions of the chest cavity. A,** Pneumothorax is air or gas in the chest cavity, usually caused by blunt injury or an open wound in the chest wall. A normal left lung is shown for comparison. **B,** Hemothorax, or blood in the pleural cavity, may be associated with pneumothorax and is a common problem associated with chest trauma or penetrating injuries.

hem/o = blood
medi/o = middle
pneum/o = air *or* lung

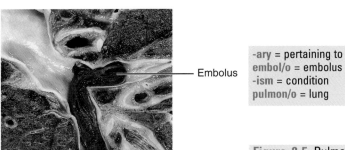

-ary = pertaining to
embol/o = embolus
-ism = condition
pulmon/o = lung

Figure 8-5 **Pulmonary embolism.** This blood clot broke loose and traveled from a lower extremity and is now located in a branch of the pulmonary artery.

pulmonary	7. Pulmonary arteries carry blood from the heart to the lungs so carbon dioxide can be exchanged for oxygen. A pulmonary embolus is an obstruction of the _____ artery or one of its branches.
pulmonary	8. Embolism is the sudden blocking of an artery by foreign material that has been brought to its site of blockage by the circulating blood. An **embolus** is often a blood clot, called a **thrombus**. The pulmonary artery is obstructed in _____ **embolism** (Figure 8-5).
rhin/o	9. Air usually first enters the respiratory passageway through the nose, which refers to the external nose as well as the nasal cavity. The two combining forms that mean nose are nas/o and _____.

nas/o = nose
para- = beside

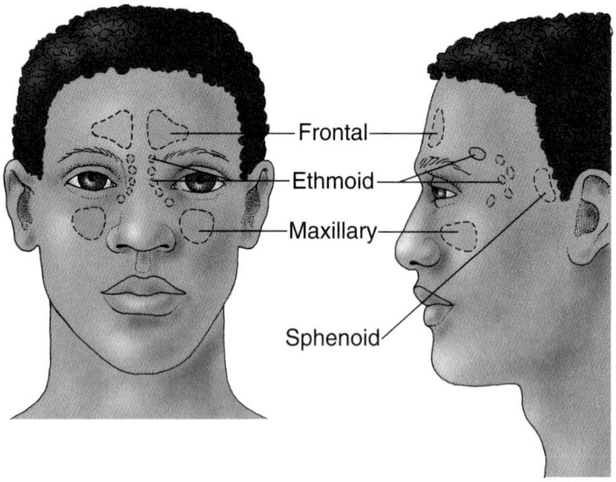

Figure 8-6 Paranasal sinuses. These air-filled, paired cavities in various bones around the nose are lined with mucous membranes. Their openings into the nasal cavity are easily obstructed.

nasal	**10.** The **nares** (singular, naris), or nostrils, are the external openings of the nose. These openings lead into two nasal cavities separated by the **nasal septum.** The partition between the two nasal cavities is the _____ septum.
nose	**11.** The **para+nasal** (para-, near or beside) **sinuses** open into the nasal cavities (Figure 8-6). The term sinus has several meanings, including canal, passage, and cavity within a bone. The paranasal sinuses are cavities within the bones of the face. Fluids from the paranasal sinuses are discharged into the _____.
sinus	**12. Sinus+itis** is inflammation of a _____, especially of a paranasal sinus.
nas/o	**13.** You learned that, in addition to rhin/o, another combining form that means nose is _____.
rhinitis	**14.** Use rhin/o to build a term that means inflammation of the nasal membrane: _____.
nose	**15. Rhino+rrhea** is a watery discharge from the _____.
nose	**16.** Air from the nose passes to the **pharynx,** commonly called the throat. **Naso+pharyng+eal** means pertaining to the _____ and pharynx.
inflammation	**17. Pharyng+itis** is _____ of the pharynx.
pharynx	**18.** The **eustachian tube,** or **auditory tube,** extends from the middle ear to the pharynx. It is sometimes called the **oto+pharyng+eal** tube, meaning a tube that connects the ear with the _____.
larynx	**19.** The lower part of the pharynx is also called the **laryngopharynx** because it is here that the pharynx divides into the **larynx** and the **esophagus.** Air passes to the _____, and food passes to the esophagus.

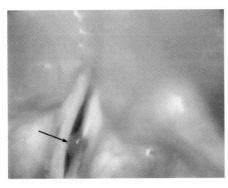

-eal, -ic = pertaining to
hem/o = blood
laryng/o = larynx
-rrhagia = hemorrhage

Figure 8-7 A laryngeal polyp. This hemorrhagic polyp *(arrow)* on the vocal cord occurs most often in adults who smoke, have many allergies, live in dry climates, or abuse their voice.

laryngitis	20. Inflammation of the larynx is _____. This condition can be caused by infectious microorganisms, allergies, irritants, or overuse of the voice.
aphonia	21. Laryngitis can result in absence of voice. In **a+phon+ia,** absence of voice, sounds cannot be produced from the larynx (phon/o means voice). Laryngitis can cause absence of voice, which is called _____.
voice	22. **Dys+phonia** means difficulty in speaking or a weak _____. Dysphonia is the same as hoarseness and may precede aphonia.
speech	23. **A+phasia** is the inability to communicate through speech, writing, or signs. It is caused by improper functioning of the brain. The combining form phas/o means speech. The term aphasia describes only one aspect of the condition, which is the absence of _____.
aphasia	24. An **a+phasic** individual is one affected by _____. Remember that in aphasia the problem does not arise in the larynx, but in the brain.
speech	25. **Dys+phasia** is a speech impairment resulting from a brain lesion. There is a lack of coordination and an inability to arrange words in their proper order. In dysphasia there is difficulty in _____.
aphonia	26. Be sure that you know the difference between aphasia and aphonia. Both can produce an absence of speech sound. Aphasia is caused by a brain dysfunction; however, aphonia is loss of audible voice. In laryngitis, for example, which is more likely to occur, aphasia or aphonia? _____
pain	27. Laryngitis can cause only minor discomfort, or the condition can become painful. **Laryng+algia** is _____ of the larynx.
glottis	28. The larynx is commonly called the voice box. The vocal apparatus of the larynx is the **glottis,** which consists of the vocal cords (or folds) and the openings between them. Muscles open and close the glottis during breathing and also regulate the vocal cords during the production of sound. Examine the structure of the larynx in Figure 8-7. This illustration also shows a **laryngeal polyp,** a small tumor-like growth on the vocal cords that can cause hoarseness. The lidlike structure that covers the larynx during the act of swallowing is called the **epiglottis** (epi-, above). The epiglottis lies above the _____.

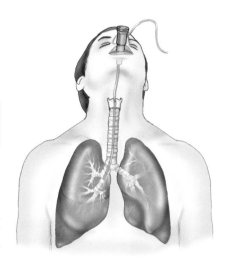

bronch/o = bronchus
-scopy = visual examination
trache/o = trachea

Figure 8-8 Bronchoscopy. Visual examination of the tracheobronchial tree using a bronchoscope. Other uses for this procedure include suctioning, obtaining a biopsy specimen or fluid, or removing foreign bodies.

trachea	29. Air passes from the larynx to the **trachea,** or windpipe. **Trache+al** pertains to the _____.
bronchitis	30. The trachea divides into two **bronchi** (singular, **bronchus**), one leading to each lung. Use bronch/o to write a word that means inflammation of the mucous membrane of the bronchi: _____.
sputum	31. Mucous membranes secrete mucus. Inflammation of the mucous membranes in bronchitis usually leads to the production of **sputum,** which can be expelled by coughing or clearing the throat. Material raised from inflamed mucous membranes of the respiratory tract and expelled by coughing is called _____.
bronchi	32. The _____ are examined in a **broncho+scopic** examination.
bronchi	33. **Tracheo+bronchial** means pertaining to both the trachea and the _____. The appearance of the trachea and bronchi in radiography probably led to the use of the term tracheobronchial tree.
bronchoscopy	34. Add a suffix to bronch/o to write a word that means a bronchoscopic examination using a **bronchoscope:** _____. This procedure may be used for obtaining a biopsy specimen, for suctioning, or for removing foreign bodies (Figure 8-8).
larynx	35. Both **bronchoscopy** and **laryngoscopy** are **endoscopic** examinations, procedures that allow visualization of organs and cavities of the body using an **endoscope.** In a laryngoscopy, the _____ is examined.
lungs	36. **Broncho+pulmon+ary** means pertaining to the bronchi and the _____.

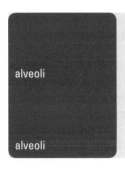

37. **Bronchi+oles** literally means little bronchi. You see that -ole means little. Bronchioles are subdivisions of the bronchi. At the ends of the bronchioles are tiny air sacs called alveoli (singular, **alveolus**). **Alveol+ar** means pertaining to the _____.

alveoli

38. In certain diseases, such as emphysema, destructive changes occur in the alveolar walls. These changes interfere with the exchange of oxygen and carbon dioxide. This gas exchange takes place by diffusion across the walls of blood capillaries and the _____.

alveoli

FINDING THE CLUE!

EXERCISE 5

Use a clue to write terms for these descriptions. Solve Question 1; each ending letter becomes the clue for the first letter of the next answer.

1. growth protruding from a mucous membrane _____
2. pertaining to the pharynx _____
3. pertaining to the larynx _____
4. painful larynx _____
5. loss of voice _____
6. loss of the power of expression of speech _____
7. pertaining to the alveoli _____
8. inflammation of the mucous membranes of the nose _____
9. inflammation of a sinus _____
10. material coughed up from the trachea, bronchi, and lungs _____

Additional diseases and disorders that affect the respiratory system are described in the following glossary list.

adult respiratory distress syndrome (ARDS) disorder characterized by respiratory insufficiency and hypoxemia.

asthma paroxysmal dyspnea accompanied by wheezing; asthma is caused by a spasm of the bronchial tubes or by swelling of their mucous membranes. A **wheeze** is a whistling sound made during respiration. **Paroxysmal** means occurring in sudden, periodic attacks or recurrence of symptoms.

atelectasis (atel/o, imperfect + -ectasis, stretching) incomplete expansion of a lung or a portion of it; airlessness or collapse of a lung that had once been expanded.

bronchiectasis (bronchi/o + -ectasis) chronic dilation of a bronchus or the bronchi accompanied by a secondary infection that usually involves the lower part of the lung.

bronchography (-graphy, recording) radiography of the bronchi after injection of a radiopaque substance. The record of the bronchi and lungs produced by bronchography is a **bronchogram**. This procedure has generally been replaced by computed tomography.

carcinoma of the lung lung cancer, the leading cause of cancer-related death. Research has consistently confirmed that smoking plays a predominant role in the development of lung cancer.

chronic obstructive pulmonary disease (COPD) disease process that decreases the lungs' ability to perform their ventilatory function. This process can result from chronic bronchitis, emphysema, chronic asthma, or chronic **bronchiolitis**. COPD is also called chronic obstructive lung disease (COLD).

emphysema chronic pulmonary disease characterized by an increase in the size of alveoli and by destructive changes in their walls, resulting in difficulty in breathing.

influenza acute, contagious respiratory infection characterized by sudden onset, chills, headache, fever, and muscular discomfort; it is caused by several different types of viruses. The 2009 H1N1 flu virus, like most influenza viruses, spreads mainly from person to person. This disease was originally called "swine flu" because the viral genetic makeup is similar to influenza viruses that normally occur in pigs.

pleuritis (pleur/o, pleura) inflammation of the pleura. It can be caused by infection, injury, or a tumor, or it can be a complication of certain lung diseases. It is characterized by a sharp pain on inspiration; it is also called **pleurisy**.

pneumoconiosis (pneum/o, lung + coni/o, dust) respiratory condition caused by inhalation of dust particles; frequently seen in people involved in occupations such as mining and stonecutting.

pulmonary embolism blockage of a pulmonary artery by foreign matter such as fat, air, tumor tissue, or a blood clot.

severe acute respiratory syndrome (SARS) infectious respiratory disease spread by close contact with an infected person and caused by a coronavirus. It is reported to have a fatality rate of approximately 3%.

silicosis (silic/o, silica) form of pneumoconiosis resulting from inhalation of the dust of stone, sand, quartz, or flint that contains silica. (Workers are frequently exposed to silica powder that is used in manufacturing processes.)

sudden infant death syndrome (SIDS) sudden, unexpected death of an apparently normal and healthy infant that occurs during sleep and with no physical or autopsy evidence of disease.

tuberculosis (TB) infectious disease caused by the bacterium *Mycobacterium tuberculosis*. It is often chronic in nature and usually affects the lungs, although it can occur elsewhere in the body. The disease is named for the **tubercles**—small, round nodules—that are produced in the lungs by the bacteria.

WRITE IT!   EXERCISE 6

Write the correct term in each blank to complete these sentences.

1. Another name for pneumonia is _____.
2. Inflammation of the lungs and the bronchi is _____.
3. A collapsed condition of the lung is called _____.
4. Inability to communicate through speech, writing, or signs because of a brain dysfunction is

   _____.
5. An infectious, sometimes fatal, respiratory disease caused by a coronavirus is called severe acute

   respiratory _____.
6. A chronic disease that is characterized by an increased size and destructive changes to the alveoli is

   _____.
7. A condition characterized by dyspnea and wheezing is _____.
8. A respiratory condition caused by inhalation of dust particles is _____.

Surgical and Therapeutic Interventions

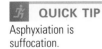 **QUICK TIP**

Asphyxiation is suffocation.

Asphyxiation requires immediate corrective measures to prevent loss of consciousness and, if not corrected, death. Removal of a foreign body in the airway may be needed before oxygen and artificial respiration are administered. One method of dislodging food or other obstructions from the windpipe is the **Heimlich maneuver** (Figure 8-9). In asphixiation, oxygen and artificial ventilation need to be promptly administered to

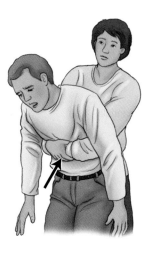

Figure 8-9 Heimlich maneuver. The rescuer grasps the choking person from behind, placing the thumb side of the fist against the victim's abdomen, in the midline, slightly above the navel and well below the breastbone. Abruptly pulling the fist firmly upward will often force the obstruction up the windpipe.

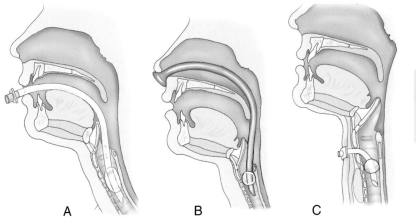

in- = inside
or/o = mouth
nas/o = nose
-stomy = formation of an opening
trache/o = trachea (windpipe)

Figure 8-10 Comparison of endotracheal intubation and a tracheostomy tube. A, Orotracheal intubation for short-term airway management. **B,** Nasotracheal intubation for short-term airway management. **C,** Tracheostomy tube for long-term airway maintenance.

prevent damage to the brain. An emergency **tracheostomy** may be necessary in upper airway obstruction. A tracheostomy requires a **tracheotomy**, an incision of the trachea through the skin and muscles of the neck overlying the trachea (usually performed for insertion of a tube to relieve tracheal obstruction). A tracheostomy is also required when prolonged mechanical ventilation is needed. A **ventilator** is a machine that is used for prolonged artificial ventilation of the lungs.

> trache/o = windpipe
> -stomy = opening
> -tomy = incision

    Endotracheal intubation is the insertion of an airway tube through the mouth or nose into the trachea. It may be used to keep an airway open, prevent aspiration of material from the digestive tract in an unconscious or paralyzed patient, permit suctioning of secretions, or provide ventilation that cannot be accomplished with a mask. **Nasotracheal intubation** and **orotracheal intubation** refer to insertion of a tube into the trachea through the nose or mouth, respectively. Compare these two types of intubation with a tracheostomy tube used for prolonged airway management (Figure 8-10).

> endo- = inside
> nas/o = nose
> or/o = mouth
> trans- = across

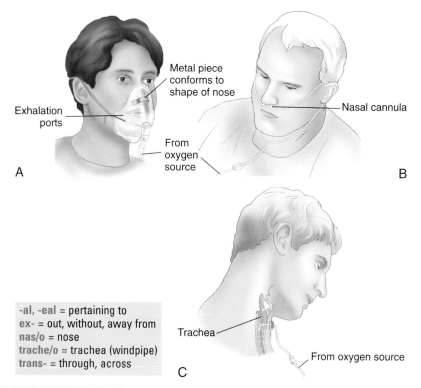

-al, -eal = pertaining to
ex- = out, without, away from
nas/o = nose
trache/o = trachea (windpipe)
trans- = through, across

Figure 8-11 Administration of oxygen. A, Simple oxygen mask is used for short-term oxygen therapy or in an emergency. **B,** Nasal cannula delivers oxygen by way of two small tubes that are inserted into the nostrils and is frequently used for long-term oxygen maintenance. **C,** Transtracheal oxygen is a more efficient long-term method of delivering oxygen and is an alternative to the nasal cannula.

In COPD or other problems in hypoxic patients, oxygen therapy may be prescribed by the physician. Oxygen is also administered during general surgery. In patients who can breathe, oxygen is often delivered through tubing using a simple face mask or nasal prongs. **Transtracheal** oxygen is more efficient and is sometimes preferred to the administration of oxygen through a mask or **nasal cannula**. Compare the three types of oxygen administration (Figure 8-11).

Several medications are used in respiratory disorders. Respiratory infections are often treated with antibiotics.

de- = reversing

- **Decongestants:** eliminate or reduce swelling or congestion
- **Anti+tussives:** prevent or relieve coughing
- **Anti+histamines:** used to treat colds and allergies
- **Broncho+dilators:** agents that cause dilation of the bronchi; used in respiratory conditions such as asthma
- **Muco+lytics:** destroy or dissolve mucus; help open the breathing passages

Seasonal influenza vaccine is recommended each year for most individuals, except in those who are allergic to eggs. A vaccine that protects against the most common cause of bacterial pneumonia is recommended for older persons, those with a chronic lung disease, or those who are immunodeficient.

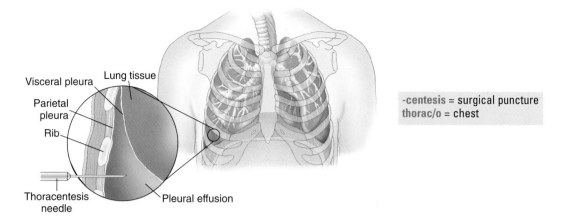

Visceral pleura
Lung tissue
Parietal pleura
Rib
Thoracentesis needle
Pleural effusion

-centesis = surgical puncture
thorac/o = chest

Figure 8-12 Insertion of the needle in thoracentesis. The insertion site depends on the location of the fluid. The term thoracocentesis is frequently shortened to thoracentesis.

Read about the following surgical procedures.

lung biopsy   removal of small pieces of lung tissue for the purpose of diagnosis. In an open lung biopsy, a segment of the lung is removed through an incision in the chest. In a **percutaneous** (per-, through + cutane/o, skin) **biopsy**, tissue is obtained by puncturing the suspected lesion through the skin. Depending on the location of the lesion, a biopsy specimen can sometimes be obtained during bronchoscopy.

pneumonectomy   (pneumon/o, lung + -ectomy, excision) surgical removal of all or part of a lung; **pneumectomy.** If a lobe of the lung is removed, it is called a pulmonary **lobectomy.**

rhinoplasty   (rhin/o, nose + -plasty, surgical repair) plastic surgery of the nose; usually performed for cosmetic reasons, but may also be necessary to provide a passage for respiration.

thoracocentesis   (thorac/o, chest + -centesis, surgical puncture) surgical puncture of the chest cavity to remove fluid; also called **thoracentesis** or thoracic **paracentesis** (Figure 8-12).

Review the following new word parts you have used in this chapter.

Additional Word Parts

Word Part	Meaning
atel/o	imperfect
coni/o	dust
embol/o	embolus
home/o	sameness
-ole	little
ox/o	oxygen
-pnea	breathing
silic/o	silica
spir/o	to breathe (sometimes, spiral)

MATCH IT!
EXERCISE 7

Match the word parts in the left column with their meanings in the right column.

_____ **1.** atel/o   **A.** breathing
_____ **2.** coni/o   **B.** dust
_____ **3.** home/o   **C.** imperfect
_____ **4.** -ole   **D.** little
_____ **5.** -pnea   **E.** sameness

BUILD IT!
EXERCISE 8

Combine the word parts to write terms for these descriptions.

1. plastic surgery of the nose (rhin/o + -plasty): _____
2. surgical puncture of the chest cavity (thorac/o + -centesis): _____
3. incision of the windpipe (trache/o + -tomy) _____
4. surgical removal of all or part of the lung (pneum/o + -ectomy) _____
5. agent that causes bronchial dilation (bronch/o + dilator) _____
6. agent that dissolves mucus (muc/o + -lytic) _____

❗ Be Careful with These!

aphonia (loss of audible voice; a vocal dysfunction) versus *aphasia* (inability to communicate through speech, writing, or signs; a brain dysfunction)
phren/o (diaphragm or mind) versus *pleur/o* (pleura)
pronunciation of *larynx* (lar´inks) and *pharynx* (far´inks) [*not* lar´nix and far´nix]

SELF TEST   Work the following exercises to test your understanding of the material in Chapter 8. Complete all the written review exercises before using Appendix VIII to check your answers.

A. MATCH IT!   Match the structures in the left column with their characteristics or functions in the right column.

_____ **1.** alveolus   **A.** branch of the trachea
_____ **2.** bronchus   **B.** muscular partition that facilitates breathing
_____ **3.** diaphragm   **C.** commonly called the throat
_____ **4.** larynx   **D.** commonly called the windpipe
_____ **5.** nose   **E.** connected with the paranasal sinuses
_____ **6.** pharynx   **F.** contains the vocal cords
_____ **7.** trachea   **G.** where oxygen and carbon dioxide exchange occurs

SELF-TEST (cont'd)

B. WRITE IT!　*Write one-word terms for each of these meanings.*

1. agent that dissolves mucus _____
2. agent used to control coughing _____
3. difficult or weak voice _____
4. direct visualization of the bronchi _____
5. incision of the trachea _____
6. inflammation of the throat _____
7. pertaining to the air sacs of the lung _____
8. record produced in bronchography _____
9. surgical repair of the nose _____
10. within the trachea _____

C. CIRCLE IT!　*Circle the one correct answer (a, b, c, or d) for each question.*

1. Mrs. Smith's doctor tells her that she has pneumonia. What is another name for her diagnosis?
   (a) congestive heart disease　(b) pneumonitis　(c) pulmonary edema　(d) pulmonary insufficiency
2. John R. is told that he has periodic absence of breathing. What is the name of his
   condition?　(a) apnea　(b) dyspnea　(c) hyperpnea　(d) hypopnea
3. What is the serous membrane that lines the walls of the thoracic cavity?
   (a) emphysema　(b) pleura　(c) rhinorrhea　(d) thrombus
4. Mrs. Sema has difficulty breathing except when sitting in an upright position. What is the term for her condition?
   (a) anoxia　(b) hyperventilation　(c) inspiration　(d) orthopnea
5. The pulmonary specialist orders a test to measure the amount of air taken into and expelled from the lungs. What
   is the name of the test?
   (a) laryngoscopy　(b) mediastinoscopy　(c) spirometry　(d) thoracometry
6. Which term means a lack of oxygen in body tissues?
   (a) anoxia　(b) dyspnea　(c) effusion　(d) orthopnea
7. Which term is another term for inspiration?
   (a) exhalation　(b) homeostasis　(c) inhalation　(d) pertussis
8. Which term means pertaining to the diaphragm?
   (a) aphasic　(b) pharyngeal　(c) phrenic　(d) thoracic
9. Which term means inflammation of the air-filled cavities in various bones around the nose?
   (a) laryngitis　(b) pleuritis　(c) tracheitis　(d) sinusitis
10. Which term means incomplete expansion of a lung or a portion of a lung?
    (a) atelectasis　(b) pneumoconiosis　(c) pulmonary edema　(d) silicosis

Continued

SELF-TEST (cont'd)

D. FINDING THE CLUE! *Use a clue to write terms for these descriptions. Solve Question 1; each ending letter becomes the clue for the first letter of the next answer.*

1. instrument used to examine an internal structure　_____
2. normal breathing　_____
3. loss of ability to communicate by speech, writing, or signs　_____
4. drug that counteracts histamine　_____
5. lidlike structure that covers the larynx　_____
6. type of pneumoconiosis　_____
7. material coughed up from the lungs　_____
8. agent that destroys mucus　_____
9. device for delivering oxygen that is placed in the nose　_____
10. one of a cluster of small air sacs at the end of a bronchiole　_____

E. READING HEALTH CARE REPORTS

MEDICAL REPORT　**County Medical Center**

666 Medical Center Drive　　**Main City, USA 63038-1000**　　**Phone:** (555) 333-3333

PHYSICAL EXAMINATION

Patient: M. A. Gordon (female, age 63)
Date: 05/04/2009
Symptoms: Fever; dyspnea; mild, productive cough; malaise; loss of appetite.
History: Bronchitis, myocardial infarction (status post-CABG 1 year ago), and deep venous thrombosis with pulmonary embolism.
Family History: Mother, age 85, with bronchiectasis; father deceased with a history of emphysema.
Physical Exam: T 100.8; P 98, R 28; BP 160/94; fine crackles bilateral lung bases with some wheezes; increased dyspnea on exertion; O_2 saturation level 92% on 2 L O_2.
Laboratory Data: WBC 24.6
Chest X-Ray: Increased right lung density; no pneumothorax or pleural effusion. Increasing rt. lung infiltrate with masslike density rt. hilum.
Diagnosis: Community-acquired pneumonia.
Treatment Plan: IV antibiotic pending sputum culture, bronchodilator such as Alupent, and expectorant such as guaifenesin.

Dr. Stephen White
Stephen White, M.D.

SELF-TEST (cont'd)

Write the terms from the report that correspond to each of these descriptions.

1. abnormal accumulation of fluid in the pleural space   _____

2. chronic dilation of the bronchi accompanied by secondary infection   _____

3. chronic pulmonary disease characterized by destructive changes in alveoli   _____

4. inflammation of the bronchi   _____

5. inflammation of the lungs   _____

6. labored or difficult breathing   _____

7. material coughed up from the bronchi or lungs   _____

8. blockage of a pulmonary artery by a substance brought by the circulating blood   _____

9. presence of air or gas in the pleural space   _____

10. therapeutic agent that relaxes the bronchioles   _____

F. SPELL IT!   *Circle all incorrectly spelled terms, and write their correct spellings.*

1. asfixiation   _____

2. endoskopic   _____

3. entubation   _____

4. polip   _____

5. pulmonik   _____

Q&E List

Use the Companion CD or audio CDs to review the terms presented in Chapter 8. Look closely at the spelling of each term as it is pronounced.

adult respiratory distress syndrome (**ə-dult´ res´pĭ-rə-tor˝e dis-tres´sin´drōm**)

alveolar (**al-ve´ə-lər**)

alveolus (**al-ve´ə-ləs**)

anoxia (**ə-nok´se-ə**)

antihistamine (**an˝te-, an´ti-his´tə-mēn**)

antitussive (**an˝te-, an˝ti-tus´iv**)

aphasia (**ə-fa´zhə**)

aphasic (**ə-fa´zik**)

aphonia (**a-fo´ne-ə**)

apnea (**ap´ne-ə**)

asphyxiation (**as-fĭk˝se-a´shən**)

asthma (**az´mə**)

atelectasis (**at˝ə-lek´tə-sis**)

auditory tube (**aw´dĭ-tor˝e tōōb**)

bradypnea (**brad´e-ne˝ə, brad-ip´ne-ə**)

bronchi (**brong´ki**)

bronchial (**brong´ke-əl**)

bronchiectasis (**brong˝ke-ek´tə-sis**)

brochiole (**brong´ke-ōl**)

bronchiolitis (**brong˝ke-o-li´tis**)

bronchitis (**brong-ki´tis**)

bronchodilator (**brong˝ko-di´la-tər, -di-la´tər**)

bronchogram (**brong´ko-gram**)

bronchography (**brong-kog´rə-fe**)

bronchopneumonia (**brong˝ko-nōō-mo´ne-ə**)

bronchopulmonary (**brong˝ko-pool´mə-nar˝e**)

bronchoscope (**brong´ko-skōp**)

bronchoscopic (**brong˝ko-skop´ik**)

bronchoscopy (**brong-kos´kə-pe**)

bronchus (**brong´kəs**)

carcinoma of the lung (**kar˝sĭ-no´mə uv thə lung**)

chronic obstructive pulmonary disease (**kron´ik ob-struk´tiv pool´mo-nar˝e dĭ-zēz´**)

decongestant (**de˝kən-jes´tənt**)

diaphragm (**di´ə-fram**)

continued

dysphasia (**dis-fa´zhə**)
dysphonia (**dis-fo´ne-ə**)
dyspnea (**disp´ne-ə, disp-ne´ə**)
edema (**ə-de´mə**)
effusion (**ə-fu´zhən**)
embolism (**em´bə-liz-əm**)
embolus (**em´bo-ləs**)
emphysema (**em˝fə-se´mə**)
endoscope (**en´do-skōp**)
endoscopic (**en˝do-skop´ik**)
endotracheal intubation (**en˝do-tra´ke-əl
    in˝too-ba´shən**)
epiglottis (**ep˝ĭ-glot´is**)
esophagus (**ə-sof´ə-gus**)
eupnea (**ūp-ne´ə**)
eustachian tube (**u-sta´ke-ən tōōb**)
exhalation (**eks˝hə-la´shən**)
expiration (**ek˝spĭ-ra´shən**)
glottis (**glot´is**)
Heimlich maneuver (**hīm´lik mə-noo´vər**)
hemothorax (**he˝mo-thor´aks**)
hyperpnea (**hi˝pər-ne´ə, hi˝pərp-ne´ə**)
hyperventilation (**hi˝pər-ven˝tĭ-la´shən**)
hypoxia (**hi-pok´se-ə**)
influenza (**in˝floo-en´zə**)
inhalation (**in˝hə-la´shən**)
inspiration (**in˝spĭ-ra´shən**)
laryngalgia (**lar˝in-gal´jə**)
laryngeal polyp (**lə-rin´je-əl pol´ip**)
laryngitis (**lar˝in-ji´tis**)
laryngopharynx (**lə-ring˝go-far´ənks**)
laryngoscopy (**lar˝ing-gos´kə-pe**)
larynx (**lar´inks**)
lobectomy (**lo-bek´tə-me**)
lung biopsy (**lung bi´op-se**)
mucolytic (**mu˝ko-lit´ik**)
nares (**na´rēz, nar´ēz**)
nasal cannula (**na´zəl kan´u-lə**)
nasal septum (**na´zəl sep´təm**)
nasopharyngeal (**na˝zo-fə-rin´je-əl**)
nasotracheal intubation (**na˝zo-tra´ke-əl
    in˝too-ba´shən**)
orotracheal intubation (**or´o-tra´ke-əl in˝too-ba´shən**)
orthopnea (**or˝thop-ne´ə**)
orthopneic (**or˝thop-ne´ik**)
otopharyngeal (**o˝to-fə-rin´je-əl**)

paracentesis (**par˝ə-sən-te´sis**)
paranasal sinuses (**par˝ə-na´zəl si´nəs-əs**)
paroxysmal (**par˝ok-siz´məl**)
percutaneous biopsy (**pur˝ku-ta´ne-əs bi´op-se**)
pharyngeal (**fə-rin´je-əl**)
pharyngitis (**far˝in-ji´tis**)
pharynx (**far´inks**)
phrenic (**fren´ik**)
pleura (**ploor´ə**)
pleural (**ploor´əl**)
pleurisy (**ploor´ĭ-se**)
pleuritis (**plōō-ri´tis**)
pneumatic (**noo-mat´ik**)
pneumectomy (**noo-mek´tə-me**)
pneumocardial (**noo˝mo-kahr´de-əl**)
pneumocentesis (**noo˝mo-sən-te´sis**)
pneumoconiosis (**noo˝mo-ko˝ne-o´sis**)
pneumohemothorax (**noo˝mo-he˝mo-thor´aks**)
pneumonectomy (**noo˝mo-nek´tə-me**)
pneumonia (**noo-mo´ne-ə**)
pneumonitis (**noo˝mo-ni´tis**)
pneumothorax (**noo˝mo-thor´aks**)
pulmonary (**pool´mo-nar˝e**)
pulmonary edema (**pool´mo-nar˝e ə-de´mə**)
pulmonary embolism (**pool´mo-nar˝e em´bə-liz-əm**)
pulmonic (**pəl-mon´ik**)
pulmonologist (**pool˝mə-nol´ə-jist**)
respiration (**res˝pĭ-ra´shən**)
respiratory (**res´pĭ-rə-tor˝e**)
rhinitis (**ri-ni´tis**)
rhinoplasty (**ri´no-plas˝te**)
rhinorrhea (**ri˝no-re´ə**)
severe acute respiratory syndrome (**sə-vēr´ ə-kŭt
    res´pĭ-rə-tor˝e sin´drōm**)
silicosis (**sil˝ĭ-ko´sis**)
sinusitis (**si˝nəs-i´tis**)
spirometry (**spi-rom´ə-tre**)
sputum (**spu´təm**)
sudden infant death syndrome (**sud´ən in´fənt deth
    sin´drōm**)
tachypnea (**tak˝ip-ne´ə, tak˝e-ne´ə**)
thoracentesis (**thor˝ə-sen-te´sis**)
thoracic (**thə-ras´ik**)
thoracocentesis (**thor˝ə-ko-sən-te´sis**)
thorax (**thor´aks**)
thrombus (**throm´bəs**)

trachea (tra´ke-ə)

tracheal (tra´ke-əl)

tracheobronchial (tra˝ke-o-brong´ke-əl)

tracheostomy (tra˝ke-os´tə-me)

tracheotomy (tra˝ke-ot´ə-me)

transtracheal (trans-tra´ke-əl)

tubercle (too´bər-kəl)

tuberculosis (too-ber˝ku-lo´sis)

ventilator (ven˝tĭ-la´tər)

wheeze (hwēz)

 Don't forget the games on the Companion CD and http://evolve.elsevier.com/Leonard/quick/ for additional review, including questions on Spanish medical terms.

Enhancing Spanish Communication

English	Spanish (pronunciation)
asphyxiation	asfixia (as-FEEC-se-ah), sofocación (so-fo-cah-se-ON)
asthma	asma (AHS-mah)
breathe	alentar (ah-len-TAR), respirar (res-pe-RAR)
chronic	crónico (CRO-ne-co)
cough	tos (tos)
diaphragm	diafragma (de-ah-FRAHG-mah)
erect, straight	derecho (day-RAY-cho)
imperfect	imperfecto (im-per-FEC-to)
influenza	gripe (GREE-pay)
lobe	lóbulo (LO-boo-lo)
nostril	orificio de la nariz (or-e-FEE-se-o day lah nah-REES)
oxygen	oxígeno (ok-SEE-hay-no)
pneumonia	neumonía (nay-oo-mo-NEE-ah)
	pulmonía (pool-mo-NEE-ah)
respiration	respiración (res-pe-rah-se-ON)
same	mismo (MEES-mo)

CHAPTER 9

Digestive System

CONTENTS

Function First
Structures of the Digestive System
    Alimentary Tract
    Accessory Organs of Digestion
Diseases, Disorders, and Diagnostic Terms
    Mouth
    Esophagus
    Stomach

Intestines
Gallbladder
Liver
Pancreas
Surgical and Therapeutic Interventions
Self-Test
Q&E List
Enhancing Spanish Communication

OBJECTIVES

After completing Chapter 9, you will be able to:

1. Recognize or write the functions of the digestive system.
2. Recognize or write the meanings of Chapter 9 word parts and use them to build and analyze terms.
3. Write terms for selected structures of the digestive system, or match them with their descriptions.
4. Write the names of the diagnostic terms and

pathologies related to the digestive system when given their descriptions, or match terms with their meanings.

5. Match surgical and therapeutic interventions for the digestive system, or write the names of the interventions when given their descriptions.
6. Spell terms for the digestive system correctly.

Function First

WORD ORIGIN

alimentum (L.)
to nourish

-ation = process

The digestive system provides the body with water, nutrients, and minerals. **Alimentation** is the process of providing **nutrition** for the body. After becoming available to the body cells, nutrients are used for growth, generation of energy, and elimination of wastes, all of which result from this process (**metabolism**).

The digestive system accomplishes its role through the following activities:

- Ingestion
- Digestion
- Absorption
- Elimination

The activities begin with **ingestion**, which in humans is the oral intake of substances into the body. Ingestion is followed by **digestion**, the mechanical and chemical conversion of food into substances that can eventually be absorbed by cells. The mechanical breakdown of food is accomplished by chewing. Chemical breakdown begins in the mouth and is completed in the stomach. **Absorption** is the process in which the digested food molecules pass through the lining of the small intestine into the blood or lymph capillaries. The final activity, **elimination**, is removal of undigested food particles. The elimination of wastes through the anus in the form of feces is called **defecation**.

WRITE IT!

EXERCISE 1

In the order in which they occur, write the names of the four digestive activities.

1. _____

2. _____

3. _____

4. _____

Use Appendix VIII to check your answers to all the exercises in Chapter 9.

Carbohydrates, proteins, and **lipids** (fats) are the three major classes of nutrients. Carbohydrates, the basic source of energy for human cells, include sugars and starches. The chemical breaking down of nutrients into simpler substances requires **enzymes**. Specific enzymes act on different types of sugars. The suffixes *-ose* (meaning sugar) and *-ase* (meaning enzyme) are generally used in the terms referring to the sugars and the enzymes that act on them. For example, **lact+ase** breaks down **lact+ose**. The eventual product of the digestion of sugars as well as starches is **glucose**, a simple sugar that is the major source of energy for the body. The enzyme that breaks down starch is **amyl+ase**. The effective enzyme that breaks down protein is called **prote+ase** or **protein+ase**. The effective enzyme that breaks down a lipid (fat) is a **lip+ase**. Lipids serve as an energy reserve.

> lact/o = milk
> -ose = sugar
> -ase = enzyme

> amyl/o = starch
> prote/o, protein/o = protein
> lip/o = fat
> -ase = enzyme

WRITE IT!

EXERCISE 2

List the three major classes of nutrients.

1. _____

2. _____

3. _____

The following table contains several word parts introduced in the material you just read, as well as some new ones often associated with the digestive tract. Word parts for structures of the digestive system are included in the next section. Commit the following word parts to memory.

Word Parts

Word Part	Meaning
-ation	action or process
bil/i, chol/e	bile
cirrh/o	orange-yellow
de-	down, from, reversing, or removing
glycos/o	sugar
-orexia	appetite
-pepsia	digestion
vag/o	vagus nerve
viscer/o	viscera

Use the electronic flashcards on the Evolve site or make your own set of flashcards using the above list. Select the word parts just presented, and study them until you know their meanings. Do this each time a set of word parts is presented.

MATCH IT!

EXERCISE 3

Match the word parts in the left column with their meanings in the right column (a choice may be used more than once).

_____ **1.** bil/i
_____ **2.** chol/e
_____ **3.** de-
_____ **4.** cirrh/o
_____ **5.** glycos/o
_____ **6.** -orexia
_____ **7.** -pepsia
_____ **8.** viscer/o

A. appetite
B. bile
C. digestion
D. down, from, reversing, or removing
E. orange-yellow
F. sugar
G. viscera

Structures of the Digestive System

The digestive system is traditionally divided into the **alimentary** canal and several organs that are considered "accessory" organs because they produce substances needed for proper digestion and absorption of nutrients. The alimentary canal is often called the digestive tract or the **alimentary tract**.

Alimentary Tract

gastr/o = stomach
intestin/o =
   intestines
-al = pertaining to

The digestive tract, basically a long, muscular tube that is lined with mucous membrane, begins at the mouth and ends at the anus. **Gastrointestinal** refers to the stomach and the intestines. The upper gastrointestinal tract (UGI) consists of the mouth, pharynx, esophagus, and stomach. The lower gastrointestinal tract (LGI) is made up of the small and large intestines.

The major organs of digestion are shown in Figure 9-1. Label the numbered blanks as you read the information that accompanies the drawing.

Become familiar with the names of the digestive organs, and recognize the parts that make up the small and large intestines. Commit the meanings of the following word parts to memory.

Word Parts: Digestive Organs

Word Part	Meaning	
cheil/o	lips	
dent/i, dent/o, odont/o	teeth	
gingiv/o	gums	mouth and teeth
gloss/o, lingu/o	tongue	
or/o, stomat/o	mouth	
esophag/o	esophagus	
gastr/o	stomach	
intestin/o, enter/o*	intestines	
duoden/o	duodenum	
jejun/o	jejunum	divisions of small intestine
ile/o	ileum	

*enter/o sometimes refers only to the small intestine.

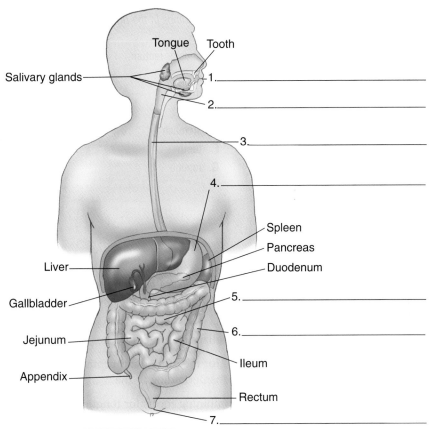

Tongue Tooth

Salivary glands—

1._____

2._____

3._____

4._____

Spleen
Pancreas
Duodenum

Liver—

5._____

Gallbladder—

6._____

Jejunum—

Ileum

Appendix—

Rectum

7._____

Figure 9-1 Structures of the digestive system. The alimentary tract, beginning at the mouth and ending at the anus, is basically a long, muscular tube. Several accessory organs (salivary glands, liver, gallbladder, pancreas) are also shown. Label the drawing as you read the following explanation. Digestion begins in the mouth *(1)* or oral cavity. The teeth grind and chew the food before it is swallowed. The pharynx *(2)*, or throat, passes the chewed food to the esophagus *(3)*, which leads to the stomach *(4)*, where food is churned and broken down chemically and mechanically. The liquid mass is passed to the small intestine *(5)*, where digestion continues and absorption of nutrients occurs. The three parts of the small intestine are shown: duodenum, jejunum, and ileum. Undigested food passes to the large intestine *(6)*, where much of the water is absorbed. It is then excreted from the anus *(7)*, the opening of the rectum on the body surface.

Word Parts: Digestive Organs—cont'd

Word Part	Meaning	
col/o, colon/o	colon or large intestine†	
append/o, appendic/o	appendix	
cec/o	cecum	
sigmoid/o	sigmoid colon	large intestine
proct/o	anus or rectum	
rect/o	rectum	
an/o	anus	

†*The colon makes up most of the large intestine. Therefore the word "colon" is sometimes used inaccurately as a synonym for the entire large intestine. In words containing col/o, the distinction between the colon and large intestine is usually not significant.*

MATCH IT!   **EXERCISE 4**

Match the word parts in the left column with their meanings in the right column (a choice may be used more than once).

_____ **1.** cheil/o
_____ **2.** enter/o
_____ **3.** gastr/o
_____ **4.** gingiv/o
_____ **5.** gloss/o
_____ **6.** lingu/o
_____ **7.** odont/o
_____ **8.** proct/o

A. anus or rectum
B. gums
C. intestines
D. lips
E. stomach
F. teeth
G. tongue

PROGRAMMED LEARNING

Remember to cover the answers (left column) with folded paper or the bookmark. Write an answer in each blank, and then check your answer before proceeding to the next frame.

mouth	1. The mouth or **oral** cavity is the beginning of the digestive tract. An oral surgeon is one who specializes in surgery of the _____.
gum	2. **Gingiva** is another name for the gum, the mucous membrane that surrounds the teeth. **Gingiv+al** means pertaining to the _____.
under	3. You have learned that combining forms for tongue are gloss/o and lingu/o. **Hypo+glossal** means _____ the tongue.
sublingual	4. Certain medications are placed under the tongue, where the medicine dissolves. Use sub- + lingu/o + -al to write an adjective that describes the use of this type of medication: _____.
teeth	5. An adult has 32 permanent teeth in a full set, 8 in each dental quadrant. **Dental** means pertaining to the teeth. Label the teeth of the lower jaw **(mandible),** called the **mandibular** arch, in Figure 9-2. The combining forms dent/i, dent/o, and odont/o all mean _____. Permanent teeth are named **incisors, cuspids** (or canines), **bicuspids,** and **molars.** The last teeth on each side of the upper and lower jaw (the third molars) are called the "wisdom teeth" because they usually erupt between 17 and 25 years of age.
teeth	6. Dentists care for the teeth and associated structures of the oral cavity. Or+al means pertaining to the mouth. The word part odont/o is used to write the names of most of the dental specialties. **Ped+odont+ics** deals with the _____ and mouth conditions of children.
orthodontist	7. **Orth+odont+ics** is the branch of dentistry concerned with tooth alignment and associated facial problems. The combining form orth/o means straight or straighten. If someone wants to have straight teeth, he or she sees a specialist in orthodontics, an _____.

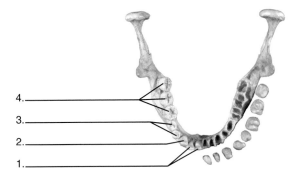

-ar = pertaining to
bi- = two
mandibul/o = mandible (lower jaw)

4.
3.
2.
1.

Figure 9-2 Designations of permanent teeth of the lower jaw (mandibular arch). Half of the teeth are removed to demonstrate the sockets. Label the teeth in one dental quadrant (1 to 4) as you read this explanation. There are two incisors *(1)*, one cuspid or canine *(2)*, two bicuspids *(3)*, and three molars *(4)*.

around	8. The tissue that supports the teeth and keeps them firmly anchored is called **peri+odont+ium.** You learned in Chapter 3 that peri- means _____. The gums are part of the periodontium.
periodontal	9. Use -al to form a word that means pertaining to the periodontium: _____.
periodontium	10. **Periodontics** is the branch of dentistry that deals with the study and treatment of the _____.
esophagus	11. Food that is swallowed passes from the mouth to the **pharynx** (throat) and then to a long tube called the _____.
stomach	12. The **esophagus** carries food to the stomach. Washing out of the stomach is called **gastric lavage.** Lavage means the irrigation or washing out of an organ, such as the stomach or bowel. Gastric lavage specifically refers to washing out of the _____. This procedure might be performed to remove poisonous material or to clean the stomach before gastric surgery.
pain	13. **Gastr+algia** and **gastro+dynia** both mean _____ of the stomach.
stomach	14. Gastro+intestinal (GI) means pertaining to the _____ and the intestines.
ileum	15. Label the three divisions of the small intestine as you read the material that accompanies Figure 9-3. The three divisions of the small intestine are the **duodenum,** the **jejunum,** and the _____.
gastroenterologist	16. **Gastro+entero+logy** is the study of the stomach, intestines, and associated structures. Write the term for a physician who specializes in gastroenterology: _____. Pain associated with digestive problems often involves examination of the abdomen. Abdominal quadrants are useful to describe location of pain in the abdomen (see Figure 5-8, p. 108).

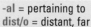

-al = pertaining to
dist/o = distant, far

Figure 9-3 The three divisions of the small intestine. Label the three parts of the small intestine (1 to 3) as you read. The first portion, the duodenum *(1)*, begins at the opening from the stomach and is the shorter section. The second section is the jejunum *(2)*, which is continuous with the third portion, the ileum *(3)*. The ileum, the distal part of the small intestine, joins with the cecum (the beginning of the large intestine).

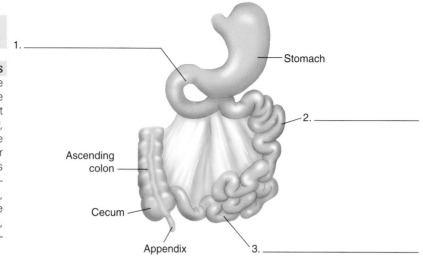

1. _____

Stomach

2. _____

Ascending colon ───

Cecum ───

Appendix

3. _____

---

mucus

17. Rhythmic muscular contraction forces food through the digestive tract. This is aided by **mucus,** secreted by the inner lining of the digestive tract, and bile (which is discussed in the next section). The slimy material, mucus, is produced by all **mucous** membranes. Remember that muc/o means _____.

ileum

18. The large intestine is much broader and shorter than the small intestine. It is composed of the **cecum, colon, rectum,** and anal canal (Figure 9-4). The first part of the large intestine is a blind pouch only a few inches long called the cecum. The **vermiform appendix,** a wormlike structure extending from the cecum, is best known for becoming inflamed. The **ileo+cecal** valve is a group of muscles that are located between the _____ and the cecum.

19. The colon makes up the major portion of the large intestine. The colon consists of four distinct parts: **ascending colon, transverse colon, descending colon,** and **sigmoid colon.** Locate the four parts of the colon using Figure 9-4. The latter part of the colon is S-shaped and thus is called the

sigmoid

_____ colon.

col/o

20. The colon makes up most of the large intestine. Thus, when speaking of the colon, one is often referring to the large intestine in general. The combining form that means colon or large intestine is _____.

rectum

21. The lower part of the large intestine, the rectum, ends in a narrow anal canal, which opens to the exterior at the **anus.** The combining form proct/o refers to the anus or the rectum. A **procto+logist is** a physician who specializes in diseases of the anus and _____ as well as disorders of the colon.

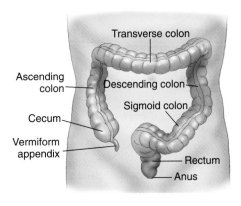

Transverse colon

Ascending colon

Descending colon

Sigmoid colon

Cecum

Vermiform appendix

Rectum

Anus

-al = pertaining to
an/o = anus
trans- = through, across

Figure 9-4 Divisions of the large intestine. The large intestine is composed of the cecum, colon, rectum, and anal canal. Note the four parts of the colon: ascending colon, transverse colon, descending colon, and sigmoid colon.

FIND IT IN NEW TERMS!

EXERCISE 5

Write the combining forms and their meanings for each of these new terms. A short definition is provided for each term.

Term/Meaning	Combining Form	Meaning
1. **anal** pertaining to the anus	_____	_____
2. **duodenal** pertaining of the duodenum	_____	_____
3. **endogastric** pertaining to the interior of the stomach	_____	_____
4. **enteral** pertaining to the small intestine	_____	_____
5. **esophageal** pertaining to the esophagus	_____	_____
6. **gastric** pertaining to the stomach	_____	_____
7. **glossal** pertaining to the tongue	_____	_____
8. **intestinal** pertaining to the intestine	_____	_____
9. **lingual** pertaining to the tongue	_____	_____
10. **rectal** pertaining to the rectum	_____	_____

Accessory Organs of Digestion

The accessory organs of digestion produce substances that are needed for proper digestion and absorption of nutrients. The liver, gallbladder, pancreas, and salivary glands are accessory organs to the digestive system (Figure 9-5). Both the liver and pancreas have additional functions in other body systems.

The liver is the largest internal organ. It performs so many vital functions that you cannot live without it. The liver produces **bile**, which breaks down fats before absorption by the small intestine. **Biliary** means pertaining to bile. Bile is continuously

bil/i = bile
-ary = pertaining to

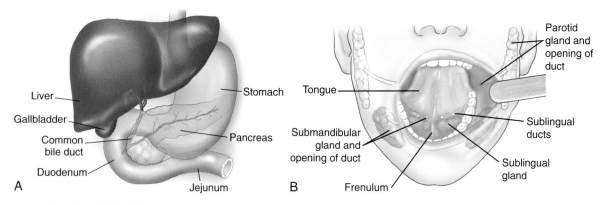

A

B

Figure 9-5 Accessory organs of digestion. A, The liver, gallbladder, and pancreas. **B,** The salivary glands (paired parotid, sublingual, and submandibular glands) consist of numerous lobes connected by vessels and ducts.

choledoch/o =
  common bile duct
-al = pertaining to

produced by the liver and is either stored by the gallbladder or transported to the small intestine for immediate use. **Cholecystic** means pertaining to the gallbladder. The main duct that conveys bile to the duodenum is the common bile duct. **Choledoch+al** means pertaining to the common bile duct.

The pancreas is a small organ with two important functions. It produces pancreatic juice, which is important in the digestion of food. The pancreas also produces **insulin,** a hormone that regulates the blood sugar level.

The **salivary** glands are located in the oral cavity. **Saliva** is produced by these glands. Saliva moistens the oral cavity and contains amy+lase, the enzyme responsible for the breakdown of starch. Because amylase is contained in saliva, starch digestion begins in the mouth.

Commit the meanings of the following word parts to memory.

Word Parts: Accessory Organs of Digestion

Word Part	Meaning
bil/i, chol/e	bile
cholecyst/o	gallbladder
choledoch/o	common bile duct
hepat/o	liver
pancreat/o	pancreas
sial/o	salivary gland

WRITE IT! **EXERCISE 6**

The first letter of each word part is given after its meaning. Use this clue to write the combining form indicated for each term.

Meaning	First Letter	Combining Form
1. common bile duct	c	_____
2. pancreas	p	_____
3. liver	h	_____
4. gallbladder	c	_____
5. salivary gland	s	_____

Diseases, Disorders, and Diagnostic Terms

Assessment of the intestinal tract has been greatly facilitated by radiology and endoscopy, revealing abnormalities such as masses, tumors, and obstructions. An **esophagram** (or **esophagogram**) is an x-ray image of the esophagus taken while the patient swallows a liquid barium suspension. This procedure is called a **barium swallow**. A **barium meal** is ingested in an upper GI series, and the radiographic examination is made as the barium passes through the esophagus, stomach, and duodenum. The lower intestinal tract is studied with a **barium enema**, a rectal infusion of barium sulfate.

The **biliary tract** is the pathway for bile flow from the liver to the bile duct and into the duodenum. A biliary calculus (**gallstone**) is a stone formed in the biliary tract, varying in size from very small to 4 or 5 cm in diameter (Figure 9-6). Biliary stones may cause **jaundice** (see Figure 3-7, p. 63), right upper quadrant pain, obstruction, and inflammation of the gallbladder (cholecystitis). The presence of stones in the gallbladder is **chole+lith+iasis**. Stones also can become lodged in the common bile duct (**choledocho+lith+iasis**). Common locations of biliary stones are illustrated in Figure 9-7.

The presence of a pancreatic stone is **pancreatolithiasis**. Other causes of obstructions include tumors. Endoscopic retrograde chol+angio+pancreato+graphy (ERCP) is an endoscopic test that provides radiographic visualization of the bile and pancreatic ducts. An endoscope is placed into the common bile duct, a radiopaque substance is instilled directly into the duct, and x-ray images are taken.

chol/e = bile
angi/o = vessel
pancreat/o = pancreas
-graphy = process of recording

The salivary ducts can be studied by injecting radiopaque substances into the ducts in a procedure called **sialography**, which may be used to demonstrate the presence of calculi in the ducts.

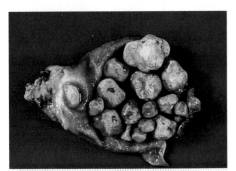

chol/e = bile
cholecyst/o = gallbladder
-ectomy = excision
-iasis = condition
lith/o = stone

Figure 9-6 Cholelithiasis, the presence of gallstones. After cholecystectomy, this photograph of an opened gallbladder shows several stones of different sizes.

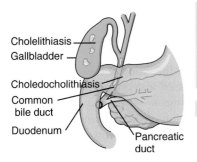

Cholelithiasis
Gallbladder
Choledocholithiasis
Common bile duct
Duodenum
Pancreatic duct

chol/e = bile
choledoch/o = common bile duct
-iasis = condition
-ic = pertaining to
lith/o = stone
pancreat/o = pancreas

Figure 9-7 Common locations of biliary calculi. Tiny stones may pass spontaneously into the duodenum. Very large stones remain in the gallbladder (cholelithiasis). Smaller stones can become lodged in the common bile duct (choledocholithiasis).

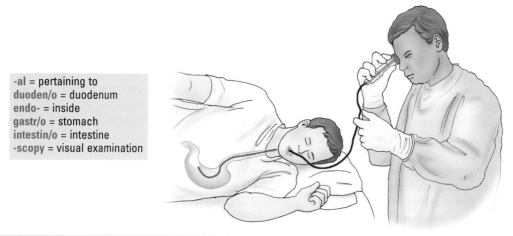

-al = pertaining to
duoden/o = duodenum
endo- = inside
gastr/o = stomach
intestin/o = intestine
-scopy = visual examination

Figure 9-8 Upper gastrointestinal endoscopy. Upper GI endoscopy is visual examination of the esophagus, stomach, and duodenum.

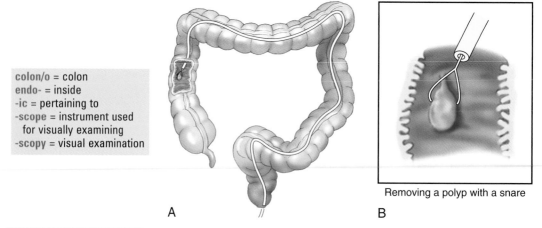

colon/o = colon
endo- = inside
-ic = pertaining to
-scope = instrument used
  for visually examining
-scopy = visual examination

Removing a polyp with a snare

A   B

Figure 9-9 Colonoscopy. A, Endoscopic examination of the colon using a flexible colonoscope. **B,** Colonic polyps can often be removed with the use of a snare (wire noose) that fits through the colonoscope.

Upper gastrointestinal endoscopy is visual examination of the esophagus, stomach, and duodenum (Figure 9-8). If the focus of the examination is the esophagus, the procedure is called **esophagoscopy**. If the stomach is the focus, the procedure is called **gastroscopy**.

Colono+scopy is the endoscopic examination of the lining of the colon with a **colonoscope**. **Coloscopy** has the same meaning but is used less often than colonoscopy. The physician may also obtain tissue biopsy specimens or remove polyps during this procedure (Figure 9-9). **Sigmoidoscopy** is inspection of the rectum and sigmoid colon with an endoscope, and **proctoscopy** is endoscopic examination of the rectum with a **proctoscope**.

proct/o = anus *or*
  rectum

BUILD IT!

EXERCISE 7

Combine the word parts to write terms for these descriptions.

1. radiographic image of the esophagus (esophag/o + -gram): _____

2. presence of stones in the gallbladder (chol/e + -lith/o + -iasis): _____

3. presence of stones in the common bile duct (choledoch/o + lith/o + -iasis): _____

4. presence of a pancreatic stone (pancreat/o + lith/o + -iasis): _____

5. radiography of the salivary ducts (sial/o + -graphy): _____

6. visual examination of the esophagus (esophag/o + -scopy): _____

7. endoscopic examination of the colon (colon/o + -scopy): _____

8. inspection of the rectum and sigmoid colon (sigmoid/o + -scopy): _____

Several blood tests, urine tests, and stool examinations are useful in assessing the organs of the digestive system, particularly liver function tests and tests for diabetes. To be accurate when referring to diabetes mellitus, it is better not to shorten the term to **diabetes** alone, although this is often done. **Diabetes mellitus** (DM) is primarily a result of resistance to insulin or lack of insulin secretion by the insulin-secreting cells of the pancreas.

Without insulin, glucose builds up in the blood and results in **hyper+glycemia**, an increased glucose level in the blood. Hyperglycemia ultimately results in the classic symptoms of diabetes mellitus:

> hyper- = increased
> glyc/o = sugar
> -emia = blood

- **Poly+phagia:** excessive hunger and uncontrolled eating
- **Poly+uria:** excessive urination
- **Poly+dipsia:** excessive thirst.

> -phagia = eating
> -uria = urination
> -dipsia = thirst

The urine sometimes contains glucose **(glycosuria)**.

Broad classifications of DM are type 1, type 2, gestational, and other types. Type 1 diabetes is genetically determined and results in absolute insulin deficiency; however, most people with this gene never develop type 1 diabetes. The specific genetic link and development of type 2 diabetes is unclear, but genetics, environmental factors, aging, and obesity may contribute to its development. Type 2 diabetes is characterized by insulin resistance rather than insufficient secretion. **Gestational diabetes mellitus**, first recognized during pregnancy, is carbohydrate intolerance, usually caused by a deficiency of insulin. It disappears after delivery of the infant but in a significant number of cases returns years later.

> glycos/o = sugar

In another dysfunction, the pancreas produces too much insulin and causes **hypo+glycemia**. In hypoglycemia the blood contains less than the normal amount of sugar.

> hypo- = less than
> normal

Carcinoma can occur in almost any organ of the gastrointestinal system, but cancers of the colon, rectum, and the oral cavity are more common. Pancreatic cancer, although uncommon, has a high mortality rate.

You are probably familiar with cholesterol, a type of lipid that generally is elevated in **hyper+lip+emia**. Sometimes the combining form, lip/o, is not used, and **hyperlipidemia** is also used to mean an increased amount of fat or lipids in the blood.

> hyper- = excessive
> lip/o = lipid
> -emia = blood

Obesity is an abnormal increase in the proportion of fat cells of the body. A person is regarded as medically obese if he or she is 20% above the desirable body weight for the person's age, gender, height, and body type.

Hyper+emesis and **dia+rrhea** can also interfere with proper nutrition. **Emesis** is also used as a word that means vomiting.

> -emesis = vomiting
> dia- = through
> -rrhea = discharge

| de- = remove |
| hydr/o = water |
| -ation = process |

Hyperemesis or diarrhea can lead to **de+hydr+ation**. Dehydration occurs when the output of body fluid exceeds fluid intake.

Emaciation is excessive leanness caused by disease or lack of nutrition. **An+orexia** is loss of appetite for food. **Anorexia nervosa**, often associated with psychologic stress or conflict, is a disorder characterized by prolonged refusal to eat that results in emaciation. **Bulimia**, is characterized by episodes of binge eating that often terminate in self-induced vomiting.

| an- = without |
| -orexia = appetite |

Either prolonged anorexia or bulimia leads to depletion of nutrients for body cells and results in **mal+nutrition**. Malnutrition can also be caused by malabsorption, the improper absorption of nutrients into the bloodstream from the intestines. **Malabsorption syndrome** is a complex of symptoms that include anorexia, weight loss, **flatulence** (excessive gas in the stomach and intestinal tract that leads to bloating), muscle cramps, and bone pain.

WRITE IT!   EXERCISE 8

Write the correct term in the blanks to complete each sentence.

1. A disorder that results from a resistance to or lack of insulin is diabetes _____.
2. The term for increased glucose in the blood is _____.
3. The term for excessive urination is _____.
4. The term for excessive thirst is _____.
5. Glucose in the urine is called _____.
6. A type of diabetes that sometimes occurs first during pregnancy is called _____ diabetes mellitus.
7. Less than the normal amount of sugar in the blood is called _____.
8. Hyperlipidemia is an increased amount of _____ in the blood.
9. Excessive vomiting is _____.
10. Excessive leanness is _____.
11. A disorder characterized by prolonged refusal to eat is _____ nervosa.
12. Binge eating often terminating in self-induced vomiting is _____.

PROGRAMMED LEARNING

Remember to cover the answers (left column) with folded paper or the bookmark. Write an answer in each blank, and then check your answer before proceeding to the next frame.

appendix	1. The vermiform (worm-shaped) appendix is attached to the cecum (see Figure 9-3). **Appendic+itis** is inflammation of the vermiform _____. It is characterized by abdominal pain followed by nausea and vomiting.
hepatitis	2. Inflammation of the liver is _____. Causes of this condition include bacterial or viral infection, parasites, drugs, and toxins.
hepatomegaly	3. When the liver becomes inflamed, it is not unusual for it also to become enlarged. Use a suffix you learned earlier to write a word that means enlargement of the liver: _____.

liver	4. **Hepatic** means pertaining to the liver. **Cirrhosis** is a chronic liver disease characterized by marked degeneration of liver cells. It might be more difficult for you to remember the meaning of cirrhosis because it does not use a familiar word part. The combining form cirrh/o is derived from a Greek word meaning orange-yellow, but you need to remember that cirrh+osis is a chronic disease of the _____.
cirrhosis	5. There are other causes of cirrhosis, but a common cause is alcohol abuse. The term for chronic liver disease characterized by marked degeneration of liver cells is _____.
liver	6. **Hepato+toxic** means toxic, or destructive, to the _____. Hepatotoxic drugs can damage the liver.
gallbladder	7. Bile is produced by the liver but stored in the _____. (*Gall* is another term for bile; thus the use of the term gallbladder.)
vessel	8. **Chol+ang+itis** is inflammation of the bile ducts, the vessels that transport bile. The combining form chol/e, meaning bile, is used to write cholangitis. The combining form angi/o means _____. (In cholangitis, the *i* in angi/o is omitted to make pronunciation easier.)
cholangiogram	9. **Cholangio+graphy** is x-ray examination of the bile ducts, usually using a contrast agent. The record of the bile ducts produced in cholangiography is called a _____.
gallbladder	10. The combining form cyst/o means bladder or sac. Whenever you see cholecyst in a word, you will know that it means _____.
cholecystitis	11. Inflammation of the gallbladder is _____.
pancreatolith	12. Stones can form in the pancreas as well as the gallbladder. Write a word that means pancreatic stone: _____.
stone	13. Saliva is produced by the salivary glands. **Sialo+lith+iasis** is the presence of a salivary _____.
digestion	14. The suffix -pepsia means _____.
"bad," poor, or abnormal	15. If **eu+pepsia** is good or normal digestion, **dys+pepsia** is _____ digestion.
viscera	16. The term **viscera** (singular, viscus) refers to large internal organs enclosed within a cavity, especially the abdominal organs. **Visceral** means pertaining to the large internal organs in the abdominal cavity. Thus, many of the digestive organs are viscera. Write the term that means large internal organs within the abdominal cavity: _____.
peritonitis	17. **Peritoneum** (periton/o + -eum, membrane) is the membrane that surrounds the viscera and lines the abdominal cavity. The peritoneum holds the viscera in position. Inflammation of the peritoneum is _____.

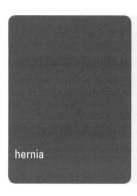

hernia

18. A hernia is protrusion of an organ through an abnormal opening in the muscle wall of the cavity that surrounds it. A weakness in the abdominal wall can result in various hernias, including umbilical hernias (those near the umbilicus), incisional hernias (herniation through inadequately healed surgery), and inguinal hernias (those in which a loop of intestine enters the **inguinal** canal, an opening in the abdominal wall for passage of the spermatic cord in males and a ligament of the uterus in females). A protrusion of an organ through an abnormal opening in the muscle wall of the cavity that contains it is called a _____. Common types of abdominal hernias are shown in Figure 5-11, p. 110.

The following list defines additional diseases and disorders affecting alimentary structures and organs of digestion.

Mouth

canker sores ulcers, chiefly of the mouth and lips.

cheilitis (cheil/o, lip + -itis, inflammation) inflammation of the lip.

gingivitis (gingiv/o, gum) inflammation of the gums.

glossitis (gloss/o, tongue) inflammation of the tongue. The tongue is painful, sometimes covered with ulcers, and swallowing is difficult.

stomatitis (stomat/o, mouth) inflammation of the mouth.

Esophagus

dysphagia (dys-, painful or difficult + phag/o, eat + -ia, condition) inability to swallow or difficulty in swallowing. This condition is often associated with such disorders as paralysis, constriction, and spasm of the esophageal muscles.

esophageal varices (esophag/o, esophagus) a complex of enlarged and swollen veins at the lower end of the esophagus that are susceptible to hemorrhage.

esophagitis inflammation of the esophagus.

gastroesophageal reflux disease (GERD) condition resulting from a backflow of the stomach contents into the esophagus. The acidic gastric juices cause burning pain in the esophagus. Repeated episodes of reflux can result in esophagitis, narrowing of the esophagus, or an esophageal ulcer. Treatment is elevation of the head of the bed, avoidance of acid-stimulating foods, and use of **antacids** (ant-, against) or antiulcer medications.

Stomach

gastritis (gastr/o, stomach) inflammation of the stomach.

gastrocele (-cele, hernia) herniation of the stomach. A common type of gastrocele is a **hiatus** or **hiatal hernia**, protrusion of a structure through the opening in the diaphragm that allows passage of the esophagus. Often the protruding structure is part of the stomach (Figure 9-10).

gastroenteritis (enter/o, intestine) inflammation of the stomach and the intestinal tract.

hyperacidity excessive amount of acid in the stomach. The condition may lead to ulceration of the stomach and is treated with antacids or anti-ulcer medications. Antibiotics are also effective in some patients.

ulcer lesion of the mucous membrane, accompanied by the sloughing (shedding) of dead tissue.

upper gastrointestinal bleeding bleeding of the upper digestive structures, sometimes evidenced by blood in the vomit (Figure 9-11, *A*).

Intestines

appendicitis (appendic/o, appendix) inflammation of the vermiform appendix.

colitis (col/o, colon) inflammation of the colon.

diverticulitis (diverticul/o, diverticulum) inflammation of a diverticulum in the intestinal tract, especially in the colon, causing stagnation, or lack of movement, of feces and pain. If diverticulitis is severe, a **diverticulectomy** is performed. A

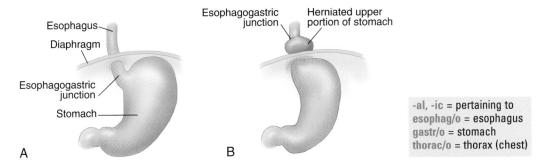

-al, -ic = pertaining to
esophag/o = esophagus
gastr/o = stomach
thorac/o = thorax (chest)

Figure 9-10 **Structural abnormality of the diaphragm in hiatal hernia. A,** Normally, muscles in the diaphragm encircle the esophagogastric junction and prevent the stomach from ascending into the thoracic cavity. **B,** Hiatal hernia, in which the upper portion of the stomach slides up and down through the opening in the diaphragm.

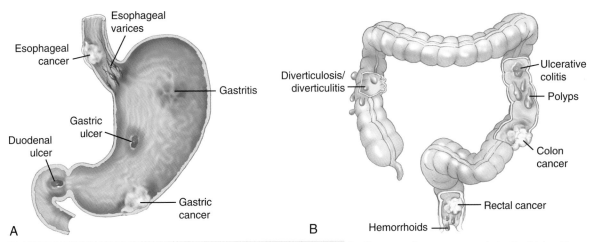

Figure 9-11 **Common causes of bleeding of the digestive tract. A,** Causes of upper gastrointestinal bleeding. **B,** Causes of lower gastrointestinal bleeding.

duoden/o = duodenum
esophag/o = esophagus
gastr/o = stomach
-itis = inflammation

col/o = colon
diverticul/o = diverticulum
-osis = condition
rect/o = rectum

diverticulum (plural, diverticula) is a small sac or pouch in the wall of an organ. **Diverticulosis** is the presence of diverticula without inflammation, a condition that affects a number of people older than 50 years and may cause few symptoms.

duodenal ulcer (duoden/o, duodenum + -al, pertaining to) an ulcer of the duodenum. Bleeding is sometimes present with this type of ulcer. Perforation can occur, which can lead to peritonitis (periton/o, peritoneum).

duodenitis inflammation of the duodenum.

enterostasis (enter/o, intestine + -stasis, stopping) stoppage or delay in the passage of food through the intestine.

hemorrhoids masses of veins in the anal canal that are unnaturally distended and lie just inside or outside the rectum. They are often accompanied by pain, itching, and bleeding.

irritable bowel syndrome (IBS) abnormally increased motility of the small and large intestines of unknown origin. Most of those affected are young adults who report diarrhea and occasionally pain in the abdomen, usually relieved by passing gas or stool. Also called functional bowel syndrome, mucous colitis, or spastic colon.

lower gastrointestinal bleeding bleeding of the lower digestive structures (see Figure 9-11, *B*).

Gallbladder

cholecystitis (cholecyst/o, gallbladder) inflammation of the gallbladder.

cholelithiasis (chol/e, gall or bile + lith/o, stone + -iasis, condition) formation or presence of gall-stones in the gallbladder or common bile duct.

cholestasis stoppage of bile excretion.

Liver

cirrhosis chronic liver disease characterized by marked degeneration of liver cells.

hepatitis (hepat/o, liver) inflammation of the liver.

hepatomegaly (-megaly, enlargement) enlargement of the liver.

Pancreas

diabetes general term for diseases characterized by excessive urination, but it usually refers to diabetes mellitus.

hypoglycemia (hypo-, below normal + glyc/o, sugar + -emia, blood) condition in which the blood glucose level is abnormally low. It can be caused by excessive production of insulin by the pancreas or by excessive injection of insulin.

pancreatitis (pancreat/o, pancreas) inflammation of the pancreas.

CIRCLE IT! **EXERCISE 9**

Choose the correct answer to complete each sentence.

1. The presence of gallstones in the gallbladder or common bile duct is (cholecystitis, cholecystography, cholelithiasis, cholestasis).
2. One type of liver disease is (cirrhosis, diverticulitis, dysphagia, splenomegaly).
3. A lesion of a mucous membrane accompanied by sloughing of dead tissue is (dysphagia, diverticulitis, a hemorrhoid, an ulcer).
4. A hiatal hernia is one type of (enterostasis, esophagitis, gastrocele, peptic ulcer).
5. Inflammation of the tongue is (cheilitis, gingivitis, glossitis, stomatitis).
6. Varicose veins of the anal canal are called (diverticula, hemorrhoids, hepatitis, hepatomegaly).

WRITE IT! **EXERCISE 10**

Write a term for each description.

1. inflammation of the esophagus _____
2. inflammation of the stomach and intestinal tract _____
3. stoppage or delay in the passage of food through the intestine _____
4. endoscopic inspection of the stomach _____
5. inflammation of the gallbladder _____
6. chronic liver disease with marked degeneration of liver cells _____

Surgical and Therapeutic Interventions

Patients who can digest and absorb nutrients but need nutritional support may receive enteral nutrition, introducing nutrients directly into the gastrointestinal tract when the patient cannot chew, ingest, or swallow food. This is accomplished by using an enteral feeding tube, including a **nasogastric** tube, a **nasoduodenal** tube, or a **nasojejunal** tube. In some patients the tube is inserted through a new opening made in the esophagus, stomach, or jejunum (**esophagostomy, gastrostomy,** or **jejunostomy,** respectively). Note the location of these types of enteral feeding tubes in Figure 9-12.

enter/o = intestine
nas/o = nose
gastr/o = stomach

Conservative approaches to weight loss for obese individuals include restricted food intake and increased exercise. An appetite-suppressing drug is an **anorexiant**. Surgical approaches for treating extreme obesity, generally used when conservative methods have failed, limit food intake or absorption by either **gastro+plasty** or **gastric bypass**. These surgeries reduce the stomach's capacity.

Several pharmaceuticals are helpful in the treatment of gastrointestinal problems, in addition to antibiotics that are used to treat infections. **Anti+diarrheals** are used to treat diarrhea and **anti+emetics** to relieve or prevent vomiting. To induce (cause) vomiting in an individual in the emergency treatment of drug overdose or certain cases of poisoning, **emetics** are used. **Laxatives** cause evacuation of the bowel and may be prescribed to correct constipation. **Purgatives** or **cathartics** are strong medications used to promote full evacuation of the bowel, as in preparation for diagnostic studies or surgery of the digestive tract.

Some forms of diabetes are treated with diet, exercise, and weight control, and other forms require glucose-lowering agents (oral agents or insulin by injection). Individuals with type 1 diabetes, as well as some with type 2 diabetes, require an outside source of insulin.

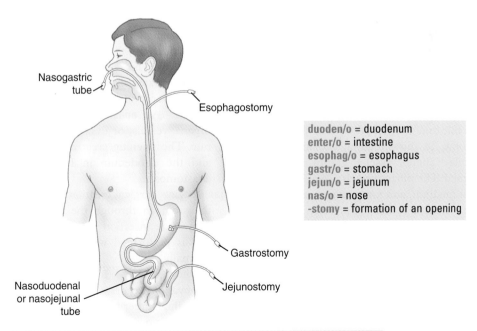

duoden/o = duodenum
enter/o = intestine
esophag/o = esophagus
gastr/o = stomach
jejun/o = jejunum
nas/o = nose
-stomy = formation of an opening

Figure 9-12 Common locations for placement of enteral feeding tubes.

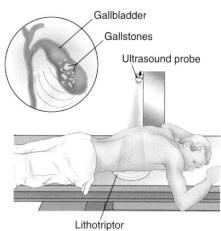

Gallbladder

Gallstones

Ultrasound probe

Lithotriptor

-ary = pertaining to
bil/i = bile
lith/o = stone
-triptor = instrument used for crushing
ultra- = beyond, excess

Figure 9-13 Biliary lithotripsy. The gallbladder is positioned over the lithotriptor. The lithotriptor is then fired, and particles slough off the gallstones until they are fragmented and can pass through the biliary ducts.

lith/o = stone
-tripsy = surgical
    crushing

lapar/o =
    abdominal wall
cholecyst/o =
    gallbladder
-ectomy = excision

Gallstones are a common disorder of the gallbladder, and nonsurgical treatments include oral drugs that dissolve stones, **laser lithotripsy**, and **shock wave lithotripsy** (Figure 9-13). Although these procedures are called lithotripsy, there is no surgical incision. The methods rely on laser or a high-energy shock wave to disintegrate the stone, and the particles pass through the biliary ducts and are eliminated. If these methods fail, cholecystectomy may be necessary. When possible, **laparoscopic chole-cystectomy** is performed. In the latter procedure, the gallbladder is excised with a laser and removed through a small incision in the abdominal wall.

The following list provides additional information about surgical procedures of the digestive organs.

appendectomy (append/o, appendix + -ectomy, excision) removal of the vermiform appendix. It is removed when it is acutely infected to prevent peritonitis, which can occur if the appendix ruptures.

cholecystectomy (cholecyst/o, gallbladder) surgical removal of the gallbladder. Exploration of the common bile duct is often performed during cholecystectomy. In this situation, cholangiography (chol/e, bile + angi/o, vessel + -graphy, recording) is performed. The biliary vessels are injected with a contrast medium, and x-ray images are taken to determine whether stones are present.

colostomy (col/o, colon + -stomy, artificial opening) creation of an artificial anus on the abdominal wall by incising the colon and drawing it out to the surface. It is performed when the feces cannot pass through the colon and out through the anus.

gastrectomy (gastr/o, stomach) surgical removal of all or part of the stomach (Figure 9-14). When the remaining portion of the stomach is joined to the duodenum, the procedure is called **gastroduo-denostomy**. This is a type of duodenal anastomosis. Translated literally, anastomosis (from the Greek word *anastomoien*) means "to provide a mouth." An **anastomosis** is the joining of two organs, vessels, or ducts that are normally separate. The opening created between the stomach and the duodenum in Figure 9-14, *B*, is an anastomosis.

gastrostomy surgical creation of a new opening into the stomach through the abdominal wall. This allows the insertion of a synthetic feeding tube and is performed when the patient cannot eat normally.

hemorrhoidectomy (hemorrhoid/o, hemorrhoid) removal of hemorrhoids by any of several means, including surgery.

ileostomy (ile/o, ileum) creation of a surgical passage through the abdominal wall into the ileum. An

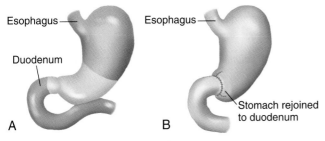

Esophagus —

Esophagus —

Duodenum

Stomach rejoined
to duodenum

A

B

-al = pertaining to
dist/o = distant from the point of attachment
duoden/o = duodenum
-ectomy = excision
gastr/o = stomach
-stomy = formation of an opening

Figure 9-14 Partial gastrectomy. A, The stomach before surgery, showing the distal acid-secreting portion *(tan).* **B,** The stomach after surgery. A new opening has been made between the stomach and the duodenum, the first part of the small intestine. This type of surgery, gastroduodenostomy, might be performed for severe chronic gastric ulcers.

ileostomy is necessary when the large intestine has been removed. Fecal material from the ileum drains through an opening called a **stoma** into a bag worn on the abdomen.

laparoscopy (lapar/o, abdominal wall + -scopy, visual examination) examination of the abdominal cavity with a laparoscope through one or more small incisions in the abdominal wall. The procedure is done for inspection of abdominal organs, particularly the ovaries and uterine tubes, and also for laparoscopic surgeries, such as a laparoscopic cholecystectomy.

liver biopsy removal of tissue from the liver for pathologic examination. A **percutaneous liver biopsy** is removal of liver tissue by using a needle to puncture the skin overlying the liver. This is considered to be a closed biopsy. (Percutaneous is derived from per-, through + cutane/o, skin + -ous, pertaining to.) An open liver biopsy involves incision of the abdominal wall to remove liver tissue for pathologic examination.

pancreatolithectomy (pancreat/o, pancreas + -lith, stone + -ectomy, excision) excision of a pancreatic stone.

vagotomy (vag/o, vagus nerve + -tomy, incision) resection (partial excision) of portions of the vagus nerve near the stomach. This procedure is performed to decrease the amount of gastric juices by severing the nerve (vagus nerve) that controls their release.

MATCH IT!

EXERCISE 11

Match the procedures in the left column with their descriptions.

_____ **1.** appendectomy
_____ **2.** cholecystectomy
_____ **3.** colostomy
_____ **4.** esophagostomy
_____ **5.** gastrectomy
_____ **6.** gastric bypass
_____ **7.** gastrostomy
_____ **8.** laparoscopy

A. an opening from the colon through the abdominal wall
B. examination of the abdominal cavity through a small incision in the abdominal wall
C. excision of the gallbladder
D. new opening into the esophagus
E. new opening into the stomach
F. removal of the vermiform appendix
G. surgery performed to reduce the stomach's capacity
H. surgical removal of the stomach

 Be Careful with These!

-orexia (appetite) versus *-pepsia* (digestion)
choledoch/o (common bile duct) versus *cholecyst/o* (gallbladder)

SELF-TEST   Work the following exercises to test your understanding of the material in Chapter 9. Complete all the exercises before using Appendix VIII to check your answers.

A. MATCH IT!   *Match the diagnostic test or procedure in the left column with the digestive structure in the right column that is the focus of study.*

_____ **1.** cholangiography   **A.** bile ducts
_____ **2.** esophagram   **B.** esophagus
_____ **3.** gastroscopy   **C.** rectum
_____ **4.** proctoscopy   **D.** salivary ducts
_____ **5.** sialography   **E.** stomach

B. MATCH IT!   *Match activities of the digestive system with their meanings.*

_____ **1.** absorption   **A.** mechanical and chemical breakdown of food
_____ **2.** digestion   **B.** oral taking of substances into the body
_____ **3.** elimination   **C.** passage of food molecules through the small intestine lining
_____ **4.** ingestion   **D.** removal of undigested food particles

C. CIRCLE IT!   *Choose the one correct answer (a, b, c, or d) for each question.*

1. Mrs. Vogel's physician tells her that she needs to see a specialist for the problem that she's been having with her colon. What is the name of the specialty practiced by the physician Mrs. Vogel should see?
(a) cardiology   (b) gastroenterology   (c) gynecology   (d) urology

2. Tests show that Cal S. has a gallstone in the common bile duct. Which of the following is a noninvasive conservative procedure to alleviate Cal's problem?
(a) cholecystostomy   (b) choledochostomy   (c) choledochojejunostomy   (d) shock wave lithotripsy

3. Linda M., a 16-year-old girl, is diagnosed as having self-induced starvation. What is the name of the disorder associated with Linda's problem?
(a) anorexia nervosa   (b) aphagia   (c) malaise   (d) polyphagia

4. Unless there is intervention for Linda's self-induced starvation, which condition will result?
(a) adipsia   (b) atresia   (c) emaciation   (d) volvulus

5. Mary suffers from GERD. The physician explains to her that radiography indicates that a portion of the stomach is protruding upward through the diaphragm. What is the name of this disorder?
(a) anorexia nervosa   (b) caries   (c) cholelith   (d) hiatal hernia

6. A 70-year-old woman has an obstruction that has led to stagnation of the normal movement of food in the intestinal tract. What is the name of this condition?
(a) duodenitis   (b) enterostasis   (c) peptic ulcer   (d) peristalsis

7. Which term means a procedure that provides radiographic visualization of the bile and pancreatic ducts?
(a) barium enema   (b) cholangiopancreatography   (c) gastrostomy   (d) sigmoidoscopy

8. Which of the following is the main source of energy for body cells?
(a) fats   (b) glucose   (c) lactose   (d) starches

9. Which of the following is a disorder characterized by episodes of binge eating that are terminated by abdominal pain, sleep, self-induced vomiting, or purging with laxatives?
(a) anorexia nervosa   (b) bulimia   (c) Crohn disease   (d) malabsorption syndrome

10. Which of the following is the name of the procedure in which the stomach is anastomosed with the duodenum?
(a) gastrectasis   (b) gastrotomy   (c) gastroduodenostomy   (d) lithotripsy

SELF-TEST (cont'd)

D. WRITE IT!   *Write one-word terms for each of these meanings.*

1. a new opening into the jejunum   _____

2. an appetite-suppressing drug   _____

3. enzyme that breaks down starch   _____

4. excessive vomiting   _____

5. excision of a pancreatic stone   _____

6. incision of the vagus nerve   _____

7. inflammation of the stomach   _____

8. pertaining to the esophagus   _____

9. poor digestion   _____

10. presence of a gallstone   _____

E. SPELL IT!   *Circle the incorrectly spelled terms, and write the correct spelling.*

1. cholangiograpfy   _____

2. enterel   _____

3. hepatik   _____

4. lithotripter   _____

5. diabetis mellitus   _____

F. WRITE IT!   *Name the three major classes of nutrients.*

1. _____

2. _____

3. _____

G. FINDING THE CLUE!   *Use a clue to write terms for these descriptions. Solve Question 1; each ending letter becomes the clue for the first letter of the next answer.*

1. artificial opening of an internal organ on the body's surface   _____

2. a connection between two vessels or ducts   _____

3. part of the colon that is S-shaped   _____

4. pouchlike herniation through the muscular wall of the colon   _____

5. the lower jaw   _____

6. normal digestion   _____

7. process of providing nutrition for the body   _____

8. pertaining to the nose and stomach   _____

9. type of ulcer often associated with stomatitis   _____

10. lower part of the large intestine   _____

Continued

H. READING HEALTH REPORTS *Read the medical report and answer the questions that follow it. Although you may be unfamiliar with some of the terms, you should be able to decide their meanings by determining the word parts.*

MEDICAL REPORT   **Mid-City Medical Center**

222 Medical Center Drive   **Main City, USA 63017-1000**   **Phone:** (555) 434-0000
                                                                    Fax: (555) 434-0001

OPERATIVE REPORT

Patient: Gloria Rush   **DOB:** 10/12/50   **Date of Surgery:** 1/12/2009
Preoperative Diagnosis: Probable neoplasm of the distal rectum
Postoperative Diagnosis: Same
Surgeon: Dr. James Miller
Anesthesiologist: Dr. Harvey Bell   **Anesthesia:** Propofol
Surgery Performed: Colonoscopy to the cecum with multiple biopsies of rectal mass.

Indications

The patient is a 55-year-old woman who has been experiencing progressive constipation and blood in the stool for 3 weeks. She also had pelvic and rectal pressure. A sonogram showed a large pelvic mass between the rectum and the vagina. She has a history of diverticulitis and cholecystectomy.

What Was Done

The patient was brought to the gastrointestinal lab and sedated with propofol, and the colonoscope was passed per anus to what appeared to be the cecum. It appeared that the ileocecal valve was visible, but due to poor preparation, the appendiceal orifice could not be identified. A hard mass was seen in the distal rectum. Multiple biopsies were taken. There were numerous small lesions in the ascending, transverse, descending, sigmoid, and rectosigmoid colon.

Treatment Plan

Patient requires an urgent exploratory laparotomy, with a probable colectomy and ileostomy.

Dr. James Miller
James Miller, M.D.

Circle the one correct answer for each question.

1. To which body structure does the diagnosis pertain?
(a) gallbladder   (b) large intestine   (c) small intestine   (d) stomach
2. Which of the following describes the rectum in the preoperative diagnosis?
(a) abnormal new growth   (b) enlarged   (c) inflamed   (d) impacted with feces
3. The patient has a history of cholecystectomy. Which organ is removed in a cholecystectomy?
(a) colon   (b) gallbladder   (c) liver   (d) small intestine
4. What structure is incised in a laparotomy?
(a) abdominal wall   (b) cecum   (c) ileum   (d) umbilicus
5. All or part of which structure is excised in a colectomy?
(a) large intestine   (b) small intestine   (c) stomach   (d) umbilicus
6. Where is the stoma created in an ileostomy?
(a) abdomen   (b) anus   (c) colon   (d) umbilicus
7. Which of the following procedures is performed in a colonoscopy?
(a) barium enema   (b) endoscopic examination   (c) liver function test   (d) radiographic examination
8. Which term in the report means inflammation of small pouches in the intestinal wall?
(a) appendiceal orifice   (b) diverticulitis   (c) neoplasm   (d) rectal mass

Q&E List

Use the Companion CD or audio CDs to review the terms presented in Chapter 9.
Look closely at the spelling of each term as it is pronounced.

absorption (**ab-sorp´shən**)
alimentary (**al˝ə-men´tər-e**)
alimentary tract (**al˝ə-men´tər-e trakt**)
alimentation (**al˝ə-men-ta´shən**)
amylase (**am´ə-lās**)
anal (**a´nəl**)
anastomosis (**ə-nas˝tə-mo´sis**)
anorexia (**an˝o-rek´se-ə**)
anorexia nervosa (**an˝o-rek´se-ə ner-vo´sə**)
anorexiant (**an˝o-rek´se-ənt**)
antacid (**ant-as´id**)
antidiarrheal (**an˝te-, an˝ti-di˝ə-re´əl**)
antiemetic (**an˝te-ə-met´ik**)
anus (**a´nəs**)
appendectomy (**ap˝en-dek´tə-me**)
appendicitis (**ə-pen˝dĭ-si´tis**)
ascending colon (**ə-send´ing ko´lon**)
barium enema (**bar´e-əm en´ə-mə**)
barium meal (**bar´e-əm mēl**)
barium swallow (**bar´e-əm swahl´o**)
bicuspids (**bi-kus´pids**)
bile (**bīl**)
biliary (**bil´e-ar-e**)
biliary tract (**bil´e-ar-e trakt**)
bulimia (**bŏŏ-le´me-ə**)
canker sores (**kang´kər sorz**)
carbohydrates (**kahr˝bo-hi´drāts**)
cathartic (**kə-thahr´tik**)
cecum (**se´kəm**)
cheilitis (**ki-li´tis**)
cholangiogram (**ko-lan´je-o-gram**)
cholangiography (**ko-lan˝je-og´rə-fe**)
cholangitis (**ko´lan-ji´tis**)
cholecystectomy (**ko´lə-sis-tek´tə-me**)
cholecystic (**ko˝lə-sis´tik**)
cholecystitis (**ko˝lə-sis-ti´tis**)
choledochal (**ko-led´ə-kəl**)
choledocholithiasis (**ko-led´ə-ko-lĭ-thi´ə-sis**)
cholelithiasis (**ko˝lə-lĭ-thi´ə-sis**)
cholestasis (**ko´lə-sta´sis**)
cirrhosis (**sĭ-ro´sis**)
colitis (**ko-li´tis**)

colon (**ko´lən**)
colonoscope (**ko-lon´o-skōp**)
colonoscopy (**ko´lən-os´kə-pe**)
coloscopy (**ko-los´ko-pe**)
colostomy (**kə-los´tə-me**)
cuspids (**kus´pids**)
defecation (**def´ə-ka´shən**)
dehydration (**de˝hi-dra´shən**)
dental (**den´təl**)
descending colon (**de-send´ing ko´lon**)
diabetes (**di˝ə-be´tēz**)
diabetes mellitus (**di˝ə-be´tēz mel´lə-təs, mə-li´tis**)
diarrhea (**di˝ə-re´ə**)
digestion (**di-jes´chən**)
diverticulectomy (**di˝vər-tik˝u-lek´tə-me**)
diverticulitis (**di˝vər-tik˝u-li´tis**)
diverticulosis (**di˝vər-tik˝u-lo´sis**)
diverticulum (**di˝vər-tik´u-ləm**)
duodenal (**doo˝o-de´nəl, doo-od´ə-nəl**)
duodenal ulcer (**doo˝o-de´nəl, doo-od´ə-nəl ul´sər**)
duodenitis (**doo-od˝ə-ni´tis**)
duodenum (**doo˝o-de´nəm, doo-od´ə-nəm**)
dyspepsia (**dis-pep´se-ə**)
dysphagia (**dis-fa´je-ə**)
elimination (**e-lim˝ĭ-na´shən**)
emaciation (**e-ma˝she-a´shən**)
emesis (**em´ə-sis**)
emetics (**ə-met´iks**)
endogastric (**en˝do-gas´trik**)
enteral (**en´tər-əl**)
enterostasis (**en˝tər-o-sta´sis**)
enzymes (**en´zīms**)
esophageal (**ə-sof´ə-je´əl**)
esophageal varices (**ə-sof´ə-je´əl văr˝ĭ-sēz**)
esophagitis (**ə-sof˝ə-ji´tis**)
esophagogram (**ə-sof´ə-go-gram**)
esophagoscopy (**ə-sof˝ə-gos´ko-pe**)
esophagostomy (**ə-sof˝ə-gos´tə-me**)
esophagram (**ə-sof´ə-gram**)
esophagus (**ə-sof´ə-gəs**)
eupepsia (**u-pep´se-ə**)
flatulence (**flat´u-ləns**)

continued

gallstone (**gawl´stōn**)

gastralgia (**gas-tral´jə**)

gastrectomy (**gas-trek´tə-me**)

gastric (**gas´trik**)

gastric bypass (**gas´trik bi´pas**)

gastric lavage (**gas´trik lah-vahzh´**)

gastritis (**gas-tri´tis**)

gastrocele (**gas´tro-sēl**)

gastroduodenostomy (**gas´´tro-doo´´o-də-nos´tə-me**)

gastrodynia (**gas´´tro-din´e-ə**)

gastroenteritis (**gas´´tro-en´´tər-i´tis**)

gastroenterologist (**gas´´tro-en´´tər-ol´ə-jist**)

gastroenterology (**gas´´tro-en´´tər-ol´ə-je**)

gastroesophageal reflux disease (**gas´´tro-ĕ-sof´´ə-je´əl re´fləks dĭ-zēz´**)

gastrointestinal (**gas´´tro-in-tes´tĭ-nəl**)

gastroplasty (**gas´tro-plas´´te**)

gastroscopy (**gas-tros´kə-pe**)

gastrostomy (**gas-tros´tə-me**)

gestational diabetes mellitus (**jes-ta´shun-al di´´ə-be´tēz mel´lə-təs, mə-li´tis**)

gingiva (**jin´jĭ-və, jin-ji´və**)

gingival (**jin´jĭ-vəl**)

gingivitis (**jin´´jĭ-vi´tis**)

glossal (**glos´əl**)

glossitis (**glos-i´tis**)

glucose (**gloo´kōs**)

glycosuria (**gli´´ko-su´re-ə**)

hemorrhoid (**hem´ə-roid**)

hemorrhoidectomy (**hem´´ə-roid-ek´tə-me**)

hepatic (**hə-pat´ik**)

hepatitis (**hep´´ə-ti´tis**)

hepatomegaly (**hep´´ə-to-meg´ə-le**)

hepatotoxic (**hep´ə-to-tok´´sik**)

hiatal hernia (**hi-a´təl hur´ne-ə**)

hiatus (**hi-a´təs**)

hyperacidity (**hi´´pər-ə-sid´ĭ-te**)

hyperemesis (**hi´´pər-em´ə-sis**)

hyperglycemia (**hi´´pər-gli-se´me-ə**)

hyperlipemia (**hi´´pər-li-pe´me-ə**)

hyperlipidemia (**hi´´pər-lip´´ĭ-de´me-ə**)

hypoglossal (**hi´´po-glos´əl**)

hypoglycemia (**hi´´po-gli-se´me-ə**)

ileocecal (**il´´e-o-se´kəl**)

ileostomy (**il´´e-os´tə-me**)

ileum (**il´e-əm**)

incisors (**in-si´zərs**)

ingestion (**in-jes´chən**)

inguinal (**ing´gwĭ-nəl**)

insulin (**in´sə-lin**)

intestinal (**in-tes´tĭ-nəl**)

irritable bowel syndrome (**ir´ĭ-tə-bəl bou´əl sin´drōm**)

jaundice (**jawn´dis**)

jejunostomy (**jĕ´´joo-nos´tə-me**)

jejunum (**jə-joo´nəm**)

lactase (**lak´tās**)

lactose (**lak´tōs**)

laparoscopic cholecystectomy (**lap´´ə-ro-skop´ik ko´´lə-sis-tek´tə-me**)

laparoscopy (**lap´´ə-ros´kə-pe**)

laser lithotripsy (**la´zer lith´o-trip´´se**)

laxative (**lak´sə-tiv**)

lingual (**ling´gwəl**)

lipase (**lip´ās, li´pās**)

lipid (**lip´id**)

liver biopsy (**liv´ər bi´op-se**)

lower gastrointestinal bleeding (**lo´ər gas´´tro-in-tes´tĭ-nəl blēd´ing**)

malabsorption syndrome (**mal´´əb-sorp´shən sin´drōm**)

malnutrition (**mal´´noo-trish´ən**)

mandible (**man´dĭ-bəl**)

mandibular (**man-dib´u-lər**)

metabolism (**mə-tab´ə-liz´´əm**)

molars (**mo´lərs**)

mucous (**mu´kəs**)

mucus (**mu´kəs**)

nasoduodenal (**na´´zo-doo´´o-de´nəl**)

nasogastric (**na´´zo-gas´trik**)

nasojejunal (**na´´zo-jə-joo´nəl**)

nutrition (**noo-trī´shən**)

obesity (**o-bēs´ĭ-te**)

oral (**or´əl**)

orthodontics (**or´´tho-don´tiks**)

orthodontist (**or´´tho-don´tist**)

pancreatitis (**pan´´kre-ə-ti´tis**)

pancreatolith (**pan´´kre-at´o-lith**)

pancreatolithectomy (**pan´´kre-ə-to-lĭ-thek´tə-me**)

pancreatolithiasis (**pan´´kre-ə-to-lĭ-thi´ə-sis**)

pedodontics (**pe-do-don´tiks**)

percutaneous liver biopsy (**pur´´ku-ta´ne-əs liv´ər bi´op-se**)

periodontal (**per´´e-o-don´təl**)

periodontics (per´´e-o-don´tiks)
periodontium (per´´e-o-don´she-əm)
peritoneum (per´´ĭ-to-ne´əm)
peritonitis (per´´ĭ-to-ni´tis)
pharynx (far´inks)
polydipsia (pol´´e-dip´se-ə)
polyphagia (pol´´e-fa´jə)
polyuria (pol´´e-u´re-ə)
proctologist (prok-tol´ə-jist)
proctoscope (prok´to-skōp)
proctoscopy (prok-tos´kə-pe)
protease (pro´te-ās)
protein (pro´tēn)
proteinase (pro´tēn-ās)
purgative (pur´gə-tiv)
rectal (rek´təl)
rectum (rek´təm)
saliva (sə-li´və)

salivary (sal´ĭ-var-e)
shock wave lithotripsy (shok wāv lith´o-trip´´se)
sialography (si´´ə-log´rə-fe)
sialolithiasis (si´´ə-lo-lĭ-thi´ə-sis)
sigmoid colon (sig´moid ko´lon)
sigmoidoscopy (sig´´moi-dos´kə-pe)
stoma (sto´mə)
stomatitis (sto´´mə-ti´tis)
sublingual (səb-ling´gwəl)
transverse colon (trans-vərs´ ko´lon)
ulcer (ul´sər)
upper gastrointestinal bleeding (up´ər
    gas´´tro-in-tes´tĭ-nəl blēd´ing)
vagotomy (va-got´ə-me)
vermiform appendix (vur´mĭ-form ə-pen´diks)
viscera (vis´ər-ə)
visceral (vis´ər-əl)

 Don't forget the games on the Companion CD and http://evolve.elsevier.com/Leonard/quick/ for additional review, including questions on Spanish medical terms.

ESPAÑOL Enhancing Spanish Communication

English	Spanish (pronunciation)
appetite	apetito (ah-pay-TEE-to)
chew, to	masticar (mas-te-CAR)
digestion	digestión (de-hes-te-ON)
gallbladder	vesícula biliar (vay-SEE-coo-la be-le-AR)
gallstone	cálculo biliar (CAHL-coo-lo be-le-AR)
gum, gingiva	encía (en-SEE-ah)
hunger	hambre (AHM-bray)
liver	hígado (EE-ga-do)
nutrition	nutrición (noo-tre-se-ON)
pancreas	páncreas (PAHN-cray-as)
rectum	recto (REK-to)
swallow	tragar (trah-GAR)
tongue	lengua (LEN-goo-ah)
tooth (teeth)	diente, dientes (de-AYN-tay, de-AYN-tays)
ulcer	ulcera (OOL-say-rah)

CHAPTER 10
Urinary System

CONTENTS

Function First
Structures of the Urinary Tract
Diseases, Disorders, and Diagnostic Terms
Surgical and Therapeutic Interventions

Self-Test
Q&E List
Enhancing Spanish Communication

OBJECTIVES

After completing Chapter 10, you will be able to:

1. Recognize or write the functions of the urinary system.
2. Recognize or write the meanings of Chapter 10 word parts and use them to build and analyze terms.
3. Write terms for selected structures of the urinary system, or match them with their descriptions.

4. Write the names of the diagnostic terms and pathologies related to the urinary system when given their descriptions, or match terms with their meanings.
5. Match surgical and therapeutic interventions for the urinary system, or write the interventions when given their descriptions.
6. Spell terms for the urinary system correctly.

Function First

The body produces wastes that are eliminated by the process of **excretion**. The body eliminates waste in several ways. The lungs and other parts of the respiratory system eliminate carbon dioxide; the digestive system rids the body of solid waste; and the skin eliminates wastes through perspiration. Through urination, the urinary system eliminates waste products that accumulate as a result of cellular metabolism. **Urin+ation** is the act of voiding.

Excretion of wastes to maintain the volume and chemical composition of blood is only one function of the urinary system. Most of the work of this body system takes place in the kidneys. The functions of the kidneys include the following:

- Maintenance of an appropriate blood volume by varying the excretion of water in the urine
- Maintenance of the chemical composition of blood by selecting certain chemicals to excrete
- Maintenance of blood pH
- Excretion of waste products of protein metabolism
- Regulation of blood pressure
- Stimulation of erythrocyte production by secreting **erythro+poietin**

> **QUICK TIP**
>
> *pH, "potential" hydrogen (hydrogen ion concentration) of a solution, its relative acidity or alkalinity*

> erythr/o = red
> -poietin = substance that causes production

Excretion of waste products by the kidneys is vital for good health. **Urea** is the final product of protein metabolism and the major nitrogenous waste product present in urine.

Uro+logy is the branch of medicine concerned with the male genital tract and the urinary tracts of both genders. A **urologist** is a physician who specializes in the practice of urology.

ur/o = urinary tract
-logy = science of

WRITE IT!
EXERCISE 1

Write a word in each blank to complete the functions of the urinary system.

1. excretion of _____ in urine to maintain blood volume

2. maintaining the chemical composition of _____

3. maintaining the blood pH, also called the "potential" _____

4. excretion of _____ products of protein metabolism

5. regulation of blood _____

6. secretion of _____ to stimulate erythrocyte production

Use Appendix VIII to check your answers to all the exercises in Chapter 10.

Many word parts in the following table are used to write terms about the urinary system. Commit the word parts and their meanings to memory.

Word Parts Associated with the Urinary System	
Word Part	**Meaning**
albumin/o	albumin
-ation	process
-esis	action, process, or result of
glycos/o	sugar
olig/o	few, scanty
ur/o	urine or urinary tract
urin/o	urine
-uria	urine or urination

Use the electronic flashcards on the Evolve site or make your own set of flashcards using the above list. Select the word parts just presented, and study them until you know their meanings. Do this each time a set of word parts is presented.

MATCH IT!
EXERCISE 2

Match the word parts in the left column with their meanings.

_____ **1.** -ation

_____ **2.** -esis

_____ **3.** glycos/o

_____ **4.** olig/o

_____ **5.** ur/o

_____ **6.** -uria

A. action, process, or result of

B. few, scanty

C. process

D. sugar

E. urine or urination

F. urine or urinary tract

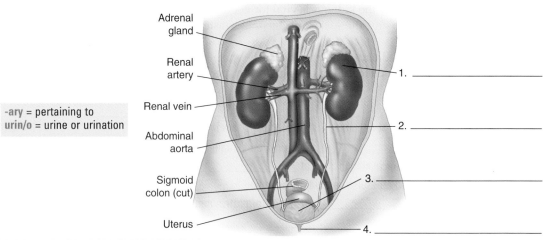

Figure 10-1 **Organs of the urinary system.** Select structures of other systems are also shown. Label the urinary structures as you read this explanation. Urine, formed in the right kidney and left kidney *(1)*, leaves by way of the ureters. Label the left ureter *(2)*. The bladder *(3)* is a temporary reservoir for the urine until it is excreted through the urethra *(4)*.

-ary = pertaining to
urin/o = urine or urination

Structures of the Urinary Tract

The urinary system is frequently called the urinary tract because its parts are arranged in a series and serve a common function to produce and eliminate urine. **Urin+ary** means pertaining to urine or the formation of urine. The urinary tract is composed of two kidneys, a ureter for each kidney, a bladder and a urethra. **Label these structures as you read the legend for Figure 10-1.**

urin/o = urine
-ary = pertaining to

The bean-shaped, purplish-brown kidneys are located in the dorsal part of the abdomen, one on each side of the spinal column. Each kidney functions independently of the other.

 QUICK TIP

Kidneys and kidney beans have similar shapes.

Urine leaves the kidneys by way of the **ureters**. Both ureters lead to the urinary bladder, where urine is stored. The filling of the bladder with urine stimulates receptors, producing the urge to urinate. Voluntary control prevents urine from being released. When this control is removed, urine is expelled through a canal called the **urethra**. The external opening of the urethra is the urinary meatus.

Combining forms for major structures of the urinary system are presented in the table. Commit these to memory.

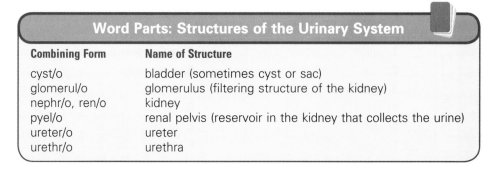

Word Parts: Structures of the Urinary System	
Combining Form	**Name of Structure**
cyst/o	bladder (sometimes cyst or sac)
glomerul/o	glomerulus (filtering structure of the kidney)
nephr/o, ren/o	kidney
pyel/o	renal pelvis (reservoir in the kidney that collects the urine)
ureter/o	ureter
urethr/o	urethra

Match the word parts in the two left columns with their meanings in the right column (a choice may be used more than once).

_____ **1.** cyst/o   _____ **4.** ren/o   **A.** bladder

_____ **2.** nephr/o   _____ **5.** ureter/o   **B.** kidney

_____ **3.** pyel/o   _____ **6.** urethr/o   **C.** renal pelvis

                                                   D. ureter

                                                   E. urethra

The adjectives **ren+al**, **ureter+al**, and **urethr+al** mean pertaining to the kidney, ureter, and urethra, respectively. **Cyst+ic** has several meanings, including pertaining to a cyst, pertaining to the gallbladder, and pertaining to the urinary bladder. The rest of the sentence must usually be read to determine the intended meaning of the word cystic. Used alone, bladder usually refers to the urinary bladder.

> cyst/o = urinary bladder *or* a cyst *or* a sac

Most of the work of the urinary system takes place in the kidneys. The other components serve to eliminate urine from the body. Anatomic features of the kidney are shown in Figure 10-2. A kidney is encased in a fibrous capsule, which provides protection for the delicate internal parts of the kidney. The ribs and muscle also provide protection from direct trauma. The renal pelvis is a funnel-shaped structure located in the center of each kidney. Each renal pelvis drains urine from the kidney to its particular ureter. Blood enters a kidney via the renal artery and leaves through the renal vein.

> fibr/o = fiber
> -ous = characterized by

Match the terms in the left column with their meanings.

_____ **1.** urinary bladder   **A.** funnel-shaped structure located in the center of each kidney

_____ **2.** renal pelvis   **B.** where urine is stored until urination

_____ **3.** ureter   **C.** tube through which urine passes from the kidney

_____ **4.** urethra   **D.** tubular passage by which urine is discharged from the bladder

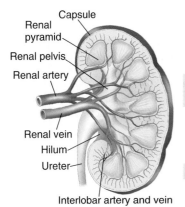

Capsule
Renal pyramid
Renal pelvis
Renal artery
Renal vein
Hilum
Ureter
Interlobar artery and vein

> inter- = between
> ren/o = kidney

Figure 10-2 The kidney (sectioned). The kidney has a convex contour with the exception of the hilum, a notch on the inner border.

A kidney contains approximately 1 million microscopic **nephrons**, its functional unit. Each nephron resembles a microscopic funnel with a long stem and tubular sections, called the **tubules** (Figure 10-3). A **glomerulus** is a cluster of blood vessels surrounded by a structure called a Bowman's capsule. The proxim+al tubule is that part of the tubule nearer the glomerulus. Follow the long twisting tubule. Notice that a tubule consists of a proximal tubule, a loop of Henle, and a dist+al tubule that opens into a collecting duct.

glomerul/o = glomerulus

proxim/o = near

dist/o = far

The kidneys constantly filter the blood, selectively reabsorb some substances, and secrete waste substances into the urine. These functions directly relate to urine formation as follows:

QUICK TIP

reabsorption, *process of being absorbed back into the blood*

- Filtering of the blood = glomerular filtration, the initial process in the formation of urine. The glomerulus allows water, salts, wastes, and most other substances, except blood cells and proteins, to pass through its thin walls.
- Selective reabsorption of some substances = tubular reabsorption. Bowman's capsule collects the substances that filter through the glomerular walls and passes them to a long, twisted tube called a tubule. As fluid passes through the tubules, substances that the body conserves, such as sugar and much of the water, are reabsorbed into the blood vessels surrounding the tubules. The water and other substances remaining in the tubule become urine.

QUICK TIP

Filtering System
1. Filter
2. Reabsorb
3. Secrete

- Secretion of substances into the urine = tubular secretion. The third process in urine formation is the secretion of some substances from the bloodstream into the renal tubule (waste products of metabolism that become toxic if they are not excreted and certain drugs, such as penicillin). These three processes—glomerular filtration, tubular reabsorption, and tubular secretion—are summarized in Figure 10-4.

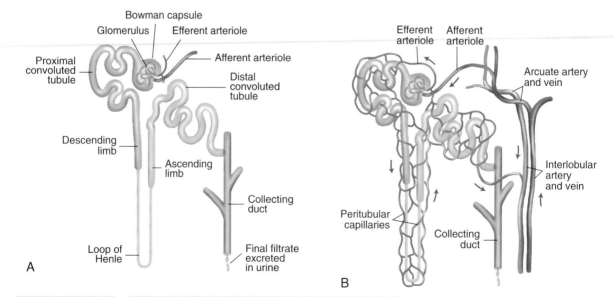

inter- = between
peri- = around

Figure 10-3 A nephron and surrounding capillaries. A, The nephron is composed of a glomerulus and tubules. **B,** As the filtrate passes through the tubular portion of the nephron, reabsorption of variable quantities of water, electrolytes, and other substances occurs across the tubule walls into blood capillaries nearby.

Waste products and some of the water remaining in the tubules after reabsorption combine to become urine, which passes to the collecting duct. Thousands of collecting ducts deposit urine in the renal pelvis, the large central reservoir of the kidney, where it drains to the bladder by way of the ureters. The bladder is a collapsible muscular bag that stores the urine until it is expelled by urination, also called voiding. Figure 10-5 is a schematic of the forming and expelling of urine.

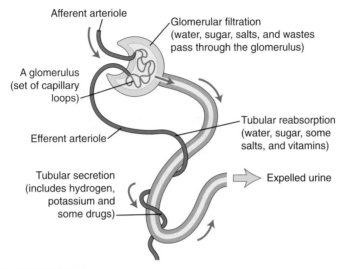

Figure 10-4 Functions of the nephron. Glomerular filtration *(upper right)*, tubular reabsorption, and tubular secretion *(lower left)*.

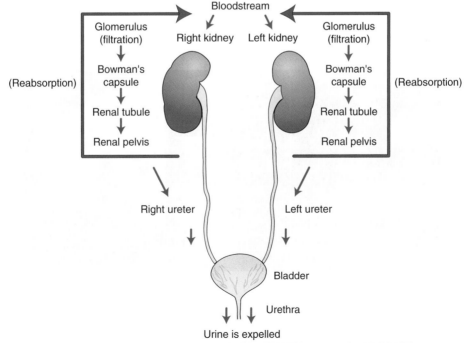

Figure 10-5 Diagram of the process of forming and expelling urine.

Anti+diuretic hormone (ADH) increases the reabsorption of water by the renal tubules, thus decreasing the amount of urine produced. **ADH is secreted by special brain cells and released as needed.**

Diseases, Disorders, and Diagnostic Terms

QUICK TIP

A urinalysis was originally called a urine analysis.

glycos/o = sugar
hemat/o = blood
py/o = pus
-uria = urine

Several urine tests are used to evaluate the status of the urinary system. A **urinalysis** (U/A, UA) is usually part of a physical examination but is particularly useful for patients with suspected urologic disorders. The complete urinalysis generally includes physical, chemical, and microscopic examinations performed in the clinical laboratory. Simple urine tests can provide valuable information about a person's health (Figure 10-6). Many substances for which urine is tested are not found in a normal urine specimen—for example, sugar, protein, and blood. The presence of one of these substances in urine is called **glycos+uria**, **protein+uria**, or **hemat+uria**, respectively. The term **albumin+uria** is sometimes used instead of proteinuria when there is a very high concentration of albumin, one type of protein, in the urine. **Py+uria** is the presence of pus in the urine.

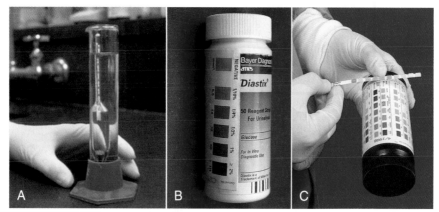

Figure 10-6 Simple urine tests. A, A urinometer is used to determine the specific gravity of a sample of urine. **B,** Glucose test strips screen for the presence of glucose in the urine. **C,** Testing urine with a Multistix, a plastic strip with reagent areas for testing various chemical constituents that may be present in the urine. These reagent strips are considered *qualitative* tests, and a positive result for an abnormal substance in the urine generally requires further testing.

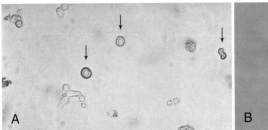 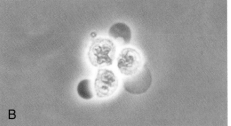

A   B

Figure 10-7 Increased number of red blood cells and white blood cells in a microscopic examination of urine. **A,** Red blood cells *(arrows).* **B,** White blood cells (the nucleated cells shown).

The microscopic study of a healthy urine sample sometimes shows a few red blood cells and white blood cells. Except in a menstruating woman, the presence of many red blood cells is abnormal (Figure 10-7, *A*). The presence of a large number of white blood cells may be indicative of an infectious or inflammatory process somewhere in the urinary tract (Figure 10-7, *B*).

Ketone bodies are end products of lipid (fat) metabolism in the body. Excessive production of ketone bodies, however, leads to **keton+uria**, the presence of ketones in the urine. Ketones are found in the urine when the body's fat stores are metabolized for energy, thus providing an excess of metabolic end products. This can occur in uncontrolled diabetes mellitus because of a deficiency of insulin. **Diabetes mellitus** is an endocrine disorder characterized by glycosuria and hyperglycemia (increased level of glucose in the blood) and results from inadequate production or use of insulin.

QUICK TIP
The onset of diabetes mellitus is sudden in children.

There are normally very few bacteria in freshly collected urine. The presence of many bacteria may indicate a urinary tract infection (UTI). If the patient has symptoms of a UTI, the physician often orders a urine culture and an antibiotic sensitivity test, to determine which drugs are effective in killing or stopping growth of the bacteria.

Urine specimens are collected according to the laboratory or physician's instructions. A *voided* specimen is one in which the patient voids (urinates) into a container supplied by the laboratory or physician's office. Because improperly collected urine may yield incorrect test results, voided urine should always be collected by using the "clean-catch midstream" technique. This technique is based on the concept that the tissues adjacent to the urethral opening must be cleansed before collection to avoid contamination of the specimen, and only the middle portion of the urine stream is collected. A catheterized urine specimen is obtained by placing a catheter in the bladder and withdrawing urine. This may be necessary to obtain an uncontaminated urine specimen. In urinary catheterization, a catheter is inserted through the urethra and into the bladder for temporary or longer-term drainage of urine. Urinary catheterization may be done to collect a urine specimen and for other reasons, including urinary testing, instillation of medications into the bladder, and drainage of the bladder during many types of surgeries or in cases of urinary obstruction or paralysis.

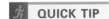
QUICK TIP
catheter = an instrument
catheterize (a verb)
catheterization (a noun)
catheterized (an adjective)

Blood urea nitrogen (BUN), a measure of the amount of urea in the blood, is directly related to the metabolic function of the liver and the excretory function of the kidneys.

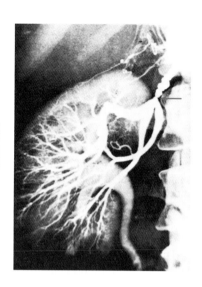

arteri/o = artery
-gram = a record
ren/o = kidney

Figure 10-8 Renal arteriogram showing stenosis of the right renal artery.

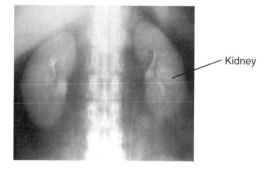

-gram = a record
nephr/o = kidney
tom/o = to cut

Kidney

Figure 10-9 Nephrotomogram. The procedure nephrotomography is helpful is assessing various planes of kidney tissue for tumors, cysts, or stones.

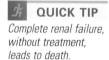

QUICK TIP

Complete renal failure, without treatment, leads to death.

A critically elevated BUN level indicates serious impairment of renal function. Another substance, creatinine, is measured in blood and urine as an indicator of kidney function.

Adequate blood circulation is essential for normal renal function, and anything that interferes with the normal circulation significantly reduces renal capabilities. **Renal angiography (renal arteriography)** is a radiographic study to assess the arterial blood supply to the kidneys. This procedure requires injection of a radiopaque contrast agent into the renal arteries by a catheter; the record produced is a **renal arteriogram**. An example of **stenosis** (constriction or narrowing) of the right renal artery is shown in Figure 10-8. A kidney scan also provides information about renal blood flow. In this procedure, radioactive material is intravenously injected and is absorbed by kidney tissue. Special equipment measures, records, and produces an image of the low-level radioactivity that is emitted.

Nephro+tomo+graphy, sectional radiographic examination of the kidneys, provides images (**nephrotomograms**) that can reveal tumors or stones (Figure 10-9). Other radiologic procedures are described in the programmed learning section, along with endoscopic examination of the urinary tract.

WRITE IT!   **EXERCISE 6**

Write a term for each description.

1. presence of albumin in the urine   _____
2. presence of blood in the urine   _____
3. presence of ketones in the urine   _____
4. presence of pus in the urine   _____
5. presence of sugar in the urine   _____
6. sectional radiographic examination of kidneys   _____
7. act of obtaining a catheterized urine specimen   _____
8. analysis of urine   _____

PROGRAMMED LEARNING

Remember to cover the answers (left column) with folded paper or the bookmark. Write an answer in each blank, and then check your answer before proceeding to the next frame.

kidney	1. **Nephro+malacia** is softening of the _____.
enlargement	2. **Nephro+megaly** is _____ of one or both kidneys. Bilateral nephromegaly is enlargement of both kidneys. Lateral pertains to a side. **Bi+lateral** (bi-, two) means pertaining to two sides—in other words, both sides.
kidneys	3. Nephromegaly and many other structural abnormalities of the kidneys (e.g., tumors or cancer, Figure 10-10) can be observed by **nephro+sonography**, which is ultrasonic scanning of the kidneys. Nephrosonography is the use of ultrasound to make a record (image) of the _____.

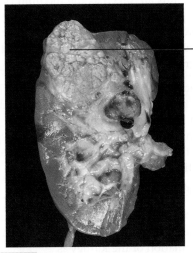

Cancerous tumor

Figure 10-10 Kidney cancer. Note the large tumor in this adult kidney that has been excised.

nephroptosis
stones
renal
kidney
renal
pyelitis
glomeruli
urogram
pyelogram
bladder
cystitis
nephritis

4. Remembering that -ptosis means sagging or prolapse, use nephr/o to write a word that means prolapse of a kidney: _____. This is also called a hypermobile (hyper-, excessive) or floating kidney. Nephroptosis can occur when the kidney supports are weakened by a sudden strain or blow, or the defect can be present at birth.

5. **Nephro+lith+iasis** is a condition marked by the presence of kidney _____.

6. **Nephro+lith** is a word, but kidney stones are usually called renal calculi. Notice that nephr/o is used more often in building medical terms, but ren/o is used to write an adjective that means pertaining to the kidney. Write that adjective: _____.

7. In a renal transplant, the recipient receives a _____ from a donor.

8. Pelvis means any basin-shaped structure or cavity. Standing alone, pelvis usually refers to the bony structure that serves as a support for the spinal column. When referring to the funnel-shaped cavity of the kidney, however, it is called the _____ pelvis.

9. Write a word that means inflammation of the renal pelvis: _____.

10. **Nephritis,** also called Bright disease, is inflammation of the kidney. The most common form of acute nephritis is **glomerulo+nephritis,** in which _____ (plural of glomerulus) of the kidney are inflamed.

11. **Intravenous uro+graphy** is a radiographic technique for examining the urinary system. Write the term for the image produced in urography: _____.

12. In intravenous urography, a contrast medium is injected intravenously, and serial x-ray films are taken as the medium passes through the urinary structures. This provides information about the structure and function of the kidney, ureters, and bladder (Figure 10-11).

Intravenous urography was formerly called intravenous **pyelography** (IVP) and the image produced was called a _____.

13. Used alone, bladder usually refers to the urinary bladder. **Cysto+scopy** is examination of the urinary bladder. In this procedure, an instrument is passed through the urethra and into the _____ (Figure 10-12). The lining of the bladder is examined by special lenses, mirrors, and a light. The instrument used in cystoscopy is a **cystoscope. Urethro+scopy** is visual examination of the urethra.

14. Inflammation of the bladder is _____.

15. Sometimes people say they have a kidney infection when they actually have cystitis, a bladder infection and a more common type of urinary tract infection. Inflammation of the kidney is _____.

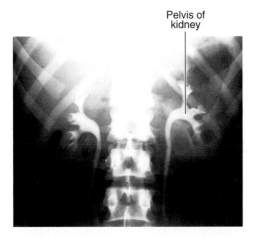

Pelvis of
kidney

-gram = a record
intra- = within
ur/o = urinary tract

Figure 10-11 Intravenous urogram. The x-ray image (radio+graph) was taken as the contrast medium is cleared from the blood by the kidneys. The renal pelvis and ureters are clearly visible, and indicate normal findings.

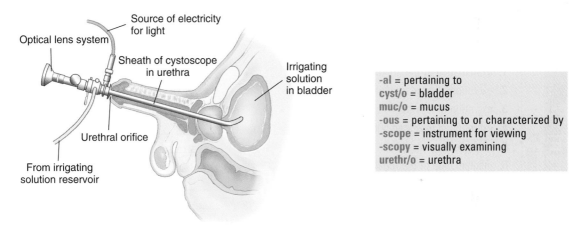

Source of electricity
for light

Optical lens system

Sheath of cystoscope
in urethra

Irrigating
solution
in bladder

Urethral orifice

From irrigating
solution reservoir

-al = pertaining to
cyst/o = bladder
muc/o = mucus
-ous = pertaining to or characterized by
-scope = instrument for viewing
-scopy = visually examining
urethr/o = urethra

Figure 10-12 Cystoscope in place inside the male bladder. In cystoscopy, the cystoscope is passed through the urethra and into the bladder. The mucous membrane is examined by means of light, mirrors, and special lenses.

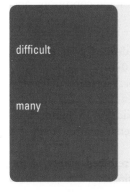

difficult

many

16. Discomfort during urination and unexplained change in the volume of urine are sometimes the earliest indications of a urinary problem. **Dys+uria** is _____ or painful urination and can be caused by a bacterial infection or an obstruction of the urinary tract.

17. **Poly+uria** is excretion of an abnormally large quantity of urine. Literal translation of polyuria is "_____ urines or urinations." You will need to remember that polyuria means excretion of an abnormally large quantity of urine. This is also called **di+ur+esis** (dia-, through + ur/o, urine + -esis, action) and can be brought about by excessive intake of fluids, the use of medications, or disease.

urination	18. Literal translation of **an+uria** is absence of _____. The precise meaning of anuria is a urine output of less than 100 mL per day.
	19. Compare the meanings of anuria and **olig+uria**. The latter means diminished capacity to form urine, or excreting less than 500 mL of urine per day. The combining form olig/o means few or scanty. Write this term that means diminished urine production of less than 500 mL per day:
oliguria	_____.
uremia	20. **Uremia** (ur/o + -emia, blood condition) is a toxic condition associated with renal insufficiency or renal failure. Urea, the chief nitrogen-containing waste product of protein metabolism, is not properly removed from the blood by the kidneys in uremia. Write the term that refers to the presence of nitrogen-containing wastes in the blood: _____. The meaning of uremia cannot be interpreted literally from its word parts, so pay particular attention to its meaning! (It might help to think of "urea in the blood," but you also need to remember that uremia is a toxic condition associated with renal insufficiency or failure.)

WRITE IT! **EXERCISE 7**

Write a term for each description.
1. examination of the urinary bladder _____
2. excretion of large quantities of urine _____
3. excretion of less than 100 mL per day _____
4. excretion of less than 500 mL per day _____
5. kidney enlargement _____
6. inflammation of the renal glomeruli _____
7. inflammation of the renal pelvis _____
8. prolapsed kidney _____
9. softening of the kidney _____
10. presence of kidney stones _____
11. toxic blood condition associated with renal failure _____
12. ultrasonic scanning of the kidneys _____

Study terms in the following list to learn more about pathologic conditions and diagnostic procedures.

cystocele (-cele, hernia) bladder hernia that protrudes into the vagina (Figure 10-13).

nephrosis (-osis, condition) condition in which there are degenerative changes in the kidneys but no inflammation.

nephrotoxic (tox/o, poison) destructive to kidney tissue.

polycystic kidney disease (poly-, many + cyst/o, cyst + -ic, pertaining to) hereditary disorder charac-terized by hundreds of fluid-filled cysts throughout both kidneys (Figure 10-14).

polyp tumor found on a mucosal surface, such as the inner lining of the bladder.

renal failure failure of the kidney to perform its essential functions. Acute renal failure (ARF) is a critical situation.

renal insufficiency (in-, not) reduced ability of the kidney to perform its functions.

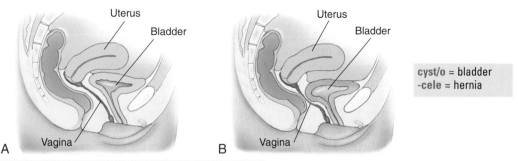

cyst/o = bladder
-cele = hernia

Figure 10-13 Normal bladder compared with cystocele. A, Normal position of the bladder in relation to other pelvic structures. **B,** A cystocele, herniation of the bladder. Note how the bladder sags and protrudes into the vagina.

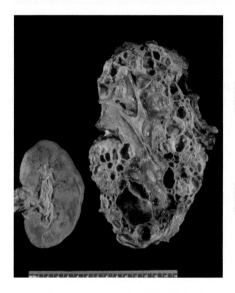

cyst/o = cyst *or* bladder
poly- = many

Figure 10-14 Normal kidney compared with polycystic kidney. The kidney on the left side of the photograph is a transplant kidney of normal size. The kidney on the right is the native kidney from a patient with adult-onset polycystic kidney disease. The diseased kidney is greatly enlarged because of the replacement of normal kidney tissue by cysts of varying sizes.

retrograde urography x-ray examination of the renal pelvis and ureter after injection of a contrast medium into the renal pelvis. In this procedure the contrast material is injected through catheters that are introduced into the ureters. (The prefix retro- means behind or backward. The use of retrograde urography provides an alternative to intravenous urography [IVU] for viewing the renal pelvis and ureters. In IVU, the contrast medium flows through the renal pelvis and ureters after reaching the kidney by way of the bloodstream. In retrograde urography, contrast medium is intro-duced through the ureter and could be considered backward or in the opposite manner of IVU.)

urinary incontinence (in-, not) inability to hold urine in the bladder.

urinary retention inability to empty the bladder.

urinary tract infection (UTI) an infection of the urinary tract.

voiding cystourethrogram (cyst/o, bladder + urethr/o, urethra) radiographic record of the bladder and urethra. After the bladder has been filled with a contrast medium, x-rays are taken while the patient is expelling urine.

Choose the one correct answer (a, b, c, or d) for each question.

1. What term means herniation of the bladder so that it protrudes into the vagina?
   (a) cystocele   (b) polyp   (c) nephromalacia   (d) nephroptosis
2. Which term means degenerative changes in the kidneys without inflammation?
   (a) nephritis   (b) nephromegaly   (c) nephrosclerosis   (d) nephrosis
3. Which of the following means an inability to hold urine in the bladder?
   (a) catheterization   (b) incontinence   (c) urinary failure   (d) urinary insufficiency
4. Which term means a tumor found on a mucosal surface?
   (a) cystocele   (b) polycystic kidney disease   (c) polyp   (d) urinary tract infection
5. Which of these terms means a radiographic record of the bladder and urethra?
   (a) cystourethrogram   (b) nephrotomogram   (c) renal angiogram   (d) urography

Surgical and Therapeutic Interventions

In a renal transplant the patient (recipient) receives a kidney from a suitable donor, often a living sibling or close relative. The donated kidney is surgically removed from the donor **(nephrectomy)**. Selected situations may allow **laparoscopic nephrectomy**, removal of the kidney through several small incisions in the abdominal wall, rather than an open surgical excision. **Immunosuppressive** therapy, the administration of agents that significantly interfere with the immune response of the recipient, are provided after renal transplantation to prevent rejection of the donor kidney.

Urinary catheterization may be used for obtaining a sterile urine sample, for instilling medication in the bladder, or for continuous drainage of the bladder, such as during surgery. Four methods (urethral, ureteral, and suprapubic catheterization and percutaneous nephrostomy) are used for urinary diversion. **Urethral catheterization** is the most common. An indwelling catheter (held securely in place by a balloon tip filled with water) is left in place for a longer period.

 QUICK TIP

Pelves is the plural of pelvis.

In **ureteral catheterization**, catheters are passed into the distal ends of the ureters from the bladder and threaded up the ureters into the renal pelves. If necessary, a ureteral catheter may be surgically inserted through the abdominal wall into the ureter.

If disease or obstruction is present, a **suprapubic catheter** can be placed in the bladder through a small incision or puncture of the abdominal wall approximately 1 inch above the symphysis pubis, the bony eminence that lies beneath the pubic hair.

The fourth means of urinary diversion is **percutaneous nephrostomy**, in which a tube is inserted on a temporary basis into the renal pelvis when a complete obstruction of the ureter is present. In a nephrostomy, a new opening is made into the renal pelvis through the overlying skin. Compare the four methods of urinary diversion shown in Figure 10-15.

Treatment for bladder cancer depends on several factors, including the size of the lesion. Radiation therapy, laser eradication of small lesions, chemotherapy, and **cystectomy** (surgical excision of the bladder) may be used. Various surgical procedures may be performed for urinary diversion if the bladder is removed. The ureters must be diverted into some type of collecting reservoir, either opening onto the abdomen or into the large intestine so that urine is expelled with bowel movements.

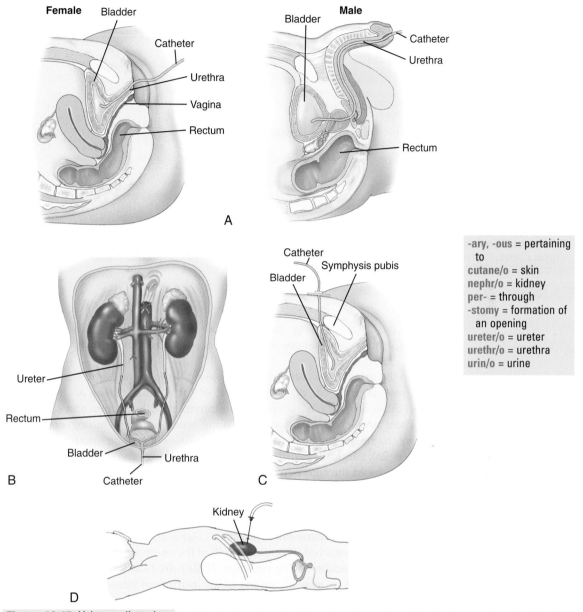

Figure 10-15 Urinary diversion. A, Urethral catheterization (female and male). **B,** Ureteral catheterization. **C,** Suprapubic catheterization. **D,** Percutaneous nephrostomy.

-ary, -ous = pertaining to
cutane/o = skin
nephr/o = kidney
per- = through
-stomy = formation of an opening
ureter/o = ureter
urethr/o = urethra
urin/o = urine

Kidney dialysis or **hemo+dia+lysis** is required if the kidneys fail to remove waste products from the blood. Kidney dialysis is the process of diffusing blood through a membrane to remove toxic materials and maintain proper chemical balance. **Peritoneal dialysis** is an alternative to hemodialysis. The peritoneum is the membrane that covers the large internal organs of the abdominal cavity and lines that cavity. In peritoneal dialysis the dialyzing solution is introduced into and removed from the peritoneal cavity.

hem/o = blood
dia- = through
-lysis = freeing or destroying

periton/o = peritoneum
-eal = pertaining to

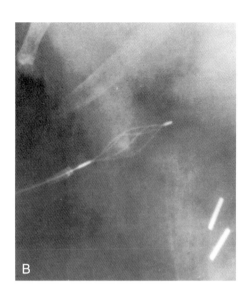

-ous = pertaining to
cutane/o = skin
nephr/o = kidney
per- = through
-stomy = artificial opening

Figure 10-16 Removal of a kidney stone. This radiograph shows a renal calculus that has been caught in a stone basket and is ready for removal. After percutaneous nephrostomy, the stone basket was maneuvered to engage the renal calculus, then both are removed through the cannula.

Diuretic means increasing urination or an agent that causes increased urination. Common substances such as tea, coffee, alcohol, and water act as diuretics.

Stones in the urinary tract are sometimes passed through the urethra, but many are too large, may be trapped, do not dissolve, or for another reason are impassable. Stones can cause urinary obstruction, which interferes with function and can be very painful. There are several methods of dealing with stones, including noninvasive litho+tripsy (high energy shock wave or laser to break the stone into fragments, see Figure 2-7, p. 26), surgically crushing a stone, or "catching" the stone in a basket that has been introduced through percutaneous nephrostomy (Figure 10-16).

Trans+urethral means through the urethra. Transurethral surgery is performed by inserting an instrument through or across the wall of the urethra, which makes it possible to perform surgery on certain organs that lie near the urethra without having an abdominal incision. In **transurethral resection** (TUR), small pieces of tissue from a nearby structure are removed through the wall of the urethra. One surgery of this type is a transurethral resection of the prostate (TURP). In TURP, surgery is performed on the **prostate** gland in men by means of an instrument passed through the wall of the urethra and is sometimes done to alleviate problems of benign prostatic hyperplasia.

The following list provides more information about surgical procedures performed on urinary structures.

trans- = through *or* across

  QUICK TIP

Note the difference in spelling of prostate and prostrate, which means lying in a facedown, horizontal position.

cystostomy (cyst/o, bladder + -stomy, new opening) surgical creation of a new opening into the bladder.

lithotripsy (lith/o, stone + -tripsy, surgical crushing) crushing of a stone. The stone may be crushed surgically or by using high-energy shock waves or a laser. A **lithotrite** is an instrument used for surgically crushing bladder stones. Renal lithotripsy using shock waves is called **extra+corpor+eal** (extra-, outside + corpor/o, body + -eal, pertaining to) shock wave lithotripsy (ESWL). After lithotripsy, the stone fragments may be expelled

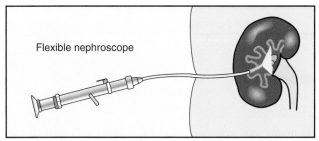

Flexible nephroscope

-ic, -ous = pertaining to
cutane/o = skin
nephr/o = kidney
opt/o = vision
per- = through
-scope = instrument for viewing
son/o = sound
ultra- = beyond or excess

Figure 10-17 One type of nephroscope. The nephroscope, a fiberoptic instrument, is inserted percutaneously into the kidney. When stones are present, an ultrasonic probe can be added. It emits high-frequency sound waves that break up the calculi.

or washed out. A **nephroscope** is sometimes used when small stones are broken up by ESWL. The nephroscope is a fiberoptic instrument that is inserted through the skin (Figure 10-17). The stone is located through the use of x-ray imaging, and its fragments are removed by suction through the scope. The use of the nephroscope to eliminate renal calculi or to examine the kidney visually is called **nephroscopy**.

nephrolithotomy (nephr/o, kidney + -tomy, incision) incision of the kidney **(nephrotomy)** for removal of a kidney stone (removal of the stone is implied in this term).

nephropexy (-pexy, surgical fixation) surgical attachment of a prolapsed kidney.

nephrostomy, pyelostomy creation of a new opening into the renal pelvis of the kidney (the opening into the renal pelvis is implied in nephrostomy). This procedure is usually done to drain urine from the kidney (see Figure 10-15, *D*).

percutaneous bladder biopsy removal of tissue from the bladder by using a needle inserted through the skin overlying the bladder; done for diagnostic purposes (percutaneous is derived from per-, through + cutane/o, skin + -ous, pertaining to).

percutaneous renal biopsy removal of tissue from the kidney using needle puncture of the skin and tissue overlying the kidney; done for diagnostic purposes.

pyelolithotomy (pyel/o, renal pelvis) surgical incision of the kidney to remove a stone from the renal pelvis (removal of the stone is implied).

ureteroplasty surgical repair of a ureter.

CIRCLE IT!   **EXERCISE 9**

Choose the one correct answer (a, b, c, or d) for each question.

1. Which term means excision of a kidney?
   (a) nephrectomy   (b) nephroscopy   (c) nephrostomy   (d) nephrotomy
2. Which of the following terms is not a type of urinary diversion?
   (a) cystitis   (b) percutaneous nephrostomy   (c) ureteral catheterization   (d) urethral catheterization
3. Which of the following terms means surgical incision of the kidney to remove a stone from the renal pelvis?
   (a) lithotripsy   (b) nephropexy   (c) nephrostomy   (d) pyelolithotomy
4. Which term means a procedure that is performed by inserting an instrument through or across the wall of the urethra?
   (a) nephroptosis   (b) transurethral resection   (c) ureterocystostomy   (d) urinary retention
5. Which term means the process of diffusing blood through a membrane to remove toxic materials and maintain proper chemical balance?
   (a) hematuria   (b) hemodialysis   (c) nephrolithotomy   (d) ureteral catheterization

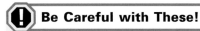

Be Careful with These!

cyt/o (cell) versus *cyst/o* (bladder or sac)
ureter/o (ureter) versus *urethr/o* (urethra)
-esis (action, process, or result of) versus *-stasis* (controlling)

SELF-TEST　　Work the following exercises to test your understanding of the material in Chapter 10. Complete all the exercises before using Appendix VIII to check your answers.

A. MATCH IT!　*Match structures in the left column with their functions in the right column*

_____ **1.** bladder
_____ **2.** nephron
_____ **3.** renal pelvis
_____ **4.** ureter
_____ **5.** urethra

A. cavity in the kidney that collects urine from many collecting ducts
B. carries urine from the bladder
C. carries urine to the bladder
D. functional unit of the kidney
E. reservoir for urine until it is expelled

B. FINDING THE CLUE!　*Use a clue to write terms for these descriptions. Solve Question 1; each ending letter becomes the clue for the first letter of the next answer.*

1. urinating　　　　　　　　　　　　　　　　　　_____
2. filtering unit of the kidney　　　　　　　　　　_____
3. narrowing　　　　　　　　　　　　　　　　　_____
4. type of laparoscopic catheterization of the bladder　_____
5. herniation of the urinary bladder into the vagina　_____
6. elimination by the act or process of excreting　　_____
7. instrument used in nephroscopy　　　　　　　　_____
8. hormone secreted by the kidney that stimulates RBC production　_____
9. functional unit of the kidney　　　　　　　　　_____
10. removal of renal calculi by cutting into the kidney　_____

C. MATCH IT!　*Choose A or B from the right column to classify the urinary substances as those normally detected in urine or as those not normally detected.*

_____ **1.** blood
_____ **2.** ketones
_____ **3.** protein
_____ **4.** sugar
_____ **5.** urea

A. normally detected in urine
B. not normally detected in urine

SELF-TEST (cont'd)

D. CIRCLE IT! *Choose the one correct response (a, b, c, or d) for each question.*

1. Which of the following means the same as nephromegaly?
(a) kidney dialysis   (b) kidney failure   (c) renal enlargement   (d) renal stone

2. Which of the following is an instrument used for surgically crushing a stone?
(a) lithotripsy   (b) lithotrite   (c) pyelogram   (d) pyelolithotomy

3. Which term means passage of a tubular, flexible instrument into a body channel or cavity for withdrawal of fluid or introduction of fluid?
(a) catheterization   (b) cystostomy   (c) lithotripsy   (d) tracheotomy

4. Which of the following means excision of a calculus from the renal pelvis?
(a) cystectomy   (b) lithotripsy   (c) pyelolithotomy   (d) tomography

5. Which term means absence of urination or production of less than 100 mL of urine per day?
(a) anuria   (b) diuresis   (c) polyuria   (d) renal failure

6. Which of the following means sugar in the urine?
(a) glycosuria   (b) ketonuria   (c) pyuria   (d) uremia

7. Which term means inflammation of the kidney?
(a) cystitis   (b) nephritis   (c) nephrosis   (d) pyelolithiasis

8. Which term means an inability to control urination?
(a) excretion   (b) incontinence   (c) stenosis   (d) uremia

9. What is the name of the instrument used in cystoscopy?
(a) cystogram   (b) cystograph   (c) cystoscope   (d) nephroscope

10. Which of the following means ultrasonic scanning of the kidney?
(a) nephroscopy   (b) nephrosonography   (c) pyelogram   (d) pyelography

E. WRITE IT! *Write one-word terms for these meanings.*

1. blood in the urine   _____

2. functional unit of the kidney   _____

3. examination of the bladder   _____

4. inflammation of the renal pelvis   _____

5. kidney dialysis   _____

6. new opening into the renal pelvis   _____

7. pertaining to the urethra   _____

8. presence of kidney stones   _____

9. surgical fixation of a prolapsed kidney   _____

10. surgical repair of a ureter   _____

SELF-TEST (cont'd)

F. READING HEALTH CARE REPORTS *Read the case report, and answer the questions that follow. Although some of the terms are new, you should be able to determine their meanings by analyzing the word parts.*

MEDICAL REPORT

Patient: M.A. Stewart (male, age 43)
Symptoms: Hematuria, dysuria
History: Cystitis, nephritis
Family History: Father—age 65 with history of BPH; mother—age 64 with history of renal calculi and pyelonephritis
Diagnostic Studies: KUB and IV urography show three small calculi in ureter
Labs: Urinalysis and urine culture show no evidence of UTI
Diagnosis: Ureteral urolithiasis
Plan: Ureteroscopy and possible lithotripsy

Circle the one correct answer (a, b, c, or d) for each question.
1. Mr. Stewart's symptom of dysuria indicates which characteristic of urine or urination?
   (a) blood   (b) decreased output   (c) difficult or painful   (d) protein
2. Which of the following conditions does his history indicate?
   (a) bladder and kidney stones   (b) inflammation of the bladder and kidney   (c) inflammation caused by trauma
   (d) frequent urinary infections
3. Which of the following is indicated in his mother's history?
   (a) kidney stones   (b) polycystic kidney   (c) renal stenosis   (d) uremia
4. Which of the following is Mr. Stewart's diagnosis?
   (a) narrowing of the ureter   (b) obstruction of the ureter   (c) stone in the ureter   (d) urinary infection
5. Which procedure is indicated by a ureteroscopy?
   (a) surgical fixation   (b) renal angiography   (c) ureteral resection   (d) visual examination

G. SPELL IT!   *Circle all incorrectly spelled terms, and write the correct spelling.*

1. cathaterized   _____
2. nefrectomy   _____
3. oliguria   _____
4. suprapubik   _____
5. urinery   _____

Q&E List

Use the Companion CD or audio CDs to review the terms presented in Chapter 10.
Look closely at the spelling of each term as it is pronounced.

albuminuria (al˝bu-mĭ-nu´re-ə)   cystectomy (sis-tek´tə-me)
anuria (an-u´re-ə)   cystic (sis´tik)
bilateral (bi-lat´ər-əl)   cystitis (sis-ti´tis)

cystocele (**sis′to-sēl**)
cystoscope (**sis′to-skōp″**)
cystoscopy (**sis-tos′kə-pe**)
cystostomy (**sis-tos′tə-me**)
diabetes mellitus (**di″ə-be′tēz mel′lə-təs, mə-li′tis**)
diuresis (**di″u-re′sis**)
diuretic (**di″u-ret′ik**)
dysuria (**dis-u′re-ə**)
erythropoietin (**ə-rith″ro-poi′ə-tin**)
excretion (**eks-kre′shən**)
extracorporeal (**eks″trə-kor-por′e-əl**)
glomerulonephritis (**glo-mer″′u-lo-nə-fri′tis**)
glomerulus (**glo-mer′u-ləs**)
glycosuria (**gli″ko-su′re-ə**)
hematuria (**he″mə-tu′re-ə, hem″ə-tu′re-ə**)
hemodialysis (**he″mo-di-al′ə-sis**)
immunosuppressive (**im″u-no-sə-pres′iv**)
intravenous urography (**in″trə-ve′nəs u-rog′rə-fe**)
ketonuria (**ke″to-nu′re-ə**)
laparoscopic nephrectomy (**lap′ə-ro-skop′ik nə-frek′tə-me**)
lithotripsy (**lith′o-trip″se**)
lithotrite (**lith′o-trīt**)
nephrectomy (**nə-frek′tə-me**)
nephritis (**nə-fri′tis**)
nephrolith (**nef′ro-lith**)
nephrolithiasis (**nef″ro-lĭ-thi′ə-sis**)
nephrolithotomy (**nef″ro-lĭ-thot′ə-me**)
nephromalacia (**nef″ro-mə-la′shə**)
nephromegaly (**nef″ro-meg′ə-le**)
nephron (**nef′ron**)
nephropexy (**nef′ro-pek″se**)
nephroptosis (**nef″rop-to′sis**)
nephroscope (**nef′ro-skōp**)
nephroscopy (**nə-fros′kə-pe**)
nephrosis (**nĕ-fro′sis**)
nephrosonography (**nef″ro-so-nog′rə-fe**)
nephrostomy (**nə-fros′tə-me**)
nephrotomogram (**nef″ro-to′mo-gram**)
nephrotomography (**nef″ro-to-mog′rə-fe**)
nephrotomy (**nə-frot′ə-me**)
nephrotoxic (**nef′ro-tok″sik**)
oliguria (**ol″ĭ-gu′re-ə**)
percutaneous bladder biopsy (**pur″ku-ta′ne-əs blad′ər bi′op-se**)
percutaneous nephrostomy (**pur″ku-ta′ne-əs nə-fros′tə-me**)
percutaneous renal biopsy (**pur″ku-ta′ne-əs re′nəl bi′op-se**)

peritoneal dialysis (**per″ĭ-to-ne′əl di-al′ə-sis**)
polycystic kidney disease (**pol″e-sis′tik kid′ne dĭ-zēz′**)
polyp (**pol′ip**)
polyuria (**pol″e-u′re-ə**)
prostate (**pros′tāt**)
proteinuria (**pro″te-nu′re-ə**)
pyelitis (**pi″ə-li′tis**)
pyelogram (**pi′ə-lo-gram**)
pyelography (**pi″ə-log′rə-fe**)
pyelolithotomy (**pi″ə-lo-lĭ-thot′ə-me**)
pyelostomy (**pi″ə-los′tə-me**)
pyuria (**pi-u′re-ə**)
renal (**re′nəl**)
renal angiography (**re′nəl an″je-og′rə-fe**)
renal arteriogram (**re′nəl ahr-ter′e-o-gram**)
renal arteriography (**re′nəl ahr″tĕr-e-og′rə-fe**)
renal failure (**re′nəl fāl′yər**)
renal insufficiency (**re′nəl in″sə-fish′ən-se**)
retrograde urography (**ret′ro-grād u-rog′rə-fe**)
stenosis (**stə-no′sis**)
suprapubic catheter (**soo″prə-pu′bik kath′ə-tər**)
transurethral resection (**trans″u-re′thrəl re-sek′shən**)
tubule (**too′būl**)
urea (**u-re′ə**)
uremia (**u-re′me-ə**)
ureter (**u-re′tər, u′rə-tər**)
ureteral (**u-re′tər-əl**)
ureteral catheterization (**u-re′tər-əl kath″ə-tur″ĭ-za′shən**)
ureteroplasty (**u-re′tər-o-plas″te**)
urethra (**u-re′thrə**)
urethral (**u-re′thrəl**)
urethral catheterization (**u-re′thrəl kath″ə-tur″ĭ-za′shən**)
urethroscopy (**u″rə-thros′kə-pe**)
urinalysis (**u″rĭ-nal′ĭ-sis**)
urinary (**u′rĭ-nar″e**)
urinary incontinence (**u′rĭ-nar″e in-kon′tĭ-nəns**)
urinary retention (**u′rĭ-nar″e re-ten′shən**)
urinary tract infection (**u′rĭ-nar″e trakt in-fek′shən**)
urination (**u″rĭ-na′shən**)
urogram (**u′ro-gram**)
urologist (**u-rol′ə-jist**)
urology (**u-rol′ə-je**)
voiding cystourethrogram (**void′ing sis″to-u-re′thro-gram**)

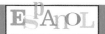 **Enhancing Spanish Communication**

English	Spanish (pronunciation)
bladder	vejiga **(vay-HEE-gah)**
catheter	catéter **(cah-TAY-ter)**
dialysis	diálisis **(de-AH-le-sis)**
excretion	excreción **(ex-cray-se-ON)**
kidney	riñón **(ree-NYOHN)**
obstruction	obstrucción **(obs-trooc-se-ON)**
renal artery	arteria renal **(ar-TAY-re-ah ray-NAHL)**
renal calculus	cálculo renal **(CAHL-coo-lo ray-NAHL)**
urea	urea **(oo-RAY-ah)**
urinalysis	urinálisis **(oo-re-NAH-le-sis)**
urinary	urinario **(oo-re-NAH-re-o)**
urination	urinación **(oo-re-nah-se-ON)**
urine	orina **(o-REE-nah)**
urology	urología **(oo-ro-lo-HEE-ah)**
vein	vena **(VAY-na)**
vessel	vaso **(VAH-so)**
voiding	urinar **(oo-re-NAR)**
water	agua **(AH-goo-ah)**

CHAPTER 11

Reproductive System

CONTENTS

Function First
FEMALE REPRODUCTIVE SYSTEM
Structures
  • *External Structures* • *Internal Structures*
Diseases, Disorders, and Diagnostic Terms
Surgical and Therapeutic Interventions
Pregnancy and Childbirth
Female Breasts

MALE REPRODUCTIVE SYSTEM
Structures
Diseases, Disorders, and Diagnostic Terms
Surgical and Therapeutic Interventions
Sexually Transmitted Diseases
Self-Test
Q&E List
Enhancing Spanish Communication

OBJECTIVES

After completing Chapter 11, you will be able to:

1. Recognize or write the functions of the reproductive system.
2. Recognize or write the meanings of Chapter 11 word parts and use them to build and analyze terms.
3. Write terms for selected structures of the female reproductive system and their associated functions, or match them with their descriptions.
4. Write the names of the diagnostic terms and pathologies related to the female reproductive system when given their descriptions, or match terms with their meanings.
5. Match surgical and therapeutic interventions for the female reproductive system, or write the names of the interventions when given their descriptions.

6. Write terms for selected structures of the male reproductive system and their associated functions, or match them with their descriptions.
7. Write the names of the diagnostic terms and pathologies related to the male reproductive system when given their descriptions, or match terms with their meanings.
8. Match surgical and therapeutic interventions for the male reproductive system, or write the names of the interventions when given their descriptions.
9. Write terms for sexually transmitted diseases, or match them with their causative agents.
10. Spell terms for the reproductive system and sexually transmitted diseases correctly.

Function First

Reproduction is the process by which genetic material is passed from one generation to the next. The major function of the reproductive system is to produce offspring. The male and female reproductive systems can be broadly organized by organs with different functions. For example, the testes and ovaries are called the **gonads,** and they function in the production of reproductive cells: spermatozoa (sperm) or ova (eggs). Singular terms for spermatozoa and ova are spermatozoon and **ovum,** respectively. The gonads also secrete important hormones. Ducts transport and receive eggs or

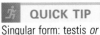

QUICK TIP
Singular form: testis *or* testicle

gon/o = genital *or* reproduction

sperm and important fluids. Still other reproductive organs produce materials that support the sperm and ova. Reproductive organs, whether male or female, or internal or external, are called the genitals or **genitalia**.

Find the terms in the material you just read and write it for these meanings.

1. another term for genitals _____

2. organs that produce either sperm or ova _____

3. singular form of ova _____

4. singular form of spermatozoa _____

5. the female gonad _____

6. the male gonad _____

7. process by which genetic material is passed from one
generation to the next _____

Use Appendix VIII to check your answers to all the exercises in Chapter 11.

Female Reproductive System

Structures

The female reproductive system aids in the creation of new life and provides an environment and support for the developing child. After birth, the female breasts produce milk to feed the child and are thus often considered part of the female reproductive system (see later section).

gynec/o = female
-logy = study of

Gyneco+logy is the study of diseases of the female reproductive organs, and a **gyneco+logist** is a specialist in the study of these diseases. Female genitalia include both external and internal structures.

The word parts in the table refer to female reproductive structures and are frequently used when discussing reproduction. Commit the word parts and their meanings to memory.

Word Parts: Female Reproductive System

Female Genitalia	Meaning	Other Word Parts	Meaning
cervic/o*	cervix	-cidal	killing
colp/o, vagin/o	vagina	cyst/o, vesic/o	bladder, cyst, or sac
gynec/o	female	genit/o	genitals
hyster/o, uter/o	uterus	gonad/o	genitals or reproduction
metr/o (occasionally metr/i)†	uterine tissue	men/o	month
		-plasia	development or formation
oophor/o, ovar/o	ovary	rect/o	rectum
salping/o	uterine tube (fallopian tube)	urethr/o	urethra
		urin/o	urine
vulv/o	vulva (external genitalia)		

Use the electronic flashcards on the Evolve site or make your own set of flashcards using the above list. Select the word parts just presented, and study them until you know their meanings. Do this each time a set of word parts is presented.

*Sometimes cervic/o means the neck.   †Sometimes metr/o and metr/i mean measure.

MATCH IT!
EXERCISE 2

Match the word parts in the two left columns with their meanings in the right column.

____ **1.** -cidal   ____ **5.** metr/o   **A.** bladder, cyst, or sac

____ **2.** colp/o   ____ **6.** oophor/o   **B.** killing

____ **3.** hyster/o   ____ **7.** salping/o   **C.** month

____ **4.** men/o   ____ **8.** vesic/o   **D.** ovary

E. uterine tissue

F. uterine tube

G. uterus

H. vagina

External Structures

The external genitalia are called the **vulva,** which includes the following structures:

- **mons pubis**
- **labia majora** (labium majus, singular)
- **labia minora** (labium minus, singular)
- **clitoris**
- openings for glands

Label these structures as you read the legend for Figure 11-1. The two pairs of skin folds protect the vaginal opening. Labia is the plural term for labium and means lips, or structures that resemble lips. Majora and minora refer to major, or larger, and minor, or smaller. **Vulv+al** and **vulv+ar** are adjectives that mean pertaining to the vulva.

> vulv/o = vulva
> -al, -ar = pertaining to

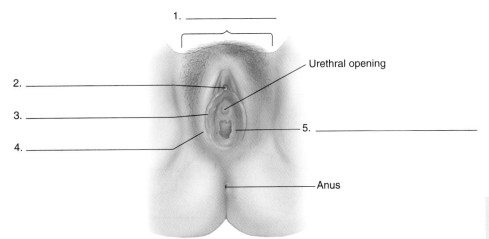

> -al = pertaining to
> urethr/o = urethra
> vagin/o = vagina

Figure 11-1 Female external genitalia. These structures are external to the vagina and are also called the vulva. The mons pubis *(1)* is a pad of fatty tissue and thick skin that overlies the front of the pubic bone. The pubic bone is the anterior portion of the hip bones. The mons pubis is covered with hair after puberty. The clitoris *(2)* is a small mass of erectile tissue and nerves that has similarities to the male penis. Two pairs of skin folds protect the vaginal opening. The smaller pair is called the labia minora *(3),* and the larger pair is called the labia majora *(4).* Small glands secrete mucus for lubrication. Openings for the glands lie near the vagina; label one of them *(5).*

MATCH IT!
EXERCISE 3

Match these female external structures with their descriptions.

_____ **1.** clitoris
_____ **2.** labia majora
_____ **3.** labia minora
_____ **4.** mons pubis
_____ **5.** vulva

A. general term for external genitalia
B. larger pair of skin folds
C. pad of fatty tissue overlying the pubic bone
D. small mass of erectile tissue
E. smaller pair of skin folds

Internal Structures

The following structures are internal genitalia:

* left ovary and associated left uterine tube
* right ovary and associated right uterine tube
* uterus
* vagina
* special glands

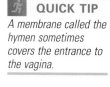

QUICK TIP

A membrane called the hymen sometimes covers the entrance to the vagina.

vagin/o = vagina

intra- = within
extra- = outside

Label the structures of the internal genitalia as you read the legend for Figure 11-2, *A.* The ovaries produce ova. The uterine tubes (also called **fallopian** tubes or oviducts) transport the ova to the uterus (womb). The **vagina,** commonly called the "birth canal," receives the sperm during intercourse. Terms that pertain to the vagina often use the adjective **vaginal.** The **uterus** provides nourishment from the time the fertilized egg is implanted until birth. A **fetus** is the latter stages of developing offspring and, in humans, is that time **in utero** after the first 8 weeks. In utero means within the uterus. **Intra+uterine** also means within the uterus, and **extra+uterine** means outside the uterus. Uterine is a frequently used adjective that means pertaining to the uterus.

1. _____
2. _____
3. _____
4. _____
5. _____

A

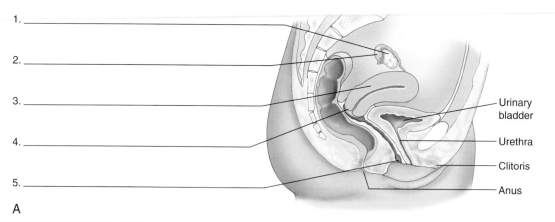

Figure 11-2 Female genitalia, midsagittal and anterior views. A, Midsagittal section. Write the names of the structures on the numbered lines as you read the following. Each ovary *(1)* produces ova and hormones. One uterine tube *(2)* is associated with each ovary. The uterus *(3)* is the muscular organ that prepares to receive and nurture the fertilized ovum. The lower and narrower part that has the outlet from the uterus is the cervix uteri *(4).* The vagina *(5)* is the canal that connects the internal and external genitalia.

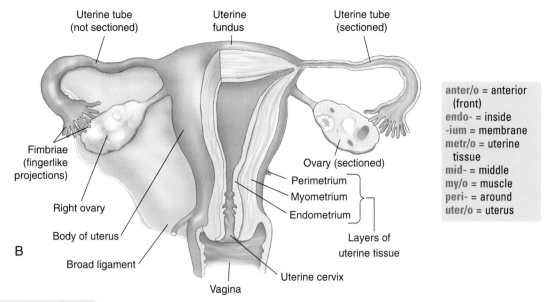

anter/o = anterior
  (front)
endo- = inside
-ium = membrane
metr/o = uterine
  tissue
mid- = middle
my/o = muscle
peri- = around
uter/o = uterus

Figure 11-2, cont'd **B,** Anterior view of the internal organs of the female reproductive system. The left ovary, the left uterine tube, and the left side of the uterus are sectioned to show their internal structure.

MATCH IT! EXERCISE 4

Match the terms in the left column with their descriptions.

_____ **1.** ovary   **A.** a gonad
_____ **2.** ovum   **B.** receives and nurtures the fertilized ovum
_____ **3.** uterine tube   **C.** receives the sperm during intercourse
_____ **4.** uterus   **D.** reproductive cell
_____ **5.** vagina   **E.** transports ova to the uterus

The cavity of the uterus has upper openings for the uterine tubes (at the uterine horns) and a lower opening into the vagina (**cervix uteri,** commonly called the cervix). The cervix is the lowermost cylindric part of the uterus (cervic/o means the neck or the cervix uteri).The adjective **cervical** pertains either to the neck itself or to the cervix, which is the neck of the uterus. Other parts of the word, or the way in which it is used, usually indicate whether cervical refers to the neck itself or the cervix.

The uterus consists of three layers of tissue. From the innermost layer to the outermost layer, the layers are called endometrium, myometrium, and perimetrium. Find these three layers of tissue in Figure 11-2, *B,* and compare their locations. The tissue that forms the lining of the uterus is called the **endo+metr+ium.** The **myometrium** is the thick muscular tissue of the uterus, and the **perimetrium** is the membrane that surrounds the uterus.

metr/o =
  measurement *or*
  uterine tissue
  (latter usage
  here)
endo- = inside
-ium = membrane
my/o = muscle
peri- = around

ovar/o = ovary

The **ovaries** are located on each side of the uterus. **Ovarian** means pertaining to one or both ovaries. Ovaries function in **ovulation** (the production of ova) and in the production of two important hormones, **estrogen** and **progesterone.** These hormones are responsible for the development and maintenance of secondary sexual characteristics, preparation of the uterus for pregnancy, and development of the mammary glands.

mamm/o = breast

men/o = month

Menstruation is the discharge of a bloody fluid from the uterus at fairly regular intervals, approximately once each month, from puberty to menopause. The **climacteric,** or **menopause,** marks the end of a woman's reproductive period. Menstruation, also called **menses,** is the sloughing off of the endometrium that has been prepared to receive a fertilized ovum but is not needed. Menstruation ceases temporarily during pregnancy and breastfeeding and permanently with the onset of menopause (unless hormones are administered).

WRITE IT!
EXERCISE 5

Write terms for these descriptions.

1. pertaining to the cervix _____
2. pertaining to one or both ovaries _____
3. pertaining to the uterus _____
4. pertaining to the vagina _____
5. pertaining to the vulva _____
6. inner lining of the uterus _____
7. membrane that surrounds the uterus _____
8. muscular tissue of the uterus _____
9. within the uterus _____
10. outside the uterus _____
11. the production of ova _____
12. another term for menses _____
13. another term for menopause _____
14. a developing human after 8 weeks in utero _____
15. another important female hormone besides estrogen _____

Diseases, Disorders, and Diagnostic Terms

The physical assessment of the female reproductive system includes examination of the breasts, the external genitalia, and the pelvis. Gynecologic and obstetric care accounts for one fifth of all visits by female patients to physicians. Throughout a female's life, annual assessment and screening for cancers of the reproductive system increase the chances that problems are detected and often corrected in their early stages. Many diagnostic procedures and treatments are available.

PROGRAMMED LEARNING

Remember to cover the answers (left column) with folded paper or the bookmark. Write an answer in each blank, and then check your answer before proceeding to the next frame.

vaginal

1. A vaginal **speculum** is an instrument that can be pushed apart after it is inserted into the vagina, to allow examination of the cervix and the walls of the vagina. A speculum is an instrument for examining body orifices (openings) or cavities. A speculum that is used to examine the vagina is a _____ speculum.

cells

2. Specimens (scrapings) for cytology can be collected during the pelvic examination. **Cyto+logy** means the study of _____.

cytology

3. **Pap smear** is an abbreviated way of saying Papanicolaou smear or test. In a Pap smear, material is collected from areas of the body that shed cells. The cells are then studied microscopically. The study of cells is called _____.

Pap

4. The term Pap smear usually refers to collection and examination of cells from the vagina and cervix (Figure 11-3), but the term may refer to collection of material from other surfaces that shed cells. Both _____ smears and biopsies are performed to detect cancer of the cervix, and both use a vaginal speculum.

dysplasia

5. It is standard practice to grade Pap smears as class I, II, III, IV, or V. Class I is normal, and class V is definitely cancer. Early diagnosis of cervical cancer is possible with the Pap test. When the Pap smear is examined microscopically, malignant cells have a characteristic appearance that indicates cancer, sometimes before symptoms appear. It may begin with **dys+plasia**, a change in shape, growth, and number of cells. This finding is not cancer, but cells of this type tend to become malignant. Write the term for this abnormality in the shape, growth, and number of cells that may be seen in a Pap smear: _____.

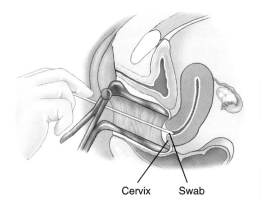

cervic/o = cervix
vagin/o = vagina

Cervix   Swab

Figure 11-3 Obtaining a cervical Pap smear by using a vaginal speculum.

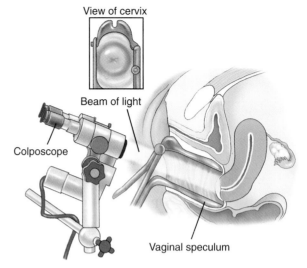

View of cervix

Beam of light

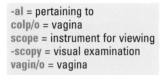

-al = pertaining to
colp/o = vagina
scope = instrument for viewing
-scopy = visual examination
vagin/o = vagina

Colposcope

Vaginal speculum

Figure 11-4 **Colposcopy.** The vagina and cervix are examined with a colposcope.

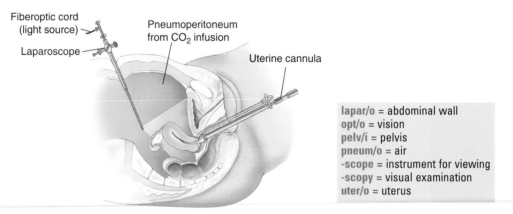

Fiberoptic cord
(light source)

Laparoscope

Pneumoperitoneum
from CO_2 infusion

Uterine cannula

lapar/o = abdominal wall
opt/o = vision
pelv/i = pelvis
pneum/o = air
-scope = instrument for viewing
-scopy = visual examination
uter/o = uterus

Figure 11-5 **Laparoscopy.** Using the laparoscope with a fiberoptic light source, the surgeon can see the pelvic cavity and the reproductive organs. Additional procedures, such as tubal sterilization or removal of the uterus or ovaries, are performed by means of a second small incision.

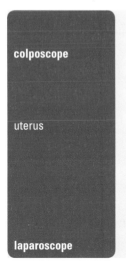

colposcope

uterus

laparoscope

6. **Colpo+scopy** involves the use of a low-power microscope to magnify the mucosa of the vagina and cervix (Figure 11-4). The instrument used is a _____.

7. Suspicious cervical or vaginal lesions may be seen during colposcopy. Some findings indicate the need for a cervical or endometrial biopsy. A cervical biopsy is removal of tissue from the cervix, and an endometrial biopsy requires collection of tissue from the lining of the _____.

8. Computed tomography and pelvic ultrasonography may be helpful in detecting masses. **Laparo+scopy** is the examination of the abdominal cavity through one or more small incisions in the abdominal wall. This surgical procedure is especially useful for inspection of structures within the pelvic cavity, as well as collection of biopsy specimens and in certain types of surgery (Figure 11-5). The name of the instrument used in laparoscopy is a _____.

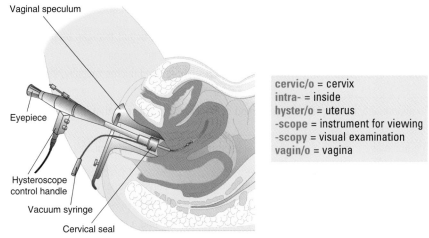

cervic/o = cervix
intra- = inside
hyster/o = uterus
-scope = instrument for viewing
-scopy = visual examination
vagin/o = vagina

Figure 11-6 Hysteroscopy. Direct visual examination of the cervical canal and uterine cavity using a hysteroscope is performed to examine the endometrium to obtain a specimen for biopsy, to excise cervical polyps, or to remove an intrauterine device.

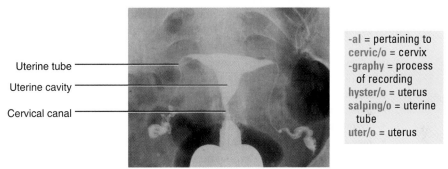

-al = pertaining to
cervic/o = cervix
-graphy = process
  of recording
hyster/o = uterus
salping/o = uterine
  tube
uter/o = uterus

Figure 11-7 Hysterosalpingogram. This x-ray image of the uterus and uterine tubes was made after the introduction of a radiopaque substance through the cervix.

---

9. Hystero+scopy is direct visual inspection of the cervical canal and uterine cavity, using an endoscope passed through the vagina (Figure 11-6). Change the suffix of hysteroscopy to write the name of the endoscope:

hysteroscope

_____.

---

10. A **hystero+salpingo+gram** is an x-ray image of the uterus and uterine tubes using a radiopaque substance introduced through the cervix (Figure 11-7). Write the name of the procedure in which a hysterosalpingogram is produced: _____.

hysterosalpingo-graphy

WRITE IT!   EXERCISE 6

Write a term in the blanks to complete each sentence.

1. A vaginal _____ is an instrument that can be pushed apart after its insertion, to allow examination of the cervix and walls of the vagina.

2. Material is collected from the vagina and cervix, then studied microscopically, in a _____ smear.

3. An abnormality in the shape, growth, and numbers of cervical cells that often tend to become malignant is called _____.

4. The procedure in which a colposcope is used to magnify the vaginal mucosa and the cervix is _____.

5. Using a hysteroscope for direct visual inspection of the cervical canal and uterine cavity is _____.

6. An x-ray image of the uterus and uterine tubes after injecting a radiopaque substance into them is _____.

Common reasons for seeking gynecologic care are pain, vaginal discharge, bleeding, and annual gynecologic examinations. A less common problem is infertility, the condition of being unable to produce offspring after a reasonable period of regular intercourse without **contraception**, the prevention of pregnancy by means of a medication, device, or method that blocks or alters the processes of reproduction. Infertility may be caused by female, male, or combined factors, and sometimes the cause cannot be identified. In women the risk for infertility increases with age.

Menstrual irregularities include the following:

- **amenorrhea:** absence of menstrual flow when it is normally expected.
- **dysmenorrhea:** painful menstruation.
- **menorrhagia:** excessive flow during menstruation.
- **metrorrhagia:** bleeding from the uterus at any time other than during the menstrual period.

Metrorrhagia literally means hemorrhage from the uterus. Menstruation, normal menstrual flow, contains the word part men/o, which means month. You will need to remember that metrorrhagia is abnormal bleeding that is not associated with menstruation.

men/o = month
-rrhea = discharge
-rrhagia = hemorrhage
metr/o = uterine tissue

QUICK TIP

men/o is used in the words menses and menstruation.

MATCH IT!   EXERCISE 7

Match the menstrual disorders with their descriptions.

___ **1.** amenorrhea   **A.** abnormally heavy or long menstrual periods

___ **2.** dysmenorrhea   **B.** absence of menstruation

___ **3.** menorrhagia   **C.** painful or difficult menstruation

___ **4.** metrorrhagia   **D.** uterine bleeding other than menstruation

The following list provides additional diseases and disorders of female reproduction.

cervical polyp fibrous or mucous stalked tumor of the cervical mucosa (lining) (*polyp* is a general term for tumors that bleed easily and are found on mucous membranes).

cervicocolpitis inflammation of the cervix and vagina.

colpitis (colp/o, vagina + -itis, inflammation) inflammation of the vagina; same as **vaginitis**.

cystocele (cyst/o, bladder + -cele, hernia) herniation or protrusion of the urinary bladder through the wall of the vagina (see Figure 10-12, B, p. 251).

endometriosis (endo-, inside + metr/i, uterine tissue + -osis, condition) condition in which tissue that somewhat resembles the endometrium is found abnormally in various locations in the pelvic cavity (Figure 11-8). Endometriosis has an unusual spelling, so be careful!

endometritis inflammation of the endometrium.

fistula abnormal, tubelike passage between two internal organs or between an internal organ and the body surface. A **rectovaginal** (rect/o, rectum) fistula is an abnormal opening between the rectum and the vagina. A **vesicovaginal** (vesic/o, bladder) fistula is an abnormal opening between the bladder and the vagina (Figure 11-9).

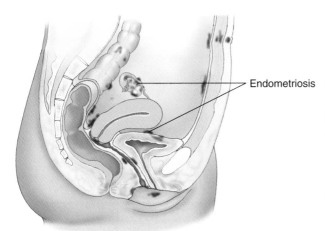

Endometriosis

endo- = inside
metr/i = uterine tissue
-osis = condition, disease
pelv/i = pelvis

Figure 11-8 Common sites of endometriosis. This abnormal location of endometrial tissue is often the ovaries and, less frequently, other pelvic structures.

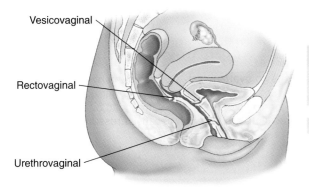

Vesicovaginal

Rectovaginal

Urethrovaginal

rect/o = rectum
urethr/o = urethra
vagin/o = vagina
vesic/o = bladder

Figure 11-9 Sites of vaginal fistulas. Abnormal openings between the vagina and the bladder, rectum, and urethra are shown. These abnormal openings are called vesicovaginal fistula, rectovaginal fistula, and urethrovaginal fistula, respectively.

hysteroptosis (hyster/o, uterus + -ptosis, sagging) prolapse of the uterus (Figure 11-10).

myoma common benign fibroid tumor of the uterine muscle.

oophoritis (oophor/o, ovary) an inflamed condition of an ovary.

oophorosalpingitis (salping/o, uterine tube) inflammation of an ovary and its uterine tube.

ovarian carcinoma cancer of an ovary, a malignancy that is rarely detected in the early stage and usually far advanced when diagnosed (Figure 11-11, *A*).

ovarian cyst sac filled with fluid or semisolid material that develops in or on the ovary, and is usually benign. Compare ovarian cancer (Figure 11-11, *A*) with a benign ovarian cyst (Figure 11-11, *B*).

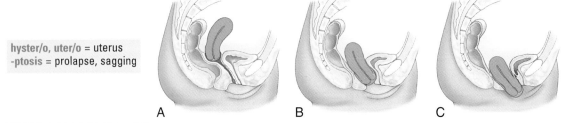

hyster/o, uter/o = uterus
-ptosis = prolapse, sagging

A   B   C

Figure 11-10 Hysteroptosis. Three stages of uterine prolapse. **A,** Grade I: uterus bulges into the vagina but does not protrude through the entrance. **B,** Grade II: cervix is visible within the vagina. **C,** Grade III: body of the uterus and the cervix protrude through the vaginal orifice.

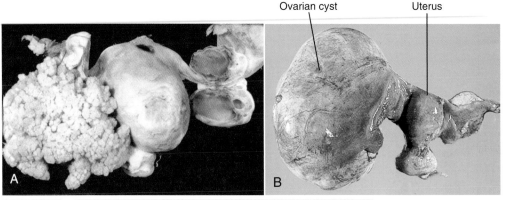

Ovarian cyst   Uterus

A   B

carcin/o = cancer
-oma = tumor

Figure 11-11 Ovarian carcinoma versus an ovarian cyst. A, Carcinoma of the ovary. The ovary is enormously enlarged by the tumor. Ovarian cancer is often far advanced when diagnosed. **B,** Ovarian cyst. This large, benign cyst is soft and surrounded by a thin capsule. Ovarian masses are often asymptomatic until large enough to cause pressure in the pelvis.

pelvic inflammatory disease (PID) infection of the upper genital organs beyond the cervix, often involving the peritoneum and intestines.

premenstrual syndrome (PMS) syndrome of nervous tension, irritability, weight gain, edema, headache, painful breasts, sleep changes, and other symptoms occurring a few days before the onset of menstruation.

salpingitis inflammation of a uterine tube.

salpingocele (-cele, hernia) hernial protrusion of a uterine tube.

uterine cancer any malignancy of the uterus, including the cervix or endometrium.

vulvitis (vulv/o, vulva) inflammation of the vulva.

MATCH IT! **EXERCISE 8**

Match the terms with their meanings.

_____ **1.** abnormal passage between two internal organs or between an internal organ and body surface

_____ **2.** prevention of pregnancy

_____ **3.** sagging of an organ

_____ **4.** tumor occurring on a mucous membrane

A. contraception
B. fistula
C. polyp
D. prolapse

CIRCLE IT! **EXERCISE 9**

Circle the correct answer to complete each sentence.

1. A word that means the same as vaginitis is (cervicitis, colpitis, salpingitis, vulvitis).

2. A condition in which tissue that somewhat resembles endometrium is found in an abnormal location in the pelvic cavity is called (endometritis, endometriosis, pelvic inflammatory disease, peritubal adhesions).

3. An examination using an instrument that magnifies the vaginal mucosa is called (colpitis, colposcopy, endometriosis, hysteroptosis).

4. Prolapse of the uterus is (extrauterine, hysterectomy, hysteroptosis, intrauterine).

5. Inflammation of the inner lining of the uterus is (colpitis, endometritis, salpingitis, vulvitis).

Surgical and Therapeutic Interventions

Refraining from sexual contact (abstinence) avoids pregnancy and sexually transmitted disease. Contraception (contra-, against) is any process or technique for preventing pregnancy in sexually active persons. Female and male **sterilization** are called tubal ligation and vasectomy, respectively. In a tubal ligation, both uterine tubes are blocked. A vasectomy is bilateral excision of the vas deferens. Both are highly effective and are recommended as a contraceptive option for people who don't want additional children. They should be considered permanent, because reversal is not always successful. Conception cannot occur after a hysterectomy, or removal of both ovaries; however, the purpose (e.g., cancer) of these surgeries is not related to contraception.

 QUICK TIP

Sterilization renders a person unable to produce children.

The Food and Drug Administration has approved a number of birth control methods or **contraceptives**, used to prevent conception, or pregnancy (Table 11-1). Oral contraceptives, contraceptive implants, contraceptive patches, and injectable contraceptives are methods that use hormones to prevent ovulation. A woman usually means she is taking oral contraceptives (OCs) when she says she is "on the pill." An intra+uterine device (IUD) is a contraceptive device that is inserted into the uterus by the physician. **Spermi+cides** are placed in the vagina to kill sperm but are not as effective as several other contraceptive methods.

Table 11-1   Effectiveness of Contraceptive Methods

Method	Action
Very Effective	
Intrauterine device (IUD) or intrauterine system (IUS)	Small plastic or metal device placed in the uterus. Cause of effectiveness is not known but may prevent fertilization or implantation. Some devices release hormones. IUD and IUS release progesterone onto the uterine lining. Used also for treating heavy menstrual periods.
Injectable contraceptives	Hormonal injections on a specific schedule prevent ovulation.
Effective	
Contraceptive patch	Transdermal patch worn on the skin.
Oral contraceptives	"Birth control pills," containing hormones, usually progestin and estrogen, that prevent ovulation.
Less Effective	
Condom (male)	Thin sheath (usually latex) worn over the penis to collect and prevent entry of semen.
Diaphragm with spermicide	Soft rubber cup that covers the uterine cervix to prevent sperm from reaching the egg.
Sponge with spermicide	Acts as barrier to sperm and releases spermicide.
Cervical cap with spermicide	Similar to diaphragm, but smaller, and covers cervix closely.
Condoms (female)	Thin sheaths placed in the vagina to prevent entry of sperm.
Coitus interruptus	Withdrawal of the penis before ejaculation.
Spermicides	Vaginal foams, creams, or jellies that are inserted into the vagina before intercourse to destroy sperm.
Calendar, or rhythm, method	Determine fertile period and practice abstinence (voluntarily avoiding sexual intercourse) during the most fertile days.

Data from www.fda.gov/fdac.

WRITE IT!   **EXERCISE 10**

Write a term in each blank space to complete the sentence.

1. Refraining from sexual intercourse is called _____.

2. A small plastic or metal device placed within the uterus to prevent contraception is an _____ device.

3. Vaginal foams, creams, or jellies that are used to destroy the sperm are _____.

4. Withdrawal of the penis before ejaculation is _____ interruptus.

5. A method of practicing abstinence during fertile periods is called the calendar or _____ method.

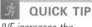 **QUICK TIP**

IVF increases the chance of multiple births.

Administration of hormones, use of vaginal medications, surgery, and counseling are some of the treatments used in correcting infertility, depending on the cause. **In vitro fertilization** (IVF) is a method of fertilizing the ova outside the body by collecting mature ova and placing them in a dish with spermatozoa before placing them in the uterus for implantation. IVF may be successful when failure to conceive is caused by insufficient numbers of sperm.

After the cause of amenorrhea is established, it is treated by surgical and pharmaceutical means (e.g., hormone replacement, stimulation of ovaries). Hormone replacement therapy (HRT) is a common intervention for women who suffer the symptoms of menopause or who are at high risk for osteoporosis, the abnormal loss of bone density and deterioration of bone tissue. There is no agreement on the value versus risk of HRT.

The following list describes several surgical interventions.

colpoplasty (colp/o, vagina + -plasty, surgical repair) plastic surgery of the vagina.

colporrhaphy (-rrhaphy, suture) suture of the vagina.

conization of the cervix excision of a cone of tissue from the cervix performed to remove a lesion from the cervix or to obtain tissue for biopsy. (This procedure is sometimes performed in conjunction with a D&C; see below.)

dilation and curettage (D&C) surgical procedure that expands the cervical opening (dilation or dilatation) so that the uterine wall can be scraped **(curettage)**.

endometrial ablation destruction of a thin layer of the uterus to stop heavy menstrual bleeding. Ablation means removal or destruction of a part.

hysterectomy (hyster/o, uterus + -ectomy, excision) surgical removal of the uterus. Removal of the uterus through the abdominal wall is called an abdominal hysterectomy, or **laparohysterectomy** (lapar/o, abdominal wall). Removal of the uterus through the vagina is called a vaginal hysterectomy.

laparoscopy (lapar/o, abdominal wall + -scopy, visually examining) abdominal exploration using a lighted instrument, the laparoscope, which allows for direct visualization of the abdominal contents (see Figure 11-5). Another instrument, a cannula, is inserted to allow movement of the uterus during the examination.

laparotomy (-tomy, incision) an abdominal operation; surgical opening of the abdomen done for various purposes.

oophorectomy (oophor/o, ovary) surgical removal of one or both ovaries.

salpingectomy (salping/o, uterine tube) surgical removal of a uterine tube.

salpingo-oophorectomy (oophor/o, ovary) removal of an ovary and its accompanying uterine tube. Bilateral salpingo-oophorectomy is removal of both ovaries and their uterine tubes.

salpingorrhaphy suture of a uterine tube.

tubal ligation sterilization by surgically binding or crushing the uterine tubes (ligation means binding or tying).

WRITE IT!
EXERCISE 11

Write terms in the blanks to complete each sentence.

1. Surgical removal of the uterus is a _____.
2. Plastic surgery of the vagina is _____.
3. Suture of the vagina is _____.
4. Removal of an ovary is _____.
5. Suture of a uterine tube is _____.
6. Tying or binding of a uterine tube for elective sterilization is a tubal _____.
7. Use of a lighted instrument to allow for direct visualization of the abdominal contents is

   _____.
8. The surgical procedure that is abbreviated D&C is dilation and _____.
9. An abdominal incision is a _____.
10. Cervical _____ is excision of a small cone of tissue from the cervix.

Pregnancy and Childbirth

Fertilization is the union of an ovum and a sperm, resulting in an embryo. Fertilization of the ovum by the sperm occurs most often in the uterine tube (Figure 11-12). **Implantation,** embedding of the fertilized ovum (called a **zygote**), usually occurs in the endometrium. Extraembryonic membranes (**amnion** and **chorion**) form around the embryo and give rise to the **placenta,** a structure through which the fetus derives nourishment during pregnancy. It is commonly called the "afterbirth" because it is expelled after delivery of the baby.

fet/o = fetus

In humans the developing embryo is called a fetus after 8 weeks. **Fetal** is an adjective that refers to the fetus. Within a few days after fertilization has occurred, a

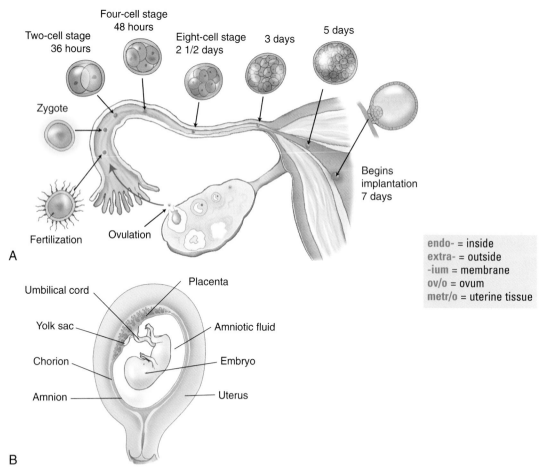

endo- = inside
extra- = outside
-ium = membrane
ov/o = ovum
metr/o = uterine tissue

Figure 11-12 Fertilization, implantation, and growth of the embryo. A, Mature ovum is released in ovulation. The ovum is fertilized by a sperm, and the product of fertilization, the zygote, undergoes rapid cell division, finally implanting in the endometrium on approximately day 7. **B,** The placenta and extraembryonic membranes (amnion and chorion) form and surround the embryo, providing nourishment and protection. The human embryonic stage begins about 2 weeks after conception and lasts until about the end of week 8, after which time the fetal stage begins.

hormone called **human chorionic gonadotropin** (HCG) is produced and can be detected in body fluids. Testing for this hormone in urine or blood can indicate whether a woman is pregnant. HCG can be detected long before other signs of pregnancy appear.

Learn the following word parts and their meanings.

Word Parts: Obstetric Terms

Word Part	Meaning
amni/o	amnion (fetal membrane)
fet/o	fetus
nat/i	birth
par/o	to bear offspring
-para	a woman who has given birth

WRITE IT! EXERCISE 12

Write combining forms for these terms.
1. amnion _____
2. birth _____
3. fetus _____
4. to bear offspring _____

Ultra+sono+graphy, also called **ultrasound,** provides an image of the developing fetus (see Figure 4-11, p. 88). Ultrasonography has many uses in obstetrics, including the detection of an embryo that has implanted outside the uterus. Such abnormal implantation is called an extrauterine or **ectopic** pregnancy. The word ectopic means located outside the usual place.

Prenatal and **postnatal** mean occurring before birth and after birth, respectively. A neonate is a newborn infant up to 6 weeks of age; this period of time is known as the **neonatal** period.

Obstetrics is the branch of medicine that specializes in the care of women during pregnancy and childbirth. The specialist is an **obstetrician. Gestation,** another word meaning pregnancy, is the period from conception to birth. Parturition is a synonym for childbirth. **Antepartum** means before childbirth, and **postpartum** means after childbirth.

The combining form par/o is often used to form words referring to the bearing of offspring. A designation showing the number of pregnancies resulting in live births is para I (or 1) or para II (or 2), but does not reflect the number of offspring in multiple births. Therefore, thinking of *para* as "birth" is acceptable if you remember that para I could represent more than one offspring. Other designations are **unipara, secundipara,** and **tripara. Nullipara** refers to a woman who has never had a viable (live) birth.

A woman who is pregnant for the first time is called **gravida** I or 1 (or **primigravida**). Gravida II or 2, III or 3, and so on designate subsequent pregnancies. Note that *gravida* refers only to pregnancy, whereas *para* designates successful pregnancies resulting in live births. A woman could be gravida III (pregnant for the third time) but para 0 (no live births, same as nullipara).

ecto- = outside
top/o = location

nat/i = birth
ne/o = new

ante- = before
post- = after

uni- = one
-para = woman who has given birth
tri- = three
nulli- = none

WORD ORIGIN
secundus (L.)
second

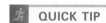
The average period of gestation (pregnancy) is 266 days from the date of fertilization, but it is clinically considered to last 280 days from the first day of the last menstrual period (LMP). The expected date of delivery (EDD) is usually calculated on the latter basis. For convenience, pregnancy is discussed in terms of the first, second, and third trimesters. A **trimester** is approximately 3 months, with the first day of the LMP to the end of 12 weeks designating the first trimester.

Labor, the process by which the child is expelled from the uterus, is that time from the beginning of cervical dilation to the delivery of the placenta. Cervical dilation, expulsion of the fetus, and expulsion of the placenta represent stages of labor. The postpartum stage, the hour or two after delivery when uterine tone is established, is sometimes included as a fourth stage of labor. The events just described are the stages of a vaginal delivery. A **cesarean section** or cesarean birth, the surgical removal of the fetus from the uterus, is performed when fetal or maternal conditions make vaginal delivery hazardous.

Fetal presentation describes the part of the fetus that is touched by the examining finger through the cervix or that has entered the mother's lower pelvis during labor. **Cephalic presentation** is normal and the most common fetal presentation. In a **breech presentation** the buttocks, knees, or feet are presented. In a **shoulder presentation** the long axis of the baby's body is across the long axis of the mother's body, and the shoulder is presented at the cervical opening. This type of presentation is also called transverse presentation. Vaginal delivery is impossible unless the baby turns spontaneously or is turned in utero. Compare the three types of presentation in Figure 11-13.

Study the following list of obstetric terms.

abruptio placentae separation of the placenta from the uterine wall after 20 or more weeks of gestation or during labor; often results in severe hemorrhage.

amnion the innermost of the membranes that surround the developing fetus. This transparent sac, also called the **amniotic** sac, holds the fetus suspended in amniotic fluid.

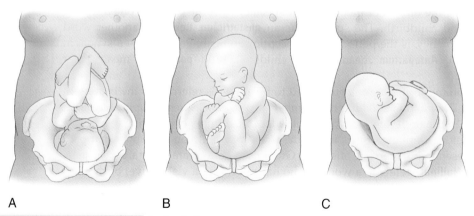

A   B   C

Figure 11-13 Fetal presentation. A, Cephalic presentation, the normal presentation of the top of the head, the brow, the face, or the chin at the cervical opening. **B,** Breech presentation. **C,** Shoulder presentation.

amniocentesis (amni/o, amnion + -centesis, puncture) **transabdominal** (through the abdomen) puncture of the amniotic sac to remove amniotic fluid. The material that is removed can be studied to detect genetic disorders or other abnormalities (see Figure 2-6, p. 26).

amniotomy (-tomy, incision) surgical rupture of the fetal membranes, performed to induce or expedite labor.

cesarean section (C-section) incision through the walls of the abdomen and uterus for delivery of a fetus.

chorionic villus sampling sampling of the placental tissue for prenatal diagnosis of potential genetic defects.

Down syndrome congenital condition characterized by mild to severe mental retardation and caused by an abnormality, usually the presence of three of chromosome 21, rather than the expected pair (Figure 11-14). Ultra-Screen is a first-trimester prenatal screening test that is designed to provide specific information about the risk of Down syndrome and other chromosomal abnormalities. The test consists of a combination of ultrasound measurement and a blood test performed between 11 weeks, 1 day and 13 weeks, 6 days of pregnancy.

episiotomy surgical procedure in which an incision is made to enlarge the vaginal opening for delivery.

erythroblastosis fetalis (erythr/o, red + blast/o, embryonic form + -osis, condition) anemia of newborns characterized by premature destruction of red blood cells and resulting from maternal-fetal blood group incompatibility, specifically involving the Rh factor and the ABO blood groups. Also called hemolytic disease of the newborn.

fetal monitoring (fet/o, fetus) assessment of the fetus in utero, usually with respect to its heartbeat (by electrocardiography).

placenta previa abnormal implantation of the placenta in the uterus so that it impinges on or covers the opening at the upper end of the uterine cervix.

MATCH IT!
EXERCISE 13

Match the terms with their meanings.

_____ **1.** antepartum

_____ **2.** gestation

_____ **3.** parturition

_____ **4.** postpartum

A. pregnancy

B. childbirth

C. before birth

D. after birth

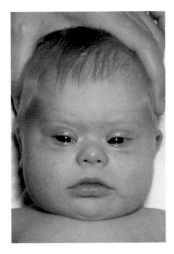

Figure 11-14 Typical facial characteristics of Down syndrome. This congenital condition, usually caused by an extra chromosome 21, is characterized by varying degrees of mental retardation and multiple defects. It can be diagnosed prenatally by amniocentesis and other methods that examine chromosomes.

Choose the correct answer for each question.

1. What is the term for a woman who has had two successful pregnancies?
   (nullipara, secundipara, tripara, unipara)
2. What is the correct term for an unborn 12-week-old developing human?
   (embryo, fetus, gestation, zygote)
3. Which term means abnormal implantation of a fertilized ovum outside the uterus?
   (abruptio placentae, cesarean section, ectopic pregnancy, transverse presentation)
4. Which term refers to the period covering the first 4 weeks after birth?
   (neonatal, obstetric, parturition, prenatal)
5. Which of the following is the normal fetal presentation?
   (breech, cephalic, shoulder, transverse)
6. Which term means the transparent sac that encloses the fetus in utero?
   (amniocentesis, amnion, congenital sac, trisomic sac)
7. Which of the following indicates a congenital condition of the newborn marked by mental retardation?
   (Down syndrome, cesarean section, ectopic pregnancy, jaundice)
8. Which term means surgical rupture of the fetal membrane?
   (amniocentesis, amniotomy, cesarean section, fetal monitoring)
9. What is the name of the structure through which the fetus receives nourishment?
   (fistula, HCG, ovary, placenta)
10. Which term means separation of the placenta from the uterine wall after 20 weeks or more of gestation or during labor?
    (abruptio placentae, episiotomy, labor, placenta previa)

Female Breasts

The female breasts are accessory reproductive organs. Each breast contains 15 to 20 lobes of glandular tissue that radiate around the nipples, which may have many smaller sections called **lobules** (Figure 11-15). The circular pigmented area of skin surrounding the nipple is the **areola.** The amount of **adipose** tissue (fat) determines the size of the breast.

mamm/o = breast
-ary = pertaining to

The female breasts are milk-producing glands and are called **mamm+ary** glands. During pregnancy, these glands undergo changes that prepare them for production of milk. Each lobe is drained by a **lactiferous** duct that has openings in the nipple.

lact/o = milk
-ation = process

Lact+ation is the secretion of milk. The production and secretion of milk is controlled by the endocrine (hormonal) and nervous systems.

Mammo+graphy is a diagnostic procedure that uses radiography to study the breast. The radiographic image produced in mammography is a **mammogram.** Breast cancer can often be diagnosed by studying a mammogram (Figure 11-16). Excluding skin cancer, breast cancer has been the most common malignancy among women in the United States for many years. Breast cancer in women is the second leading cause of cancer death, after lung cancer. Treatment of breast cancer may require **lumpectomy** (removal of the lump or tumor), **chemotherapy,** radiation therapy, hormone therapy, or **mast+ectomy.**

mast/o = breast
-ptosis = sagging or prolapse
-pexy = surgical fixation
-plasty = surgical repair

Mastalgia and **mastodynia** mean pain in the breast; **mammalgia** also means painful breast. **Mastitis** means inflammation of the breast.

Mastoptosis means sagging breasts. A surgical procedure to lift the breasts is **mastopexy.** Augmentation **mammoplasty** is plastic surgery to increase the size of the female breast (see Figure 2-8, p. 30). Reduction mammoplasty is plastic surgery to reduce the size of the breast.

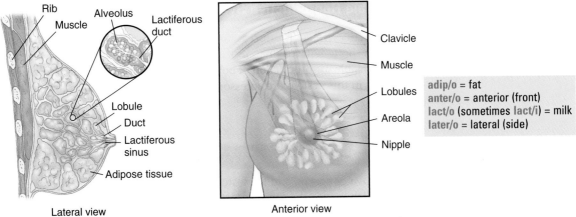

Rib
Muscle
Alveolus
Lactiferous duct
Lobule
Duct
Lactiferous sinus
Adipose tissue

Lateral view

Clavicle
Muscle
Lobules
Areola
Nipple

Anterior view

adip/o = fat
anter/o = anterior (front)
lact/o (sometimes lact/i) = milk
later/o = lateral (side)

Figure 11-15 Structure of the adult female breast, lateral and anterior views. The breasts are mammary glands and function as part of both the endocrine and reproductive systems. The amount of adipose tissue determines the size of the breasts, but not the amount of milk that can be produced. The nipple contains the openings of the lactiferous, or milk, ducts. Breasts are prepared for milk production during pregnancy. After childbirth, interactions between the nervous system, hormones, and the breasts result in expression of milk.

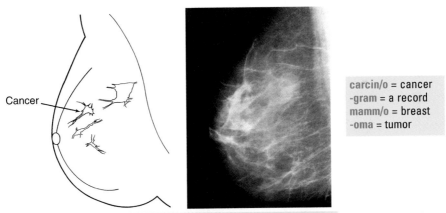

Cancer

carcin/o = cancer
-gram = a record
mamm/o = breast
-oma = tumor

Figure 11-16 Mammogram, including a drawing, of cancer of the breast. The light areas that are visible on the mammogram indicate carcinoma.

MATCH IT!
EXERCISE 15

Match terms in the left column with those in the right column.

_____ **1.** mammary
_____ **2.** mastectomy
_____ **3.** mammography
_____ **4.** mastoptosis

A. pertaining to the breast
B. radiographic examination of the breast
C. sagging breasts
D. surgical removal of a breast

Male Reproductive System

The male reproductive system produces, sustains, and transports spermatozoa; introduces sperm into the female vagina; and produces hormones. The testes, the male gonads, are responsible for production of both sperm and hormones. All other organs, ducts, and glands in this system are accessory reproductive organs that transport and sustain the sperm.

Structures

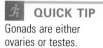

QUICK TIP

Gonads are either ovaries or testes.

Gonads produce ova or sperm, and the testes are the male gonads. **Testes** is the plural form of testis, which means the same as **testicle.**

Write the names of the structures in the blank lines (*1* to *12*) on Figure 11-17 as you read the following information. The **penis** *(1)* transfers sperm to the vagina. The **prepuce** *(2)*, a loose fold of skin, covers the **glans penis** *(3)*.

Only one **testis** *(4)* is shown in Figure 11-17. After sperm are produced by the testis, they are stored in the **epididymis** *(5)*. The testes and epididymis are contained in a pouch of skin called the **scrotum** *(6)*.

Each **ductus deferens** *(7)*, also called the **vas deferens,** begins at the epididymis, continues upward, and enters the abdominopelvic cavity. Each ductus deferens joins a duct from the seminal vesicle *(8)* to form a short ejaculatory duct *(9)*, which passes through the prostate gland *(10)*. Ejaculation is the expulsion of semen from the urethra *(11)*. Paired **bulbourethral** glands *(12)* contribute an alkaline, mucus-like fluid to the semen.

Several important word parts refer to male reproductive organs. Commit the meanings of the word parts in the table on the next page to memory.

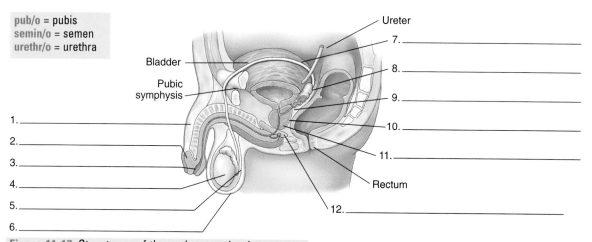

pub/o = pubis
semin/o = semen
urethr/o = urethra

Ureter
Bladder
Pubic symphysis
Rectum

1.____
2.____
3.____
4.____
5.____
6.____
7.____
8.____
9.____
10.____
11.____
12.____

Figure 11-17 Structures of the male reproductive system. The structures that are already labeled lie near, but are not part of, the male reproductive system.

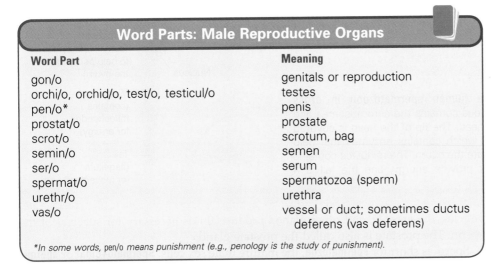

Word Parts: Male Reproductive Organs

Word Part	Meaning
gon/o	genitals or reproduction
orchi/o, orchid/o, test/o, testicul/o	testes
pen/o*	penis
prostat/o	prostate
scrot/o	scrotum, bag
semin/o	semen
ser/o	serum
spermat/o	spermatozoa (sperm)
urethr/o	urethra
vas/o	vessel or duct; sometimes ductus deferens (vas deferens)

*In some words, pen/o means punishment (e.g., penology is the study of punishment).

WRITE IT! EXERCISE 16

Write combining forms for the following.

1. genitals or reproduction _____
2. penis _____
3. prostate _____
4. scrotum _____
5. semen _____
6. sperm _____
7. testes _____
8. vas deferens _____

The testes produce an important male hormone, **testosterone,** that induces and maintains male secondary sex characteristics. In addition, the testes are responsible for **spermato+genesis,** the formation of mature functional sperm. Human sperm are produced in vast numbers after puberty. Each sperm has a head with a nucleus, a neck, and a tail that provides propulsion (Figure 11-18). The formation of sperm is also influenced by hormones produced by the brain and the pituitary gland. **Semen,** also called seminal fluid, is a mixture of sperm cells and secretions. Although millions of sperm are ejaculated in semen, only one sperm fertilizes an ovum. The production of sperm outside the body cavity is necessary for viability of the sperm. The testes develop in the abdominal cavity of the fetus and normally descend through the inguinal canal into the scrotum shortly before birth (sometimes shortly after birth).

spermat/o = sperm
-genesis = formation

Sperm leave the male's body in semen, the fluid that is discharged from the penis at the height of sexual excitement. **Seminal vesicles** serve as a reservoir for semen until it is discharged. The combining form vesic/o means bladder, cyst, or sac. The term *vesicle,* however, means a small sac containing fluid or a small, blister-like elevation on the skin containing serous fluid. Seminal vesicles refer to small sacs that store semen, whereas vesicular rash refers to an eruption of blisters on the skin. The seminal

semin/o = semen

WORD ORIGIN
semen (L.) seed

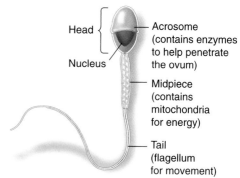

Head
Acrosome
(contains enzymes
to help penetrate
the ovum)

Nucleus

Midpiece
(contains
mitochondria
for energy)

Tail
(flagellum
for movement)

Figure 11-18 The human spermatozoon in cross section. The nucleus contains the chromosomes and is located in the head. The tip of the head is covered by an acrosome, which contains enzymes that help the sperm penetrate the ovum. The midpiece contains mitochondria that provide energy, and the tail is a typical flagellum.

vesicles, the **prostate,** and other glands produce fluids necessary for survival of the sperm. The prostate is also called the prostate gland.

-cidal = killing

Sperm is short for **spermatozoa,** the mature male sex cells. **Spermato+cidal** or **spermi+cidal** refers to the killing of sperm. Contraceptive foams and creams are spermicidal, and as such are designed to prevent pregnancy.

FIND IT IN NEW TERMS!

EXERCISE 17

Write the meaning of the combining forms in these terms.

Term	Meaning of Combining Form
1. penile	_____
2. prostatic	_____
3. scrotal	_____
4. seminal	_____
5. testicular	_____

Diseases, Disorders, and Diagnostic Terms

benign prostatic hyperplasia (BPH) (hyper-, increase + -plasia, formation) nonmalignant, noninflammatory enlargement of the prostate, most common among men older than 50 (Figure 11-19).

cryptorchidism (crypt/o, hidden + orchid/o, testis + -ism, condition) undescended testicles; failure of the testicles to descend into the scrotum before birth.

hydrocele (hydr/o, water + -cele, hernia) accumulation of fluid in a saclike cavity, especially serous tumors of the testes or associated parts. Serous (ser/o, serum + -ous, pertaining to) means resembling serum or producing or containing serum (Figure 11-20).

orchiditis or **orchitis** (orchid/o or orchi/o, testis + -itis, inflammation) inflammation of a testis. (Notice the spelling of orchitis. In joining orchi/o + -itis, one *i* is dropped to avoid double *i.*)

prostatic carcinoma slowly progressing cancer of the prostate; typically detected by a prostate-specific antigen (PSA) test and rectal examination. Treatment is by surgery, radiation therapy, or hormones.

prostatitis inflammation of the prostate.

testicular torsion (testicul/o, testicle) axial rotation of the spermatic cord, which cuts off the blood supply to the testicle (see Figure 11-20).

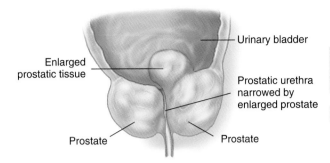

-ic = pertaining to
prostat/o = prostate
urin/o = urine

Figure 11-19 Benign prostatic hyperplasia. As the prostate (shown in cross section) enlarges, it extends upward into the bladder, and inward, obstructing the outflow of urine from the bladder.

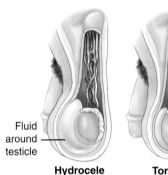

Twisted spermatic cord and blood vessels

-ar = pertaining to
-cele = hernia
hydr/o = water
testicul/o = testicle

Fluid around testicle

Hydrocele   **Torsion**

Figure 11-20 Hydrocele and testicular torsion.

Write a term in the blanks to complete each sentence.

1. A term for undescended testicles is _____.

2. A nonmalignant, noninflammatory enlargement of the prostate is benign prostatic

_____.

3. The term that means inflammation of the prostate is _____.

4. A synonym for orchiditis is _____.

5. Accumulation of fluid in the testicle is called a(n) _____.

Surgical and Therapeutic Interventions

circumcision surgical removal of the end of the foreskin that covers the head of the penis. This is usually performed shortly after birth for hygienic or religious reasons.

orchidectomy (orchid/o, testes, + -ectomy, excision) surgical removal of a testicle (often done to treat malignancy of a testicle). Excision of both testes is **castration. Orchiectomy** is a synonym for orchidectomy.

orchidoplasty (-plasty, surgical repair) plastic surgery of the testis, particularly the surgery performed to correct a testicle that has not descended properly into the scrotum.

orchiopexy (-pexy, surgical fixation) surgical fixation of an undescended testicle in the scrotum. Also called **orchidopexy**.

orchiotomy (-tomy, incision) incision and drainage of a testis.

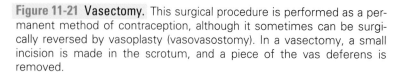

contra- = against
-ectomy = excision
-plasty = surgical repair
vas/o = vas deferens

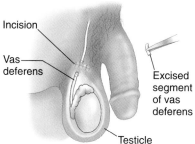

Figure 11-21 Vasectomy. This surgical procedure is performed as a permanent method of contraception, although it sometimes can be surgically reversed by vasoplasty (vasovasostomy). In a vasectomy, a small incision is made in the scrotum, and a piece of the vas deferens is removed.

prostatectomy (prostat/o, prostate) removal of all or part of the prostate.

transurethral microwave thermotherapy (trans-, across + urethr/o, urethra; therm/o, heat) (TUMT) treatment of BPH performed through the urethra using microwave energy to raise the temperature selectively and destroy prostatic tissue.

transurethral needle ablation (TUNA) treatment of BPH performed through the urethra using low-level radio frequency energy. *Ablation* is a general term for excision or removal of a growth or any part of the body.

transurethral prostatectomy partial or complete removal of the prostate gland by passing a cystoscope through the urethra. It is also called **transurethral resection** of the prostate (TURP). Resection is a term that means excision of all or part of a structure.

vasectomy (vas/o, vas deferens) removal of all or a segment of the vas deferens, usually done bilaterally to produce sterility (Figure 11-21).

vasovasostomy (-stomy, new opening) surgically reconnecting the ends of the severed ductus deferens, done to correct an obstruction or as a form of vasectomy reversal.

WRITE IT! **EXERCISE 19**

Write a term in each blank to complete these sentences.

1. The term for surgical fixation of an undescended testicle is _____.

2. Surgical removal of the end of the foreskin that covers the head of the penis is _____.

3. Surgical removal of a segment of the ductus deferens is a _____.

4. Surgical removal of a testicle is _____.

5. Surgical removal of all or part of the prostate is called a _____.

6. A general term for excision or removal of a growth or any part of the body is _____.

Sexually Transmitted Diseases

urethr/o = urethra
vagin/o = vagina

genit/o = genitals
-ur/o = urinary tract

A disease acquired through sexual contact is a sexually transmitted disease (STD), sometimes called venereal disease (venereal was named for Venus, goddess of love). Generally, STDs cause one of these problems: male **urethr+itis,** female lower genitourinary tract infection, and vagin+itis. The term **genito+urin+ary** (GU) pertains to the genitals and the urinary organs.

Study Table 11-2 to learn the names and characteristics of several STDs. You may want to refer to the table to complete Exercises 20 and 21.

Table 11-2 Sexually Transmitted Diseases and Their Causes

Disease of the Genitals*	Causative Agent	Characteristics
Bacterial		
Gonorrhea (Figure 11-22)	*Neisseria gonorrhoeae*; commonly called **gonococcus** (GC)	Males: Urethral discharge, dysuria Females: Often asymptomatic
Syphilis	*Treponema pallidum* (a **spirochete**)	Primary stage: Painless **chancre** (Figure 11-23) Secondary stage: Rash Late: Only about one third of untreated cases progress to syphilitic involvement of viscera, cardiovascular system, and central nervous system
Chlamydial infection	*Chlamydia trachomatis*	Males: Urethritis, dysuria, frequent urination Females: Mild symptoms to none; one of the most common STDs in North America, frequent cause of pelvic inflammatory disease (PID) and sterility
Chancroid (nonsyphilitic venereal ulcer)	*Haemophilus ducreyi*	Painful ulceration of the genitals

Continued

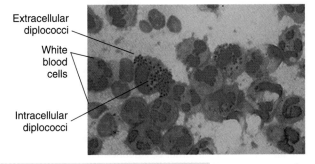

-ar = pertaining to
cellul/o = cell
dipl/o = double
extra- = outside
gon/o = reproduction or genitals
intra- = within

Extracellular diplococci

White blood cells

Intracellular diplococci

Figure 11-22 Gram-negative intracellular diplococci. The presence of gram-negative intracellular diplococci in a urethral smear is usually indicative of gonorrhea in males. The same finding in females is considered presumptive and is generally followed by culture to confirm the diagnosis. Note also the presence of many extracellular diplococci.

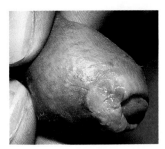

Figure 11-23 Syphilitic chancre. The lesion of primary syphilis generally occurs about 2 weeks after exposure. The chancre is not usually located on the glans penis but can be located on the foreskin. Scrapings from the ulcer show spirochetes, the causative organism of syphilis, when examined microscopically using special illumination.

Table 11-2   Sexually Transmitted Diseases and Their Causes—cont'd

Disease of the Genitals*	Causative Agent	Characteristics
Nonspecific genital infection	Various organisms, not all of which are bacteria	Males: Nongonococcal urethritis Females: PID, cervicitis
Viral		
Acquired immuno-deficiency syndrome (AIDS)	Human immuno-deficiency virus (HIV)	A fatal late stage of infection with HIV that involves profound immunosuppression. To be diagnosed as having AIDS, one must be infected with HIV and have a clinical disease that indicates cellular immunodeficiency, or have a specified level of markers in the blood, including certain T lymphocytes. Characterized by opportunistic infections and malignant neoplasms that rarely affect healthy individuals, especially **Kaposi sarcoma** (Figure 11-24). Transmitted by infected body fluids (sexual contact, blood and blood products, breast milk).
Herpes genitalis (genital herpes)	Herpes simplex type 2 (HSV-2)	Blisters and ulceration of the genitalia, fever, and dysuria (Figure 11-25)

Continued

hem/o = blood
-oma = tumor
-rrhagic = pertaining to hemorrhage (-rrhage + -ic)

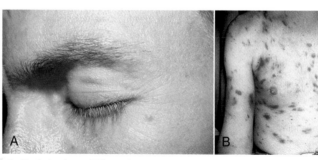

Figure 11-24 Kaposi sarcoma. A, Early lesion of Kaposi sarcoma. **B,** Advanced lesions of Kaposi sarcoma. Note widespread hemorrhagic plaques and nodules.

-al, -ar = pertaining to
genit/o = genitals
vulv/o = vulva

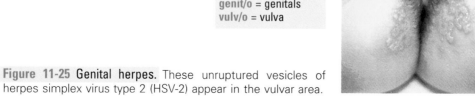

Figure 11-25 Genital herpes. These unruptured vesicles of herpes simplex virus type 2 (HSV-2) appear in the vulvar area.

Table 11-2 Sexually Transmitted Diseases and Their Causes—cont'd

Disease of the Genitals*	Causative Agent	Characteristics
Viral–cont'd		
Condyloma acuminatum (genital warts)	Human **papillomavirus** (HPV)	Cauliflower-like genital and anal warts (Figure 11-26); infection puts females at high risk for cervical cancer. A vaccine is available that prevents infection with the two types of HPV responsible for most cervical cancer cases.
Hepatitis B, C, and D	Hepatitis B, C, and D viruses (HBV, HCV, and HDV)	These inflammatory conditions of the liver are separate diseases acquired by sexual contact, contaminated blood, or use of contaminated needles or equipment. Diseases vary from mild symptoms to serious complications. Hepatitis B vaccine is available for those at high risk; hepatitis B immune globulin provides postexposure passive immunity.
Protozoal		
Trichomoniasis	*Trichomonas vaginalis*	Females: Frothy discharge of varying severity Males: Often asymptomatic
Fungal		
Candidiasis	*Candida albicans*	Vulvovaginitis: white patches, cheeselike discharge
Parasitic		
Pubic lice	*Phthirus pubis*	Severe itching, redness, and inflammation of the skin and mucous membranes

Although diseases of the genitals are given emphasis here, many of the organisms can infect other organs.

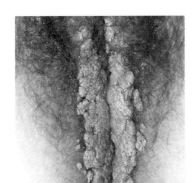

genit/o = genitals
vulv/o = vulva

Figure 11-26 Genital warts. Severe vulvar warts. The growth may be solitary, or a cauliflower-like group in the same area of the genitalia as shown in this example.

WRITE IT!

EXERCISE 20

Write a term in each blank to complete these sentences.

1. An STD caused by a gonococcus is _____.

2. Where are intracellular diplococci of gonorrhea located relative to the cell, within or outside?

_____

3. A lesion that is characteristic of the primary stage of syphilis is called a _____.

4. A disease that may be asymptomatic in females but is one of the most common STDs in North America is a _____ infection.

5. A late-stage infection with HIV is called acquired _____ syndrome.

6. A malignant lesion of AIDS that is rarely seen in healthy individuals is _____ sarcoma.

7. A viral infection that causes blisters and ulceration of the genitalia is _____ genitalis.

8. Cauliflower-like genital and anal warts are characteristic of the infection commonly called genital _____.

9. HBV, HCV, or HDV causes an inflammatory condition of the liver called _____.

10. The STD caused by *Trichomonas vaginalis* is _____.

11. Inflammation of the vulva and vagina accompanied by a cheeselike discharge is characteristic of _____.

12. A parasitic STD that causes severe itching, redness, and inflammation of the skin and mucous membranes is pubic _____.

MATCH IT!

EXERCISE 21

Choose the category of causative agent in the right column to classify these STDs.

_____ **1.** AIDS
_____ **2.** candidiasis
_____ **3.** chlamydial infection
_____ **4.** genital herpes
_____ **5.** genital warts
_____ **6.** gonorrhea
_____ **7.** hepatitis B, C, or D
_____ **8.** syphilis
_____ **9.** trichomoniasis

A. bacteria
B. fungi
C. protozoa
D. virus

 Be Careful with These!

cervic/o can refer to the uterine cervix or the neck.
metr/o can mean uterine tissue, but sometimes means measure.
vas/o means vessel or duct, but sometimes specifically means the ductus deferens.

SELF-TEST   Work the following exercises to test your understanding of the material in Chapter 11. Complete all the exercises before using Appendix VIII to check your answers.

A. LABEL IT!   *Label the diagram with the following combining forms that correspond to numbered lines 1 through 5 (the first one is done as an example): cervic/o, colp/o, hyster/o, oophor/o, salping/o.*

1. *oophor/o*
2. _____
3. _____
4. _____
5. _____

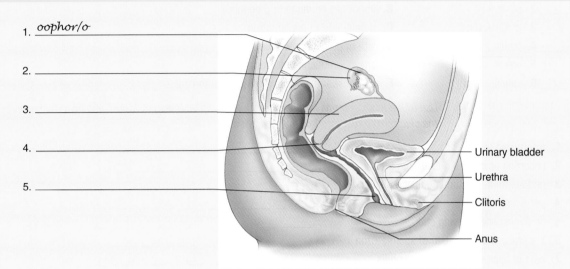

Urinary bladder
Urethra
Clitoris

Anus

Label the diagram with the following combining forms that correspond to numbered lines 6 through 11 (the first one is done as an example): orchi/o, pen/o, prostat/o, scrot/o, urethr/o, vas/o.

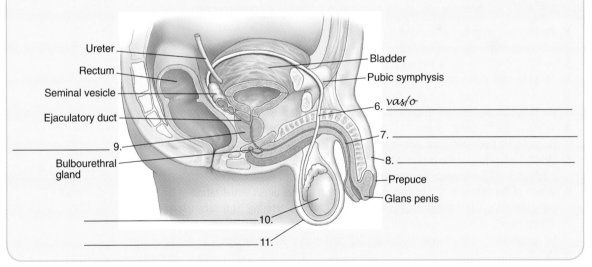

Ureter
Rectum
Seminal vesicle
Ejaculatory duct
_____ 9.
Bulbourethral gland

Bladder
Pubic symphysis
6. *vas/o* _____
7. _____
8. _____
Prepuce
Glans penis

10. _____
11. _____

Continued

SELF-TEST   (cont'd)

B. MATCH IT!   *Match the terms on the left with the descriptions in the right column.*

_____ **1.** ovary	**A.** afterbirth
_____ **2.** placenta	**B.** important hormone of pregnancy
_____ **3.** progesterone	**C.** normal site of implantation
_____ **4.** testis	**D.** site of production of ova
_____ **5.** uterus	**E.** site of production of sperm
_____ **6.** vagina	**F.** where sperm are received during intercourse

C. FINDING THE CLUE!   *Use a clue to write terms for these descriptions. Solve Question 1; each ending letter becomes the clue for the first letter of the next answer.*

1. a fertilized ovum   _____

2. occurring or located outside the uterus   _____

3. endometrium located in unusual places   _____

4. pertaining to semen   _____

5. producing or conveying milk   _____

6. the process of formation of spermatozoa   _____

7. type of bacteria that causes syphilis   _____

8. outside the usual place   _____

9. undescended testicle   _____

10. sagging breasts   _____

D. CIRCLE IT!   *Choose the one correct response (a, b, c, or d) for each question.*

1. Which term refers to the lining of the uterus?
  (a) cervix uteri   (b) endometrium   (c) myometrium   (d) perimetrium

2. Which of the following is the hormone tested for in a pregnancy test?
  (a) BPH   (b) EDD   (c) HCG   (d) LMP

3. Which of the following is a genetic disorder in which the fetus has an extra chromosome?
  (a) Down syndrome   (b) endometriosis   (c) erythroblastosis fetalis   (d) hemolytic anemia

4. Which of the following is abnormal placement of the placenta in the uterus?
  (a) abruptio placentae   (b) cesarean section   (c) ectopic pregnancy   (d) placenta previa

5. Which term refers to the normal presentation of the fetus during labor?
  (a) breech   (b) cephalic   (c) shoulder   (d) transverse

6. Which of the following is a lighted instrument that allows direct visualization of the abdominal contents?
  (a) colposcope   (b) dilation and curettage   (c) fetal monitoring   (d) laparoscope

7. Which branch of medicine specializes in the care of women during pregnancy and childbirth?
  (a) gynecology   (b) internal medicine   (c) obstetrics   (d) pediatrics

8. Which hormone has the primary responsibility of induction and maintenance of male sexual characteristics?
  (a) amnion   (b) estrogen   (c) testosterone   (d) uterine

SELF-TEST   (cont'd)

9. Which term means a woman who has never given birth to a viable offspring?
   (a) nullipara (b) secundipara (c) tripara (d) unipara
10. What are reproductive organs called?
   (a) genitalia (b) gonadotropin (c) uteri (d) vulva
11. What is the name of the transparent sac that encloses the fetus in utero?
   (a) amniocentesis sac (b) amniotic sac (c) congenital membrane (d) trisomic membrane
12. Which term is the same as pregnancy?
   (a) climacteric (b) dysmenorrheal (c) fistula (d) gestation
13. Which term means an abnormal tubelike passage?
   (a) adhesion (b) colposcopy (c) fistula (d) polyp
14. Which of the following means childbirth?
   (a) gestation (b) neonatality (c) obstetrics (d) parturition
15. What is the term for a tumor found on a mucous membrane?
   (a) curettage (b) Pap (c) polyp (d) ovum
16. A chancre is characteristic of the primary stage of which disease?
   (a) chancroid (b) chlamydial infection (c) syphilis (d) trichomoniasis
17. Which of the following is characterized by cauliflower-like genital and anal warts?
   (a) candidiasis (b) condyloma acuminatum (c) gonorrhea (d) nonspecific genital infection
18. Which of the following is a parasitic STD that causes severe itching, redness, and inflammation?
   (a) chancroid (b) papillomavirus (c) pubic lice (d) syphilis
19. Which of the following means direct visual inspection of the cervical canal and uterine cavity?
   (a) colposcopy (b) hysteroscopy (c) laparoscopy (d) mammography
20. Which of the following means destruction of a thin layer of the uterus?
   (a) chorionic villus sampling (b) endometrial ablation (c) hysterectomy
   (d) transurethral resection

E. WRITE IT!   *Write one word for each of the following.*

1. a newborn   _____
2. attachment of a fertilized ovum to the endometrium   _____
3. deliberate rupture of the fetal membranes to induce labor   _____
4. incision made to enlarge the vaginal opening for delivery   _____
5. menopause   _____
6. painful menstruation   _____
7. pertaining to the cervix uteri   _____
8. prolapse of the uterus   _____
9. surgical puncture of the amnion   _____
10. release of an ovum from the ovary   _____

Continued

SELF-TEST (cont'd)

F. READING HEALTH CARE REPORTS   *Read the laboratory report and answer the questions that follow the report.*

MEDICAL REPORT   **Mid-City Medical Center**

222 Medical Center Drive   **Main City, USA 63017-1000**   **Phone:** (555) 222-0000
    Fax: (555) 222-0001

LABORATORY REPORT

Date of Report: 2/2/2009
Name of Patient: Esra Esselman
SS #: 498-04-0003
Specimen Received 1/27/2009: Vaginal swab
Findings: Gram stain of the material showed the presence of both intracellular and extracellular gram-negative diplococci. *Neisseria gonorrhoeae* grown in culture.

1. What is meant by intracellular and extracellular diplococci? _____
2. What is the name of the sexually transmitted disease that is implied? _____
3. What is the common name of the organism that causes this disease? _____

G. SPELL IT!   *Circle all incorrectly spelled terms, and write their correct spelling.*

1. cervicokolpitis   _____
2. epididymis   _____
3. korionic   _____
4. sistocele   _____
5. sifilis   _____

Q&E List
Use the Companion CD or audio CDs to review the terms presented in Chapter 11.
Look closely at the spelling of each term as it is pronounced.

abruptio placentae **(ab-rup´she-o plə-sen´te)**
acquired immunodeficiency syndrome **(ə-kwīrd´**
  im´´u-no-də-fish´ən-se sin´drōm)
adipose **(ad´ĭ-pōs)**
amenorrhea **(ə-men´´o-re´ə)**
amniocentesis **(am´´ne-o-sen-te´sis)**
amnion **(am´ne-on)**

amniotic **(am´´ne-ot´ik)**
amniotomy **(am´´ne-ot´ə-me)**
antepartum **(an´´te-pahr´təm)**
areola **(ə-re´o-lə)**
benign prostatic hyperplasia **(bə-nīn´ pros-tat´ik**
  hi-pər-pla´zhə)
breech presentation **(brēch pre´´zən-ta´shən)**

bulbourethral gland (**bul˝bo-u-re˝thrəl gland**)

candidiasis (**kan˝dĭ-di˝ə-sis**)

castration (**kas-tra˝shən**)

cephalic presentation (**sə-fal˝ik pre˝zən-ta˝shən**)

cervical (**sur˝vĭ-kəl**)

cervical polyp (**sur˝vĭ-kəl pol˝ip**)

cervicocolpitis (**sur˝vĭ-ko-kol-pi˝tis**)

cervix uteri (**sur˝viks u˝tər-i**)

cesarean section (**sə-zar˝e-ən sek˝shən**)

chancre (**shang˝kər**)

chancroid (**shang˝kroid**)

chemotherapy (**ke˝mo-ther˝ə-pe**)

chlamydial infection (**klə-mid˝e-əl in-fek˝shən**)

chorion (**kor˝e-on**)

chorionic villus sampling (**kor˝e-on˝ik vil˝əs
   sam˝pling**)

circumcision (**sur˝kəm-sizh˝ən**)

climacteric (**kli-mak˝tər-ik**)

clitoris (**klit˝ə-ris, kli˝tə-ris, klĭ-tor˝is**)

colpitis (**kol-pi˝tis**)

colpoplasty (**kol˝po-plas˝te**)

colporrhaphy (**kol-por˝ə-fe**)

colposcope (**kol˝po-skōp**)

colposcopy (**kol-pos˝kə-pe**)

condyloma acuminatum (**kon˝də-lo˝mə
   ə-ku˝mĭ-nāt˝um**)

conization of the cervix (**kon˝ĭ-za˝shən ov
   thə sur˝viks**)

contraception (**kon˝trə-sep˝shən**)

contraceptive (**kon˝trə-sep˝tiv**)

cryptorchidism (**krip-tor˝kĭ-diz˝˝əm**)

curettage (**ku˝rə-tahzh˝**)

cystocele (**sis˝to-sēl**)

cytology (**si-tol˝ə-je**)

dilation and curettage (**di-la˝shən and ku˝rə-tahzh˝**)

Down syndrome (**doun sin˝drōm**)

ductus deferens (**duk˝təs def˝ər-enz**)

dysmenorrhea (**dis-men˝ə-re˝ə**)

dysplasia (**dis-pla˝zhə**)

ectopic (**ek-top˝ik**)

endometrial ablation (**en˝do-me˝tre-əl ab-la˝shən**)

endometriosis (**en˝do-me˝tre-o˝sis**)

endometritis (**en˝do-me-tri˝tis**)

endometrium (**en˝do-me˝tre-əm**)

epididymis (**ep˝ĭ-did˝ə-mis**)

episiotomy (**ə-piz˝e-ot˝o-me**)

erythroblastosis fetalis (**ə-rith˝ro-blas-to˝sis fĕ-tă˝ləs**)

estrogen (**es˝trə-jen**)

extrauterine (**eks˝trə-u˝tər-in**)

fallopian (**fə-lo˝pe-ən**)

fertilization (**fur-tĭ-lĭ-za˝shən**)

fetal (**fe˝təl**)

fetal monitoring (**fe˝təl mon˝ĭ-tər-ing**)

fetus (**fe˝təs**)

fistula (**fis˝tu-lə**)

genitalia (**jen˝ĭ-tāl˝e-ə**)

genitourinary (**jen˝ĭ-to-u˝rĭ-nar-e**)

gestation (**jes-ta˝shən**)

glans penis (**glanz pe˝nis**)

gonads (**go˝nads**)

gonococcus (**gon˝o-kok˝əs**)

gonorrhea (**gon˝o-re˝ə**)

gravida (**grav˝ĭ-də**)

gynecologist (**gi˝nə-kol˝ə-jist, jin˝ə-kol˝ə-jist**)

gynecology (**gi˝nə-kol˝ə-je, jin˝ə-kol˝ə-je**)

hepatitis (**hep˝ə-ti˝tis**)

herpes genitalis (**hur˝pēz jen-ĭ-tal˝is**)

human chorionic gonadotropin (**hu˝mən kor˝e-on˝ik
   go˝nə-do-tro˝pin**)

hydrocele (**hi˝dro-sēl**)

hysterectomy (**his˝tər-ek˝tə-me**)

hysteroptosis (**his˝tər-op-to˝sis**)

hysterosalpingogram (**his˝tər-o-sal-ping˝go-gram**)

hysterosalpingography (**his˝tər-o-sal˝ping-gog˝rə-fe**)

hysteroscope (**his˝tər-o-skōp˝**)

hysteroscopy (**his˝tər-os˝kə-pe**)

implantation (**im˝plan-ta˝shən**)

intrauterine (**in˝trə-u˝tər-in**)

in utero (**in u˝tər-o**)

in vitro fertilization (**in ve˝tro fur˝tĭ-lĭ-za˝shən**)

Kaposi sarcoma (**kah˝po-she, kap˝o-se sahr-ko˝mə**)

labia majora (**la˝be-ə mă-jor˝ə**)

labia minora (**la˝be-ə mi-nor˝ə**)

lactation (**lak-ta˝shən**)

lactiferous (**lak-tif˝ər-əs**)

laparohysterectomy (**lap˝ə-ro-his˝tə-rek˝tə-me**)

laparoscope (**lap˝ə-ro-skōp˝**)

laparoscopy (**lap˝ə-ros˝kə-pe**)

laparotomy (**lap˝ə-rot˝ə-me**)

lobule (**lob˝ūl**)

lumpectomy (**ləm-pek˝tə-me**)

mammalgia (**mə-mal˝jə**)

continued

mammary (**mam´ər-e**)

mammogram (**mam´ə-gram**)

mammography (**mə-mog´rə-fe**)

mammoplasty (**mam´o-plas´´te**)

mastalgia (**mas-tal´jə**)

mastectomy (**mas-tek´tə-me**)

mastitis (**mas-ti´tis**)

mastodynia (**mas´´to-din´e-ə**)

mastopexy (**mas´to-pek-se**)

mastoptosis (**mas´´to-to´sis**)

menopause (**men´o-pawz**)

menorrhagia (**men´´ə-ra´jə**)

menses (**men´sēz**)

menstruation (**men´´stroo-a´shən**)

metrorrhagia (**me´´tro-ra´jə**)

mons pubis (**monz pu´bis**)

myoma (**mi-o´mə**)

myometrium (**mi-o-me´tre-əm**)

neonatal (**ne´´o-na´təl**)

neonate (**ne´o-nāt**)

nonspecific genital infection (**non´´spə-sif´ik jen´ĭ-təl in-fek´shən**)

nullipara (**nə-lip´ə-rə**)

obstetrician (**ob´´stə-trĭ´shən**)

obstetrics (**ob-stet´riks**)

oophorectomy (**o´´of-ə-rek´tə-me**)

oophoritis (**o´´of-ə-ri´tis**)

oophorosalpingitis (**o-of´´ə-ro-sal´´pin-ji´tis**)

orchidectomy (**or´´kĭ-dek´tə-me**)

orchiditis (**or´´kĭ-di´tis**)

orchidopexy (**or´kĭ-do-pek´´se**)

orchidoplasty (**or´kĭ-do-plas´´te**)

orchiectomy (**or´´ke-ek´tə-me**)

orchiopexy (**or´ke-o-pek´´se**)

orchiotomy (**or´´ke-ot´ə-me**)

orchitis (**or-ki´tis**)

ovarian (**o-var´e-ən**)

ovarian carcinoma (**o-var´e-ən kahr´´sĭ-no´mə**)

ovarian cyst (**o-var´e-ən sist**)

ovaries (**o´və-rēs**)

ovulation (**ov´´u-la´shən**)

ovum (**o´vəm**)

Pap smear (**pap smēr**)

papillomavirus (**pap´´ĭ-lo´mə-vi´´rəs**)

parturition (**pahr´´tu-rĭ´shən**)

pelvic inflammatory disease (**pel´vik in-flam´ə-tor´´e dĭ-zēz´**)

penis (**pe´nis**)

perimetrium (**per´´ĭ-me´tre-əm**)

placenta (**plə-sen´tə**)

placenta previa (**plə-sen´tə pre´ve-ə**)

postnatal (**pōst-na´təl**)

postpartum (**pōst-pahr´təm**)

premenstrual syndrome (**pre-men´stroo-əl sin´drōm**)

prenatal (**pre-na´təl**)

prepuce (**pre´pūs**)

primigravida (**pri´´mĭ-grav´ĭ-də**)

progesterone (**pro-jes´tə-rōn**)

prostate (**pros´tāt**)

prostatectomy (**pros´´tə-tek´tə-me**)

prostatic carcinoma (**pros-tat´ik kahr´´sĭ-no´mə**)

prostatitis (**pros´´tə-ti´tis**)

pubic lice (**pu´bik līs**)

rectovaginal (**rek´´to-vaj´ĭ-nəl**)

salpingectomy (**sal´´pin-jek´tə-me**)

salpingitis (**sal´´pin-ji´tis**)

salpingocele (**sal-ping´go-sēl**)

salpingo-oophorectomy (**sal-ping´´go-o´´of-ə-rek´tə-me**)

salpingorrhaphy (**sal´´ping-gor´ə-fe**)

scrotum (**skro´təm**)

secundipara (**se´´kən-dip´ə-rə**)

semen (**se´mən**)

seminal vesicles (**sem´ĭ-nəl ves´ĭ-kəls**)

shoulder presentation (**shōl´dər pre´´zən-ta´shən**)

speculum (**spek´u-ləm**)

spermatocidal (**sper´´mə-to-si´dəl**)

spermatogenesis (**sper´´mə-to-jen´ə-sis**)

spermatozoa (**sper´´mə-to-zo´ə**)

spermicidal (**sper´´mĭ-si´dəl**)

spermicide (**sper´mĭ-sīd**)

spirochete (**spi´ro-kēt**)

sterilization (**ster´´ĭ-lĭ-za´shən**)

syphilis (**sif´ĭ-lis**)

testes (**tes´tēz**)

testicle (**tes´tĭ-kəl**)

testicular torsion (**tes-tik´u-lər tor´shən**)

testis (**tes´tis**)

testosterone (**tes-tos´tə-rōn**)

transabdominal (**trans´´ab-dom´ĭ-nəl**)

transurethral microwave thermotherapy (**trans´´u-re´thrəl mi´kro-wāv thur´´mo-ther´ə-pe**) transurethral needle ablation (**trans˝u-re´thrəl ne´dəl ab-la´shən**)

transurethral prostatectomy (**trans˝u-re´thrəl pros´tə-tek´tə-me**)

transurethral resection (**trans˝u-re´thrəl re-sek´shən**)

trichomoniasis (**trik˝o-mo-ni´ə-sis**)

trimester (**tri-mes´tər**)

tripara (**trip´ə-rə**)

tubal ligation (**too´bəl lĭ-ga´shən**)

ultrasonography (**ul˝trə-sə-nog´rə-fe**)

ultrasound (**ul´trə-sound**)

unipara (**u-nip´ə-rə**)

urethritis (**u˝rə-thri´tis**)

uterine cancer (**u´tər-in kan´sər**)

uterus (**u´tər-əs**)

vagina (**və-ji´nə**)

vaginal (**vaj´ĭ-nəl**)

vaginitis (**vaj˝ĭ-ni´tis**)

vas deferens (**vas def´ər-ens**)

vasectomy (**və-sek´tə-me**)

vasovasostomy (**vas˝o-, va˝zo-va-zos´tə-me**)

vesicovaginal (**ves˝ĭ-ko-vaj´ĭ-nəl**)

vulva (**vəl´və**)

vulval (**vul´vəl**)

vulvar (**vul´vər**)

vulvitis (**vəl-vi´tis**)

zygote (**zi´gōt**)

 Don't forget the games on the Companion CD and http://evolve.elsevier.com/Leonard/quick/ for additional review activities, including questions on Spanish medical terms.

E*SPAÑOL* Enhancing Spanish Communication

English	Spanish (pronunciation)
birth	nacimiento (**nah-se-me-EN-to**)
childbirth	parto (**PAR-to**)
circumcision	circuncisión (**ser-coon-se-se-ON**)
conception	concepción (**con-sep-se-ON**)
condom	condón (**con-DON**)
contraception	contracepción (**con-trah-cep-se-ON**)
diaphragm	diafragma (**de-ah-FRAHG-mah**)
erection	erección (**ay-rec-se-ON**)
foam	espuma (**es-POO-mah**)
hormone	hormona (**or-MOH-nah**)
impotency	impotencia (**im-po-TEN-se-ah**)
intercourse, sexual	cópula (**CO-poo-lah**)
menopause	menopausia (**may-no-PAH-oo-se-ah**)
menstruation	menstruación (**mens-troo-ah-se-ON**)
newborn	recién nacida (**ray-se-EN nah-SEE-dah**)
nipple	pezón (**pay-SONE**)
nutrition	nutrición (**noo-tre-se-ON**)
ovarian	ovárico (**o-VAH-re-co**)
ovary	ovario (**o-VAH-re-o**)

English	Spanish (pronunciation)
parturition	parto (**PAR-to**)
penis	pene (**PAY-nay**)
pregnancy	embarazo (**em-bah-RAH-so**)
pregnant	embarazada (**em-bah-rah-SAH-dah**)
prostate	próstata (**PROS-ta-tah**)
prostatic	prostático (**pros-TAH-te-co**)
prostatitis	prostatitis (**pros-ta-TEE-tis**)
reproduction	reproducción (**ray-pro-dooc-se-ON**)
rhythm method	método de ritmo (**MAY-to-do day REET-mo**)
sexual	sexual (**sex-soo-AHL**)
sterile	estéril (**es-TAY-reel**)
symptom	síntoma (**SEEN-to-mah**)
testicle	testículo (**tes-TEE-coo-lo**)
vagina	vagina (**vah-HEE-nah**)

CHAPTER 12

Integumentary System

CONTENTS

Function First
Structures of the Integumentary System
  Layers of the Skin
  Accessory Skin Structures
Diseases, Disorders, and Diagnostic Terms
  Skin Lesions
  Injuries to the Skin
  Skin Disorders
  Disorders of Accessory Skin Structures

Surgical and Therapeutic Interventions
Self-Test
Q&E List
Enhancing Spanish Communication

OBJECTIVES

After completing Chapter 12, you will be able to:

1. Recognize or write the functions of the integumentary system.
2. Recognize or write the meanings of Chapter 12 word parts and use them to build and analyze terms.
3. Write terms for select structures of the integumentary system, or match them with their descriptions.

4. Write the names of the diagnostic terms and pathologies related to the integumentary system when given their descriptions, or match terms with their meanings.
5. Match surgical and therapeutic interventions for the integumentary system or write the names of the interventions when given their descriptions.
6. Spell terms for the integumentary system correctly.

Function First

The integumentary system is the skin and its appendages, hair, nails, sweat glands, and sebaceous glands. The skin is the **integument**, or external covering of the body. We are more familiar with the skin than many other organs because it is external. Skin has the following important functions:

- Covers the body and protects the underlying tissues from harmful light rays, drying out, and invasion by microbes
- Helps control body temperature
- Has receptors that receive stimuli from the environment
- Has sweat glands that excrete water and salts

 QUICK TIP

When you see sebaceous, think of sebum, the oily secretion of the skin.

WORD ORIGIN

integument (L.) a covering

299

WRITE IT!

EXERCISE 1

Write an answer in each blank to complete these sentences.

1. The skin is the external covering and is called the _____.

2. The skin protects the underlying tissues from drying out, harmful light rays, and invasion of

_____.

3. Skin structures called _____ receive stimuli from the environment.

4. The sweat glands help control body temperature and excrete water and _____.

Use Appendix VIII to check your answers to all the exercises in Chapter 12.

Structures of the Integumentary System

WORD ORIGIN

derma (Gk), *cutis* (L.)
skin

---

epi- = above
sub- = below
cutane/o = skin
-ous = pertaining to
adip/o = fat

Layers of the Skin

The skin consists of two main parts: the **epi+dermis** and the **dermis**. Remembering that epi- means above, it is easy to remember that the epidermis is located above the dermis. Label Figure 12-1 as you read the following information. The epidermis (1) is the thin outer layer. The dermis (2) is the thick layer under the epidermis. A layer of **sub+cutane+ous adipose tissue** (3) is located under the dermis. **Cutaneous** means pertaining to the skin, and subcutaneous means beneath the skin. **Adipose** means fatty, because adip/o means fat. The subcutaneous adipose tissue is composed of fat that serves as insulation and a cushion against shock.

adip/o = fat
cutane/o, derm/a
   = skin
epi- = above *or*
   upon
pil/o = hair
seb/o = sebum
sub- = under

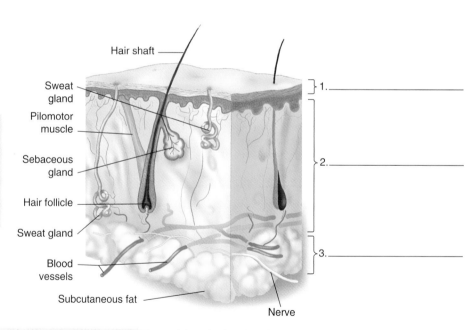

Hair shaft

Sweat gland

Pilomotor muscle

Sebaceous gland

Hair follicle

Sweat gland

Blood vessels

Subcutaneous fat

Nerve

1. _____

2. _____

3. _____

Figure 12-1 Layers and structures of the skin. The epidermis *(1)*, the thin outer layer, is composed of four to five layers. Underneath the epidermis is the thicker dermis *(2)*, which is composed of connective tissue containing lymphatics, nerves, blood vessels, hair follicles, sebaceous glands, and sweat glands. Beneath the dermis is a layer of subcutaneous adipose tissue *(3)*.

When it is intact, the skin serves as protection from microorganisms. The outermost part of the epidermis contains nonliving cells that are constantly being shed and replaced. The primary component of these nonliving cells is **keratin**, a **sclero+protein**, which is insoluble in most solvents. The dermis contains numerous blood vessels, nerves, and glands. Hair follicles are also embedded in this layer. The upper region of the dermis has many finger-like projections that result in ridges on the outermost layer of the skin. The ridge patterns on the fingertips and thumbs (fingerprints) are unique to each person.

scler/o = hard

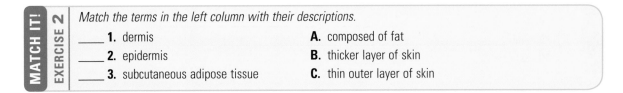

MATCH IT! EXERCISE 2

Match the terms in the left column with their descriptions.

____ **1.** dermis
____ **2.** epidermis
____ **3.** subcutaneous adipose tissue

A. composed of fat
B. thicker layer of skin
C. thin outer layer of skin

Commit the word parts in the following table to memory.

Word Parts: Integumentary System	
Combining Forms	**Meaning**
adip/o, lip/o	fat
axill/o	axilla (armpit)
bacter/i, bacteri/o	bacteria
cutane/o, derm/a, derm/o, dermat/o	skin
erythemat/o	erythema or redness
follicul/o	follicle
ichthy/o	fish
kerat/o*	horny tissue (tissue containing keratin)
onych/o, ungu/o	nail
pil/o, trich/o	hair
seb/o	sebum
seps/o	infection
sept/o	infection or septum
xer/o	dry
Suffixes	
-cidal	killing
-static	keeping stationary

Use the electronic flashcards on the Evolve site or make your own set of flashcards using the above list. Select the word parts just presented, and study them until you know their meanings. Do this each time a set of word parts is presented.

*Sometimes kerat/o means cornea.

WRITE IT! **EXERCISE 3**

Write combining forms for these meanings.

1. dry _____
2. erythema or redness _____
3. fat _____ or _____
4. fish _____
5. follicle _____
6. hair _____ or _____
7. horny tissue _____
8. infection _____ or _____
9. nail _____ or _____
10. sebum _____

Accessory Skin Structures

pil/o = hair
motor = mover,
    pertaining to
    motion

The accessory skin structures include the hair, nails, sebaceous glands, and sweat glands. Locate these structures in Figure 12-1. **Pilomotor muscles** cause erection of the hairs of the skin in response to a chilly environment, emotional stimulus, or skin irritation.

axill/o = axilla

Hair protects the scalp from injury. Hair in the nostrils and external ear canal protects these structures from dust and insects. Eyebrows and lashes protect the eyes. **Axilla** means armpit. Hair develops in the **axillary** region at puberty.

seb/o = sebum

Sweat glands are also called **sudoriferous glands**. Certain sweat glands produce perspiration when they are stimulated by increased temperature or emotional stress. Although elimination of waste in the form of **perspiration** is a function of the sweat glands, their principal function is to help regulate body temperature.

QUICK TIP

kerat/o also refers to the cornea, the transparent structure at the front of the eye.

Sebaceous glands generally arise from the hair follicles and produce **sebum**, the oily substance that inhibits the growth of bacteria and is responsible for lubrication of the skin. The hair **follicles** are tiny tubes of epidermal cells that contain the root of the hair shaft. Sebaceous glands are found in all areas of the body that have hair.

kerat/o = horny
    tissue

Fingernails and toenails are composed of keratin, a hard, fibrous protein. When kerat/o is used in discussions pertaining to the skin, it means hard or horny tissue. **Ungual** means pertaining to the nail.

ungu/o = nail

WRITE IT! **EXERCISE 4**

Write an answer in each blank to complete these sentences.

1. Hair, nails, sebaceous glands, and sweat glands are the _____ skin structures.
2. A term that means pertaining to the armpit is _____.
3. Sweat glands are _____ glands.
4. Another term for sweat is _____.
5. Glands that produce sebum are called _____ glands.
6. A term that means pertaining to the nail is _____.

Diseases, Disorders, and Diagnostic Terms

The skin is a reflection of the general health of a person, and it can communicate information to the trained observer. Normal skin has an even tone that is free of lesions, bruises, or signs of inflammation. Skin changes may be related to specific skin diseases but also may reflect an underlying systemic disorder.

Skin Lesions

A skin **lesion** is any visible, localized abnormality of the skin, such as a wound, rash, or sore. This includes spots that appear on the skin, as well as swellings and changes of shape, such as an underlying tumor. Perhaps you are familiar with the benign skin lesions of **seborrheic keratosis** that are often seen in older persons. Some lesions of this type are deeply pigmented (Figure 12-2).

  Primary lesions are initial reactions to an underlying problem that alters one of the structural components of the skin. Both a cyst and a **nodule** cause a raised area of the overlying skin, but the **cyst** is filled with fluid or a semisolid material (Figure 12-3). See other primary lesions of the skin in Figure 12-4 and read the characteristics of each type. **Macules** (e.g., freckles) are small and nonraised, unlike **papules** (e.g., moles). A **plaque** (e.g., dandruff) is elevated and appears as a large patch. Blisters or fluid-filled lesions include **vesicles, bullae**, and pustules. Vesicles are smaller than bullae, and

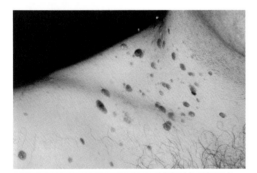

kerat/o = horny tissue
-rrhea = flow or discharge
seb/o = sebum

Figure 12-2 Seborrheic keratoses, benign skin lesions. Numerous seborrheic keratoses are present, some of which are deeply pigmented with melanin. The large lesions show the characteristic stuck-on appearance.

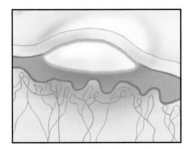

A **cyst** is a sac filled with fluid or semi-solid material.

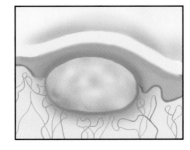

A **nodule** is a marble-like, solid lesion more than 1 cm wide and deep.

Figure 12-3 Differentiation of two types of lesions (seen here in cross section).

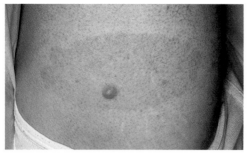

Macules
Nonraised, discolored spots less than 1 cm in diameter

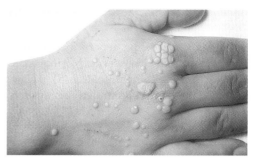

Papules
Elevated lesion less than 1 cm in diameter

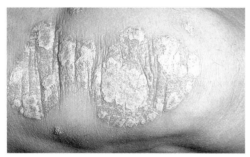

Plaques
Elevated and circumscribed patches more than 1 cm in diameter

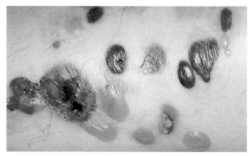

Bullae
Blisters greater than 1 cm and filled with clear fluid

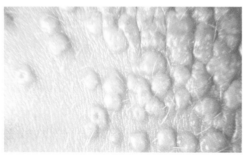

Vesicles
Blisters less than 1 cm and filled with clear fluid

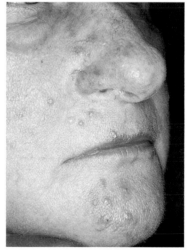

Pustules
Vesicles filled with cloudy fluid or pus

Figure 12-4 Primary lesions of the skin. These are initial reactions to an underlying problem that alters one of the structural components of the skin.

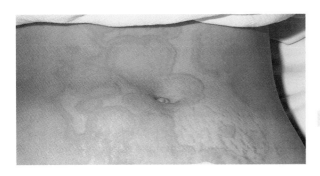

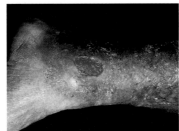

Figure 12-5 **Wheals.** This elevated, irregularly shaped lesion is seen in urticaria (hives), an allergic skin eruption. Notice the irregular shapes of the lesions.

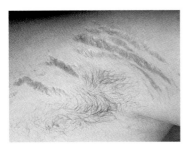

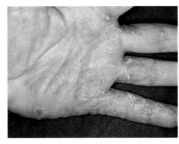

Atrophy
Wasting of the epidermis; skin appears thin and transparent

Ulcer
Irregularly shaped erosions that extend into the dermis

Fissures
Deep linear splits through the epidermis into the dermis

Figure 12-6 **Secondary lesions of the skin.** Atrophy of the skin, ulcers, and fissures result from changes in the initial skin lesion.

pustules are filled with cloudy fluid or pus. **Wheals** (Figure 12-5), often seen in an allergic skin eruption, are elevated and irregularly shaped lesions. A memory aid for primary skin lesions follows:

Primarily **be**cause **m**y **n**ew **p**ick-**up pl**odded, I **pa**id for a **V W**.
Primary: **b**ulla, **c**yst, **m**acule, **n**odule, **pu**stule, **pl**aque, **pa**pule, **v**esicle, **w**heal

Match the skin lesions in the left column with their descriptions.

_____ **1.** bulla
_____ **2.** macule
_____ **3.** papule
_____ **4.** pustule
_____ **5.** vesicle

A. blister, larger than 1 cm
B. blister less than 1 cm, filled with clear fluid
C. discolored spot, not elevated
D. small elevated lesion
E. fluid-filled sac containing pus

Secondary lesions of the skin are changes in the appearance of the primary lesion and can occur with normal progression of a disease. Atrophy of the skin, ulcers, and fissures are secondary lesions (Figure 12-6). **Atrophy** of the skin (e.g., stretch marks) is characterized by thinning with the loss of skin markings. **Ulcers** are deep, irregular erosions that extend into the dermis. Athlete's foot produces linear cracks in the epidermis and is an example of a **fissure**. **Scales**, not shown in the illustration, are dried fragments of sloughed epidermis that are whitish and irregular in size and shape.

 QUICK TIP
Secondary lesions:
    atrophy
    ulcer
    fissure
    scales

Injuries to the Skin

QUICK TIP

Examples of wounds:
laceration
incision
puncture
abrasion
contusion
burn

a- = without
sept/o = infection
-ic = pertaining to

A wound is a physical injury involving a break in the skin, usually caused by an act or accident rather than a disease. The trauma (injury) to the skin and underlying tissues requires healing to repair the defect. If damage to the skin is severe, a scar remains after healing of a wound. Excessive overgrowth of unsightly scar tissue, called a **keloid**, occurs in some individuals, especially blacks. A **laceration** is a torn, jagged wound, whereas an **incision** is a smooth-edged wound produced by a sharp instrument. Surgical incisions generally heal faster than other wounds because they are performed under a+sept+ic conditions, and because minimal damage is done by the sharp instruments used. **Aseptic** means free of pathogenic organisms. A puncture is a wound made by piercing. An **abrasion** results when skin is scraped or rubbed away by friction. A **contusion** (bruise) is caused by a blow to the body that does not break the skin.

MATCH IT! **EXERCISE 6**

Match the injuries to the skin in the left column with their descriptions.

_____ **1.** abrasion   **A.** a bruise

_____ **2.** contusion   **B.** skin is scraped or rubbed away by friction

_____ **3.** incision   **C.** smooth-edged wound produced by a sharp instrument

_____ **4.** laceration   **D.** torn, jagged wound

_____ **5.** puncture   **E.** wound made by piercing

Burns are tissue injuries resulting from excessive exposure to heat, electricity, chemicals, radiation, or gases. The extent of the injury is determined by the amount of exposure and the nature of the agent that caused the burn. In the past, burns were classified as first-, second-, third-, and fourth-degree injuries. Currently, the American Burn Association recommends categorizing a burn injury according to the depth of tissue destruction, as a superficial burn, a deep partial-thickness burn, a full-thickness burn, or a deep full thickness burn (Figure 12-7). These were formerly called first-degree, second-degree, third-degree, and fourth degree burns. In addition to the burn depth, burn severity includes factors such as the size and location of the burn, mechanism of the injury, duration and intensity of the burn, and the age and health of the patient. TBSA refers to the total body surface area that is burned. Very young and older persons are most at risk. Severe burns often require skin grafting, often from the patient's own body. In a **skin graft**, skin is implanted to cover areas where skin has been lost.

WRITE IT! **EXERCISE 7**

Write a word to complete each of these sentences.

1. Only the epidermis is damaged in a _____ partial-thickness burn.

2. In a deep partial-thickness burn, damage does not extend beyond the layer of skin called the

_____.

3. Underlying bone and muscle are damaged in a _____ full-thickness burn.

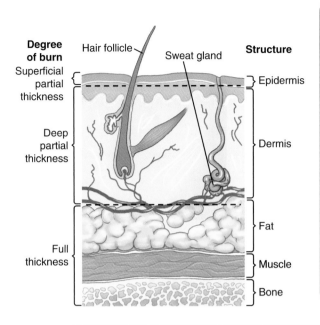

	Dermal Layers	Appearance
Type of Burn	**Involved**	**of Skin**
Partial-Thickness Burn		
Superficial (first degree)	Only the epidermis	Red, no immediate blisters, but may blister after 24 hours
Deep (second degree)	Extends into the dermis	Red and moist, blistered
Full-Thickness Burn		
(third degree)	Throughout the dermis and epidermis, sometimes into subcutaneous fat layer	Hard, dry, and leathery White, deep red, yellow, brown to black
Deep Full-Thickness Burn		
(fourth degree)	No skin layers remain. Underlying bone and muscle are damaged.	Wound is blackened and depressed. Muscle and bone are exposed.

Figure 12-7 Cross-section of skin indicating the degree of burn and structures involved.

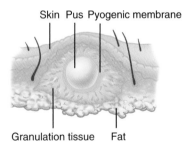

-genic = produced in
py/o = pus

Figure 12-8 An abscess. The pus is contained within a thin, pyogenic membrane that is surrounded by harder granulation tissue, the tissue's response to the infection.

Skin Disorders

abscess cavity that contains pus caused by an infectious microorganism and surrounded by inflamed tissue (Figure 12-8).

acne vulgaris disease of the skin that is common where sebaceous glands are numerous (face, upper back, and chest); acne.

albinism (albin/o, white + -ism, condition) absence of normal pigmentation, present at birth, caused by a defect in **melanin** precursors. The person affected with albinism is an **albino** (see Figure 3-5, p. 61).

cellulitis acute infection of the skin and subcutaneous tissue characterized most often by local heat, redness, pain, and swelling.

contact dermatitis skin rash resulting from exposure to an irritant or to a sensitizing agent that initiates an allergic response, such as poison ivy and allergic reaction to nickel in jewelry (see Figure 2-12, p. 37).

cyanosis (cyan/o, blue + -osis, condition) bluish discoloration of the skin and mucous membranes (see Figure 3-6, p. 62).

dermatitis (dermat/o, skin + -itis, inflammation) inflammatory condition of the skin.

discoid lupus erythematosus (DLE) chronic disorder, primarily of the skin, characterized by lesions that are covered with scales. The disorder was so named because of the reddish facial rash that

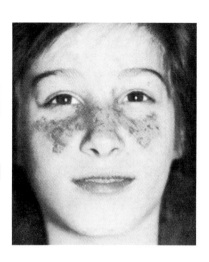

erythemat/o = erythema *or* redness
lupus = wolf

Figure 12-9 Characteristic "butterfly rash" of lupus erythematosus. *Lupus* is the Latin term for wolf, the name perhaps originated from the rash over the nose and cheeks, which resembles a wolf's snout. The rash is usually red, and thus the term erythematosus, from the Greek *erythēma*, meaning redness.

necr/o = dead
-osis = condition

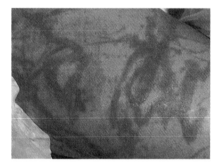

Figure 12-10 Tissue necrosis. Necrosis that resulted from contact with the stinging structures on the tentacles of a jellyfish.

appears in some patients (Figure 12-9), giving them a wolflike appearance. Erythemat/o means **erythema**, a redness or inflammation of the skin or mucous membranes. Also called cutaneous lupus erythematosus.

frostbite damage to skin, tissues, and blood vessels as a result of prolonged exposure to cold.

furuncle localized skin infection originating in a gland or hair follicle and characterized by pain, redness, and swelling. Also called a boil.

hypopigmentation decreased tissue pigmentation, but not complete absence of skin color as in albinism.

ichthyosis (ichthy/o, fish) any of several generalized skin disorders marked by skin that is dry and scaly, resembling fish skin.

lipoma (lip/o, fat + -oma, tumor) benign tumor consisting of mature fat cells.

malignant melanoma (melan/o, black + -oma, tumor) any of a group of malignant tumors that

originate in the skin and that are composed of **melanocytes** (see Figure 2-3, *B*, p. 21).

mycodermatitis (myc/o, fungus) inflammation of the skin caused by a fungus.

necrosis death of areas of damaged or diseased tissue or bone surrounded by healthy tissue (Figure 12-10).

onychomycosis any fungal infection of the nails.

pediculosis infestation by lice and named for a genus of sucking lice, *Pediculus.* There are head lice, body lice, and pubic lice.

petechiae tiny, purple or red spots appearing on the skin as a result of tiny hemorrhages within dermal or submucosal layers (Figure 12-11, *A*).

psoriasis common chronic skin disorder characterized by circumscribed red patches covered by thick, dry, silvery scales (Figure 12-11, *B*).

scabies contagious dermatitis caused by the itch mite that is transmitted by close contact.

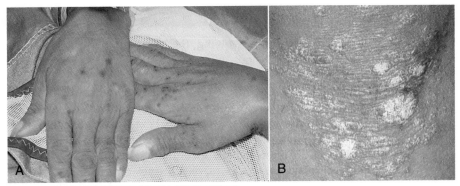

Figure 12-11 Common benign disorders of the skin. A, Petechiae appear on the skin as a result of tiny hemorrhages beneath the surface. **B,** Psoriasis is characterized by circumscribed red patches covered by thick, dry, silvery scale.

scleroderma (scler/o, hard + -derma, skin) chronic hardening and thickening of the skin.

skin cancer any of several **neoplasms** of the skin; the most common and most curable malignancies.

urticaria skin eruption characterized by wheals of varying shapes and sizes with well-defined margins and pale centers. Its causes include drugs, foods, and insect bites. Also called **hives** (see Figure 12-5).

xerosis (xer/o, dry) minor irritation of the skin characterized by excessive dryness, which can lead to scaling, thinning, and injury.

Disorders of Accessory Skin Structures

acne vulgaris skin disease characterized by blackheads (the result of blocked hair follicles becoming infected with bacteria), whiteheads, and pus-filled lesions.

folliculitis inflammation of a hair follicle.

hidradenitis (hidr/o, sweat + aden/o, gland + -itis, inflammation) inflammation of a sweat gland caused by occlusion (closing off) of the pores with subsequent bacterial infection of the gland.

onychopathy any disease of the nails.

seborrhea (seb/o, sebum + -rrhea, discharge) excessive production of sebum.

seborrheic dermatitis inflammatory condition of the skin that begins with the scalp but may involve other areas, particularly the eyebrows; commonly called dandruff.

trichosis (trich/o, hair + -osis, condition) any abnormal condition of hair growth, including baldness or excessive hair growth in an unusual place.

MATCH IT! EXERCISE 8

Match the skin disorders in the left column with their descriptions.

____ **1.** abscess   **A.** a boil
____ **2.** albinism   **B.** benign tumor composed of fat cells
____ **3.** cyanosis   **C.** bluish discoloration of the skin
____ **4.** furuncle   **D.** cavity that contains pus
____ **5.** ichthyosis   **E.** congenital absence of normal pigment
____ **6.** lipoma   **F.** dry and scaly skin, resembling fish skin
____ **7.** mycodermatitis   **G.** excessive dryness of the skin
____ **8.** onychomycosis   **H.** fungal infection of the nails
____ **9.** petechiae   **I.** inflammation of the skin caused by a fungus
____ **10.** xerosis   **J.** tiny, purple or red spots on the skin

Surgical and Therapeutic Interventions

Most surgical procedures involving the skin are performed to repair or treat damaged skin, remove lesions, or penetrate the skin to allow diagnostic or other procedures.

Wound irrigation is the flushing of an open wound using a medicated solution, water, sterile saline (balanced salt solution), or an antimicrobial liquid preparation. This is done to cleanse and remove debris and excessive drainage. Superficial wounds often heal without suturing. Deep wounds that are located where movements open the wound edges are often stapled or sutured.

top/o = place

Topical medications are drugs placed directly on the skin. Topical antimicrobial agents and dressings are often applied to prevent infection when the skin has been broken. **Bacterio+static** means inhibiting the growth of bacteria, whereas **bactericidal** means killing bacteria. **Asepsis** means the absence of germs (its literal translation is the absence of infection), such as in the description of a wound that is not infected. The opposite of asepsis is **sepsis**, which means infection or contamination. An infected wound is described as **septic**.

bacteri/o, bacter/i = bacteria
-cidal = killing
-static = keeping stationary

trans- = across *or* through
derm/o = skin

Transdermal drug delivery is a method of applying a drug to unbroken skin. The drug is absorbed through the skin and then enters the circulatory system. Transdermal delivery is used particularly for estrogen and nicotine, and to deliver drugs to prevent motion sickness. Unfortunately, not all medications can be administered transdermally.

adip/o, lip/o = fat

Lipo+suction, also called suction-assisted lipectomy, removes adipose tissue with a suction pump device and is used primarily as cosmetic surgery to remove or reduce localized areas of fat, particularly in the neck, arms, legs, and belly (Figure 12-12).

Collagen injections use an insoluble protein, collagen, to enhance the lips or fatten sunken facial skin. The injections are nonsurgical means of smoothing out facial lines and wrinkles but require ongoing treatments to maintain the improvements achieved. Ongoing treatments are also necessary for injections of minute doses of the *Clostridium botulinum* toxin (e.g., Botox) administered by a physician (Figure 12-13). The injections reduce contractions of the muscles that cause persistent frown lines, especially those between the brows. The toxin was used to treat several spastic muscle disorders long before it was used for cosmetic effects.

Treatment of acne vulgaris includes the use of topical and oral antibiotics, special skin washes, and other products (e.g., Retin-A) that produce a mild, superficial peel of the epidermis. The latter products also improve the appearance of aged or sun-damaged skin. Superficial scars, wrinkles, blemishes, and sun-damaged areas of the

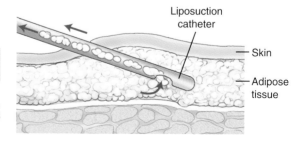

adip/o, lip/o = fat
-ectomy = excision

Figure 12-12 Liposuction. This procedure, also called suction lipectomy, removes adipose tissue with a suction pump device.

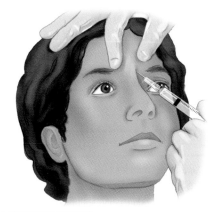

Figure 12-13 Injections to reduce facial lines. Injecting botulinum toxin (Botox) to reduce frown lines between the brows.

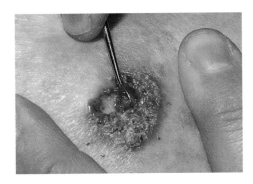

Figure 12-14 Curettage. A curet (or curette) is used to scrape material from the surface of a wound. Curettage is performed to obtain tissue for either microscopic examination or culture, or to clear unwanted material from areas of chronic infection.

outermost layers of the skin can be reduced or removed by laser, chemical peels, or physical sanding of the skin. The top layers peel away, and new, smoother skin layers replace the old ones. One technique, dermabrasion, is included in the following list of additional surgical or therapeutic terms pertaining to the skin.

derm/a = skin

antimicrobial medicine applied to broken skin to prevent infection.

antiperspirants compounds that act against or inhibit perspiration.

aspiration the act of withdrawing fluid from a cyst with a syringe.

biopsy removal of a small piece of tissue for microscopic examination to confirm or establish a diagnosis; abbreviated Bx or bx.

cryosurgery use of subfreezing temperature to destroy tissue.

curettage scraping of material from a surface to remove abnormal tissue (Figure 12-14).

debridement removal of foreign material and dead or damaged tissue, especially from a wound.

dermabrasion treatment for the removal of superficial scars on the skin by the use of revolving wire brushes or sandpaper.

electrolysis (electr/o, electricity + -lysis, destruction) destruction of a substance by passing electrical current through it. Laser treatments are sometimes used to destroy the hair follicles when hair is growing in an undesirable place.

electrosurgery surgery performed with electrical instruments that operate on high-frequency electric current and are often used to destroy skin lesions.

MATCH IT **EXERCISE 9**

Match the terms in the left column with their descriptions.

_____ **1.** cryosurgery   **A.** physical sanding of the skin

_____ **2.** curettage   **B.** removal of localized areas of fat

_____ **3.** dermabrasion   **C.** scraping a surface to remove abnormal tissue

_____ **4.** liposuction   **D.** use of subfreezing temperatures to destroy tissue

---

🛑 Be Careful with These!

macule (nonraised, discolored spot) versus *papule* (elevated lesion <1 cm in diameter)
vesicles (blisters <1 cm) versus *bullae* (blisters >1 cm)
cyst (sac filled with fluid or semisolid material) versus *nodule* (solid lesion >1 cm wide and deep)

SELF-TEST   Work the following exercises to test your understanding of the material in Chapter 12. Complete all the exercises before using Appendix VIII to check your answers.

A. WRITE IT! *List four functions of the integumentary system.*

1. _____

2. _____

3. _____

4. _____

B. WRITE IT! *Write the names of the two skin layers and describe them, as well as the underlying fatty tissue.*

1. _____

2. _____

3. _____

C. FINDING THE CLUE! *Use a clue to write terms for these descriptions. Solve Question 1; each ending letter becomes the clue for the first letter of the next answer.*

1. tiny, purple or red dot on the skin   _____

2. skin is scraped or rubbed away   _____

3. solid, marble-like lesion   _____

4. redness of the skin or mucous membrane   _____

5. cavity that contains pus   _____

6. type of gland that produces sweat   _____

7. excessive production of sebum   _____

8. skin disease common on the face   _____

9. destruction using electrical current   _____

10. dermatitis caused by the itch mite   _____

SELF-TEST (cont'd)

D. MATCH IT! *Match the skin lesions in the left column with their descriptions.*

_____ **1.** bulla	**A.**	blister, larger than 1 cm
_____ **2.** cyst	**B.**	blister, smaller than 1 cm
_____ **3.** fissure	**C.**	cracklike lesion of the skin
_____ **4.** macule	**D.**	discolored spot, not elevated
_____ **5.** papule	**E.**	fluid-filled sac containing pus
_____ **6.** pustule	**F.**	sac filled with clear fluid
_____ **7.** vesicle	**G.**	solid elevation, less than 0.5 cm in diameter

E. CIRCLE IT! *Choose the one correct answer (a, b, c, or d) to each question.*

1. In describing a burn by thickness, which type of burn is characterized by immediate blisters?
(a) deep partial-thickness (b) deep full-thickness (c) full-thickness (d) superficial partial-thickness

2. Which term means the death of areas of tissue or bone surrounded by healthy parts?
(a) atrophy (b) erosion (c) fissure (d) necrosis

3. Which procedure destroys tissue by using very cold temperatures?
(a) cryosurgery (b) curettage (c) dermabrasion (d) liposuction

4. Which of the following terms is *not* an accessory skin structure?
(a) adipose (b) hair (c) nails (d) sebaceous glands

5. Which term means scraping of material from a surface to remove abnormal tissue?
(a) aspiration (b) curettage (c) electrosurgery (d) fissure

6. Which term means an acute infection of the skin and subcutaneous tissue characterized by local heat, redness, pain, and swelling?
(a) cellulitis (b) contact dermatitis (c) ichthyosis (d) lipoma

7. Which term means pertaining to the skin?
(a) abrasion (b) abscess (c) cutaneous (d) dermatitis

8. Which of the following is a general term for any visible, localized abnormality of the skin?
(a) abrasion (b) abscess (c) lesion (d) wound

9. Which of the following is a skin eruption characterized by wheals?
(a) lupus erythematosus (b) malignant melanoma (c) pediculosis (d) urticaria

10. Which of the following is a primary component of epidermis?
(a) adipose (b) keratin (c) plaque (d) sebum

F. WRITE IT! *Write one-word terms for each of these meanings.*

1. a boil _____

2. torn, jagged wound _____

3. absence of pigment in the skin, hair, and nails _____

4. another name for a bruise _____

5. any disease of the nails _____

6. benign, fatty tumor _____

7. chronic hardening and thickening of skin _____

8. excessive dryness of the skin _____

9. inflammation of a sweat gland _____

10. pertaining to the nails _____

SELF-TEST (cont'd)

G. READING HEALTH CARE REPORTS   *Find the correct terms in the medical report to match the descriptions that follow the report.*

MEDICAL REPORT   **Mid-City Medical Center**

| **222 Medical Center Drive** | **Main City, USA 63017-1000** | **Phone:** (555) 434-0000 |
| | | **Fax:** (555) 434-0001 |

CONSULTATION

Name of Patient: Michael Turner   **Date:** 2/4/2009

Reason for Plastic Surgery Consultation: Hypertrophic scarring and keloid formation, left upper extremity and neck.

History of Present Illness: 34-year-old black male who suffered 25% TBSA full- and partial-thickness flame burns to bilateral upper extremities and neck after tripping and falling into a camp fire four months ago. Patient was treated with Silvadene dressing changes and split-thickness skin grafts to the bilateral upper extremities and neck, with right and left thighs as donor sites. Donor sites were treated with a single layer of petrolatum gauze and have healed well. Right upper extremity graft site has healed without sepsis or excessive scarring. Left upper extremity and neck show hypertrophic scarring and keloid formation despite wearing of elastic pressure bandage.

Medical History: Unremarkable except for onychomycosis of the toenails.

Family History: Mother age 68 with melanoma; father age 70 with high blood pressure and seborrheic dermatitis.

Allergies: Neomycin ointment

Impression: Keloid formation, left upper extremity and neck.

Plan: Surgery to correct keloid formation, left upper extremity and neck.

Thank you for this consultation.

David M. Crane
David M. Crane, M.D.

ara:DMC
2/7/2009

1. an overgrowth of collagenous scar tissue at the site of a wound _____
2. areas of skin removed from one site and transplanted to another site _____
3. infection _____
4. the classification of the type of burn _____
5. fungal condition of the nails _____

H. SPELL IT!   *Circle all incorrectly spelled terms, and write the correct spellings.*

1. anteperspiratant _____   4. integumant _____
2. axilary _____   5. petechie _____
3. follikle _____

Q&E List

Use the Companion CD or audio CDs to review the terms presented in Chapter 12.
Look closely at the spelling of each term as it is pronounced.

abrasion (ə-bra´zhən)
abscess (ab´ses)
acne vulgaris (ak´ne vəl-ga´ris)
adipose (ad´ĭ-pōs)
albinism (al´bĭ-niz-əm)
albino (al-bi´no)
antimicrobial (an´´te-, an´´ti-mi-kro´be-əl)
antiperspirant (an´´te-, an´´ti-pur´spər-ant´´)
asepsis (a-sep´sis)
aseptic (a-sep´tik)
aspiration (as´´pĭ-ra´shən)
atrophy (at´rə-fe)
axilla (ak-sil´ə)
axillary (ak´sĭ-lar´´e)
bactericidal (bak-ter´´ĭ-si´dəl)
bacteriostatic (bak-tĕr´´e-o-stat´ik)
biopsy (bi´op-se)
bullae (bul´e)
cellulitis (sel´u-li´tis)
contact dermatitis (kon´takt dur´´mə-ti´tis)
contusion (kən-too´zhən)
cryosurgery (kri´o-sər´jər-e)
curettage (ku´´rə-tahzh´)
cutaneous (ku-ta´ne-əs)
cyanosis (si´´ə-no´sis)
cyst (sist)
debridement (da-brēd-maw´)
dermabrasion (dur´´mə-bra´zhən)
dermatitis (dur´´mə-ti´tis)
dermis (dur´mis)
discoid lupus erythematosus (dis´koid loo´pəs
   er´´ə-them´´ə-to´sis)
electrolysis (e´´lek-trol´ə-sis)
electrosurgery (e-lek´´tro-sər´jər-e)
epidermis (ep´´ĭ-dur´mis)
erythema (er´´ə-the´mə)
fissure (fish´ər)
follicle (fol´ĭ-kəl)
folliculitis (fə-lik´´u-li´tis)
frostbite (frost´bīt)
furuncle (fu´rung-kəl)

hidradenitis (hi´´drad-ə-ni´tis)
hives (hīvz)
hypopigmentation (hi´´po-pig´´mən-ta´shən)
ichthyosis (ik´´the-o´sis)
incision (in-sizh´ən)
integument (in-teg´u-mənt)
keloid (ke´loid)
keratin (ker´ə-tin)
laceration (las´´ər-a´shən)
lesion (le´zhən)
lipoma (lip-o´mə)
liposuction (lip´´o-suk´shən)
macule (mak´ūl)
malignant melanoma (mə-lig´nənt mel´´ə-no´mə)
melanin (mel´ə-nin)
melanocyte (mel´ə-no-sĭt, mə-lan´o-sĭt)
mycodermatitis (mi´´ko-der´´mə-ti´tis)
necrosis (nə-kro´sis)
neoplasm (ne´o-plaz-əm)
nodule (nod´ūl)
onychomycosis (on´´ĭ-ko-mi-ko´sis)
onychopathy (on´´ĭ-kop´ə-the)
papule (pap´ūl)
pediculosis (pə-dik´´u-lo´sis)
perspiration (pur´´spĭ-ra´shən)
petechiae (pə-te´ke-e)
pilomotor muscle (pi´´lo-mo´tər mus´əl)
plaque (plak)
psoriasis (sə-ri´ə-sis)
pustule (pus´tūl)
scabies (ska´bēz)
scales (skālz)
scleroderma (sklĕr´´o-der´mə)
scleroprotein (sklĕr´´o-pro´tēn)
sebaceous gland (sə-ba´shəs gland)
seborrhea (seb´´o-re´ə)
seborrheic dermatitis (seb´´o-re´ik dur´´mə-ti´tis)
seborrheic keratosis (seb´´o-re´ik ker´´ə-to´sis)
sebum (se´bəm)
sepsis (sep´sis)
septic (sep´tik)

continued

skin cancer (**skin kan´sər**)

skin graft (**skin graft**)

subcutaneous adipose tissue (**sub´´ku-ta´ne-əs ad´ĭ-pŏs tish´oo**)

sudoriferous gland (**soo´´do-rif´ər-əs gland**)

topical medication (**top´ĭ-kəl med´´ĭ-ka´shən**)

transdermal (**trans-dur´məl**)

trichosis (**tri-ko´sis**)

ulcer (**ul´sər**)

ungual (**ung´gwəl**)

urticaria (**ur´´tĭ-kar´e-ə**)

vesicle (**ves´ĭ-kəl**)

wheals (**hwēlz, wēlz**)

xerosis (**zēr-o´sis**)

  Don't forget the games on the Companion CD and http://evolve.elsevier.com/Leonard/quick/ for additional review activities, including questions on Spanish medical terms.

E͡SPA͡ÑOL Enhancing Spanish Communication

English	Spanish (pronunciation)
axilla	sobaco (**so-BAH-co**)
bruise	contusión (**con-too-se-ON**), moretón (**mo-ray-TON**)
eyebrow	ceja (**SAY-hah**)
eyelash	pestaña (**pes-TAH-nyah**)
hives	roncha (**RON-chah**)
incision	incisión (**in-se-se-ON**), corte (**COR-tay**)
nails	uñas (**OO-nyahs**)
perspiration	sudor (**soo-DOR**)
skin	piel (**pe-EL**)
suture	sutura (**soo-TOO-rah**)
ulcer	ulcera (**OOL-say-rah**)

CHAPTER 13

Nervous System and Psychologic Disorders

CONTENTS

Function First
Structures of the Nervous System
  Organization of the Nervous System
  Central Nervous System
  Peripheral Nervous System and the Sense Organs
Diseases, Disorders, and Diagnostic Terms
  Psychologic Disorders

Surgical and Therapeutic Interventions
Self-Test
Q&E List
Enhancing Spanish Communication

OBJECTIVES

After completing Chapter 13, you will be able to:

1. Recognize or write the functions of the nervous system.
2. Recognize or write the meanings of Chapter 13 word parts and use them to build and analyze terms.
3. Write terms for select structures of the nervous system, or match them with their descriptions.
4. Write the names of the diagnostic terms and pathologies related to the nervous system when given their descriptions, or match terms with their meanings.
5. Match the names of psychologic disorders with their descriptions.
6. Match surgical and therapeutic interventions for the nervous system or write the names of the interventions when given their descriptions.
7. Spell terms for the nervous system and psychologic disorders correctly.

Function First

Each of the body systems has specific functions, yet all are interrelated and work together to sustain life. It has been said that the human body is more complex than the greatest computer. The nervous system keeps us in touch with both our internal and external environments. Serving as the control center and communications network, the nervous system stores and processes information, stimulates movement, and detects change. In addition, working with the endocrine system, the nervous system helps maintain homeostasis, a dynamic equilibrium of the internal environment of the body.

The nervous system affects both psychologic and physiologic functions. The study of behavior and the function and processes of the mind is called psycho+logy. The nervous system influences other body systems; for example, damage to certain nerves may result in respiratory arrest.

Sensory, or **afferent**, receptors detect changes that occur inside and outside the body and convey them to the brain. Some receptors monitor changes in the outside

> home/o = sameness
> -stasis = controlling

 QUICK TIP
Physiologic pertains to function; *psychologic* pertains to the mind.

> physi/o = nature

Nervous system

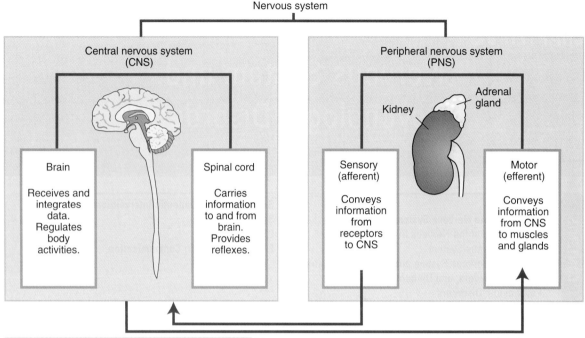

Figure 13-1 Major divisions of nervous system. Note that the peripheral nervous system contains both afferent (sensory) and efferent (motor) nerves.

environment, such as in room temperature, and other receptors monitor changes within the body, such as in body temperature. Integrative functions create sensations, produce thoughts and memory, and make decisions based on what is received from the sensory receptors. The nervous system responds by sending motor, or **efferent**, signals from the brain to muscles and glands to cause an effect. The interrelation of these activities is usually explained in a diagram, as shown in Figure 13-1. The part of the nervous system under conscious or voluntary control is called the **somatic** nervous system. The part of the nervous system that relates to involuntary or automatic body functions is called the **autonomic nervous system.**

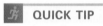

QUICK TIP

Somatic usually pertains to the body, as distinguished from the mind.

aut/o = self

WRITE IT!   **EXERCISE 1**

Write a word in each blank to complete these sentences.

As the control center and communication network, the nervous system has several functions:

- stores and processes (1) _____;
- stimulates (2) _____;
- detects (3) _____ in both the internal and external environment;
- works with the endocrine system to maintain (4) _____(internal equilibrium)

Receptors that detect internal or external changes are called sensory or (5) _____ receptors. Motor or (6) _____ signals to muscles and glands bring about an effect. The part of the nervous system under voluntary control is the (7) _____ nervous system, and the part that relates to involuntary body functions is the (8) _____ nervous system.

Use Appendix VIII to check your answers to all the exercises in Chapter 13.

Structures of the Nervous System

Organization of the Nervous System

Two major divisions of the nervous system are the **central nervous system** (CNS) and the **peripheral nervous system** (PNS). The CNS, the control center, includes the brain and spinal cord. The second division, the PNS, consists of the various nerve processes that connect the brain and spinal cord with receptors, muscles, and glands. The PNS consists of nerves that carry impulses toward as well as away from the CNS, allowing the brain to detect sensations within the body, as well as respond to sensations outside the body. Study Figure 13-1 again until you are sure you understand the relationship between these two parts of the nervous system.

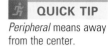
QUICK TIP
Peripheral means away from the center.

> **WRITE IT!**
> **EXERCISE 2**
> *Write the names of the two major divisions of the nervous system.*
> 1. _____
> 2. _____

The nervous system is composed of two types of cells: **neurons** and glial (neuroglial) cells. The two types of cells have different functions.

- Neurons conduct impulses either to or from the nervous system (Figure 13-2). Note the **cytoplasmic** projections: a single axon and several dendrites that project from the cell body. **Dendrites** transmit impulses to the cell body and the **axon** carries impulses away from the cell body. Many axons are surrounded by a white fatty covering called a **myelin sheath.** These fibers conduct nerve impulses faster than axons that lack the myelin sheath. The outermost layer of the axon is called the **neurilemma** (or neurolemma).
- **Neuroglia**, or **glia**, are the supporting tissue cells of the nervous system. Neuroglial cells provide special support and protection. If glial cells are destroyed, they can replace themselves; however, if an axon is destroyed, it cannot be replaced.

WORD ORIGIN
glia (Gk) glue

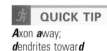
QUICK TIP
Axon **a**way;
dendrites towar**d**

QUICK TIP
Neuroglia is composed of glial cells.

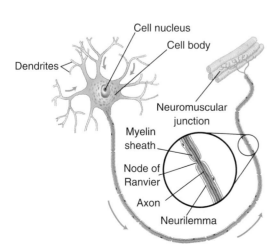

neur/o = nerve
muscul/o = muscle
myel/o = spinal cord

Figure 13-2 Structure of a typical neuron. The basic parts of a neuron are the cell body, a single axon, and several dendrites. Arrows indicate the direction that an impulse travels to or from the cell body. Some axons are surrounded by a segmented myelin sheath. The myelinated regions provide much faster conduction of the nerve impulse than parts of the axon that are not myelinated.

WRITE IT! **EXERCISE 3**

Write a term in each blank to complete these sentences.

1. The _____ nervous system includes the brain and spinal cord.
2. The _____ nervous system consists of nerves that carry impulses toward, as well as away from, the brain and spinal cord.
3. A nerve cell that has dendrites and an axon is called a _____.
4. The supporting structure of nervous tissue is composed of _____ cells.

Commit the word parts in the following table to memory.

Word Parts: Nervous System and Psychologic Disorders

Combining Forms	Meaning	Combining Forms	Meaning
aut/o	self	nerv/o, neur/o	nerve
cerebell/o	cerebellum	phren/o	mind or diaphragm
cerebr/o,* encephal/o	brain	physi/o	nature
cervic/o	neck (sometimes cervix uteri)	retin/o	retina
		sacr/o	sacrum
coccyg/o	coccyx (tailbone)	spin/o	spine
crani/o	cranium (skull)	thorac/o	thorax (chest)
dendr/o	tree	vascul/o	vessel
dur/o	dura mater		
gli/o	neuroglia or a sticky substance	**Prefix**	
		agora-	open marketplace
kerat/o	cornea; hard or horny		
lumb/o	lower back	**Suffixes**	
mening/o	meninges	-asthenia	weakness
ment/o, psych/o	mind	-esthesia	sensation, perception
myel/o	bone marrow or spinal cord	-lexia	words, phrases
		-orexia	appetite

Use the electronic flashcards on the Evolve site or make your own set of flashcards using the above list. Select the word parts just presented, and study them until you know their meaning. Do this each time a set of word parts is presented.

Sometimes cerebr/o means cerebrum.

MATCH IT! **EXERCISE 4**

Match the terms in the left column with their descriptions.

_____ 1. aut/o   **A.** brain
_____ 2. cerebr/o   **B.** cornea
_____ 3. cervic/o   **C.** lower back
_____ 4. crani/o   **D.** mind
_____ 5. dendr/o   **E.** neck
_____ 6. kerat/o   **F.** self
_____ 7. lumb/o   **G.** skull
_____ 8. myel/o   **H.** spinal cord
_____ 9. phren/o   **I.** tree
_____ 10. vascul/o   **J.** vessel

WRITE IT!

EXERCISE 5

Write the meanings of these word parts.

1. agora- _____

2. -asthenia _____

3. cerebell/o _____

4. coccyg/o _____

5. dur/o _____

6. encephal/o _____

7. gli/o _____

8. -lexia _____

9. ment/o _____

10. physi/o _____

Central Nervous System

The central nervous system consists of the brain and spinal cord, both encased in bone—the skull (or **cranium**), and the spinal column, respectively. The principal structures of the brain are shown in Figure 13-3. Major structures are the **cerebrum,** which is approximately seven eighths ($\frac{7}{8}$) of the total weight of the brain, the **diencephalon,** the **cerebellum,** and the brainstem. The **hypothalamus** (located beneath the **thalamus**) communicates directly with the pituitary gland, which is discussed in Chapter 14. Different lobes of the brain are identified with speech, vision, movement of the body, and so forth. Additional protection for the brain and spinal cord is provided by **cerebrospinal fluid** (CSF) and three membranes that are collectively called the **meninges.** The brainstem (midbrain, **pons,** and **medulla oblongata**) connects the cerebrum with the spinal cord.

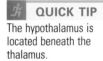

QUICK TIP
The hypothalamus is located beneath the thalamus.

di- = twice *or* two
encephal/o = brain
hypo- = beneath
mid- = middle
spin/o = spine

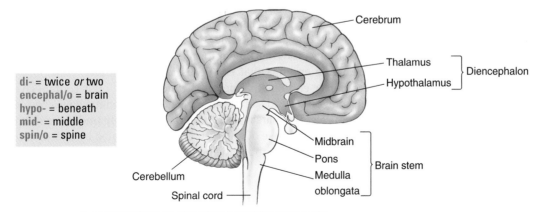

Figure 13-3 Principal structures of the brain (midsagittal view). The brainstem consists of the midbrain, the pons, and the medulla. Its lower end is a continuation of the spinal cord. The diencephalon is above the brainstem and consists of the thalamus and the hypothalamus. The cerebrum is about $\frac{7}{8}$ of the total weight of the brain and spreads over the diencephalon. The cerebellum is inferior to the cerebrum.

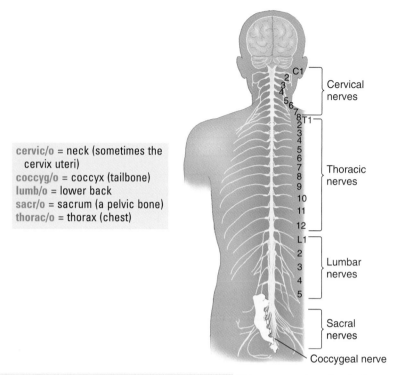

cervic/o = neck (sometimes the cervix uteri)
coccyg/o = coccyx (tailbone)
lumb/o = lower back
sacr/o = sacrum (a pelvic bone)
thorac/o = thorax (chest)

Figure 13-4 The spinal cord and emerging nerves. Thirty-one pairs of spinal nerves arise from the spinal cord and are named and numbered according to the region and level of the spinal cord from which they emerge.

Peripheral Nervous System and the Sense Organs

cervic/o = neck
thorac/o = chest
lumb/o = lower back
sacr/o = sacrum
coccyg/o = coccyx

The peripheral nervous system is the part of the nervous system that is outside the central nervous system. The PNS consists of both sensory nervous tissue and motor nervous tissue. Thirty-one pairs of nerves emerge from the spinal cord and are named and numbered as **cervical, thoracic, lumbar, sacral,** and **coccygeal** nerves (Figure 13-4).

Special sense organs—the eyes, the ears, the skin, the mouth, and the nose—have receptors that detect sensations, and the information is then transmitted to the brain. The receptors are nerve endings that enable us to see, hear, feel, taste, and smell.

chem/o = chemical

therm/o = heat

phot/o = light

Chemoreceptors are nerve endings that detect chemicals. Taste buds contain chemoreceptors for sweet, sour, bitter, and salty tastes. The nose and tongue have chemoreceptors that detect chemicals. **Thermoreceptors** located immediately under the skin detect changes in temperature. The sense of touch and pain are initiated by special receptors that are widely distributed throughout the body. The eyes contain **photoreceptors** and are responsible for vision.

MATCH IT!
EXERCISE 6

Match the terms in the left column with their descriptions.

____ **1.** chemoreceptors   **A.** nerve cells that are receptive to light

____ **2.** photoreceptors   **B.** nerve cells that detect changes in temperature

____ **3.** thermoreceptors   **C.** nerve cells that detect sweet, sour, bitter, and salty tastes

The structures of the eye and ear are shown in Figure 13-5. It is important to recognize the names associated with these structures. **Lacrim+al** means pertaining to tears. The lacrimal gland produces tears that keep the eye moist. If more lacrimal fluid is produced than can be removed, we say that the person is tearing, or crying. **Lacrimation** refers to the production and discharge of tears. The **nasolacrimal** duct carries tears to the nasal cavity and explains why a runny nose often accompanies crying. The lens of the eye is located just posterior to the pupil and is responsible for focusing the light rays to produce a perfect image. The **cornea** is the convex, transparent structure at the front of the eyeball. Corneal conditions are the leading cause of visual problems in the United States. The cornea was one of the first organs transplanted, and rejection of the transplanted tissue is uncommon. The **retina,** located in the posterior part of the eye, contains photoreceptors (rods and cones). It is continuous with the optic nerve, which carries the impulse to the cerebrum and enables vision.

lacrim/o = tear
-al = pertaining to

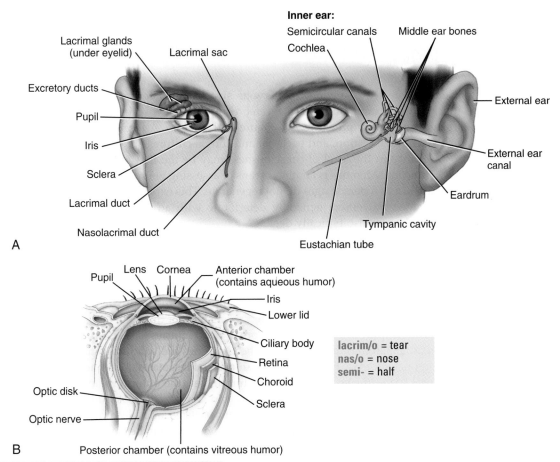

lacrim/o = tear
nas/o = nose
semi- = half

Figure 13-5 Structures of the ear and eye. A, Major structures of the eye and ear. Note that the eustachian (auditory) tube joins the middle ear cavity and the back of the throat and serves to adjust the air pressure in the ear to the external atmospheric pressure. **B,** Structures of the eyeball, transverse section.

The ears have receptors that detect touch, pain, heat, and cold, but the receptors that enable us to hear usually come to mind when we think of the ear as a sense organ. We also depend on our ears for our sense of **equilibrium,** or balance. Anatomically, the ear is divided into the external ear, middle ear, and inner ear (see Figure 13-5). The outer ear collects sound waves and directs them into the ear. The middle ear is an air-filled cavity that contains the eardrum and three tiny bones that transmit vibrations of the eardrum to fluids in the inner ear. The **cochlea** in the inner ear contains receptors that enable us to hear. The **semicircular canals** enable us to maintain a sense of balance.

MATCH IT!
EXERCISE 7

Choose A or B from the right column to classify these structures as part of the ear or the eye.

_____ **1.** cochlea   _____ **4.** cornea   **A.** ear
_____ **2.** lacrimal gland   _____ **5.** semicircular canals   **B.** eye
_____ **3.** retina

Diseases, Disorders, and Diagnostic Terms

cerebr/o = brain
spin/o = spine

Certain illnesses involving the nervous system may require chemical analysis and microscopic examination of the cerebrospinal fluid, obtained by spinal puncture (usually a lumbar puncture; see Figure 6-21, p. 157). A large number of leukocytes may indicate infection, and bacterial and fungal cultures are done if indicated.

A change in the level of consciousness may be the first indication of a decline in CNS function. Memory is another means of assessing neurologic function. Nerve cells that are lost as a person ages do not regenerate. This explains why balance, reflex, and coordinated movement generally deteriorate with advancing age. Vision, hearing, taste, and smell also typically decline.

electr/o = electric
encephal/o = brain
-graphy = recording

Electro+encephalo+graphy is the recording and analysis of the electrical activity of the brain (see Figure 3-9, p. 69). The record obtained is an **electroencephalogram.** The diagnosis of brain death may require electroencephalography to demonstrate that electrical activity of the brain is absent.

Magnetic resonance imaging (MRI), computed tomography (CT), and scans using radioisotopes are used to assess structural changes of the brain and spinal cord. CT is especially helpful in diagnosing tumors or head injuries (see Figure 4-9, p. 87). Three types of hematomas associated with head injuries are subdural, epidural, and intra-cerebral hematomas (Figure 13-6). In an **epidural hematoma.** blood accumulates in the epidural space, the space outside the dura mater (the outermost and toughest of the three meninges surrounding the brain and spinal cord). Accumulation of blood beneath the dura mater is called a **subdural hematoma,** and bleeding occurs within the brain in an **intracerebral hematoma.** All hematomas within the skull are serious and can result in compression of the brain, so they are removed whenever possible.

epi- = on, upon
dur/o = dura mater
sub- = under
intra- = within

vascul/o = vessel

 QUICK TIP
Cerebrovascular accident is CVA, stroke, or a stroke syndrome.

In a **cerebro+vascul+ar** accident (CVA), normal blood supply to the brain is disrupted. CVA results in insufficient oxygen to brain tissue and is caused by hemorrhage, occlusion (closing), or constriction of the blood vessels that normally supply oxygen to the brain. Paralysis, weakness, speech defect, and other complications, as

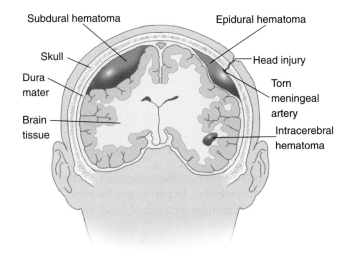

cerebr/o = brain
dur/o = dura mater
epi- = upon
hemat/o = blood
intra- = within
mening/o = meninges
-oma = tumor
sub- = under

Figure 13-6 Hematomas. Three types associated with head injuries: subdural hematoma, epidural hematoma, and intracerebral hematoma.

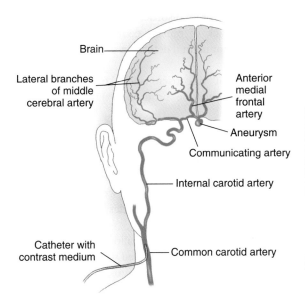

angi/o = vessel
anter/o = anterior, front
cerebr/o = brain
-graphy = recording
later/o = side
medi/o = middle

Figure 13-7 Cerebral aneurysm. Diagram of an aneurysm and the major cerebral arteries visible in cerebral angiography.

well as death, may occur. Some types of strokes are often preceded by warning signs, such as a **transient ischemic attack** (TIA), which is caused by a brief interruption in cerebral blood flow. Ischemic refers to deficient blood circulation. TIA symptoms often include disturbance of normal vision, dizziness, weakness, and numbness.

Disorders that interfere with CSF flow, such as brain tumors, can cause **hydrocepha-lus,** or accumulation of fluid in the skull. The fluid accumulation usually causes increased intracranial pressure. When this happens in an infant, before the cranial bones fuse, the skull enlarges (see Figure 5-14, p. 115). In an older child or adult, the pressure damages the soft brain tissue.

A cerebral aneurysm (localized dilation of the wall of a cerebral artery) may require cerebral angiography for diagnosis (Figure 13-7). A danger of a cerebral aneurysm is rupture, which results in a hemorrhagic stroke.

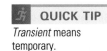

QUICK TIP
Transient means temporary.

hydr/o = water
cephal/o = head

Write a one-word term for each of these descriptions.
1. common name for a cerebrovascular accident _____
2. fluid accumulation in the skull _____
3. the recording of the electrical activity of the brain _____
4. type of hematoma in which blood accumulates beneath the dura mater _____
5. type of hematoma in which blood accumulates outside the dura mater _____
6. type of hematoma in which bleeding occurs within the brain _____

Fractures as well as excessive bending or extension of the spine can result in spinal cord injuries. These spinal injuries include excessive hyperflexion (beyond normal bending), hyperextension (beyond normal maximum extension), and vertical compression (Figure 13-8).

The following list provides information on additional diseases and disorders related to the nervous system.

akinesia (a-, no + kinesi/o, movement + -ia, condition) complete or partial loss of muscle movement.

anesthesia (an-, no + esthesi/o, feeling) partial or complete loss of sensation with or without loss of consciousness; results from disease, injury, or administration of an anesthetic.

aphagia (a-, no + -phagia, eating) inability or refusal to swallow. It is characterized by abstention from eating because swallowing is painful.

aphasia (-phasia, speech) an abnormal neurological condition in which there is absence or impairment of the ability to communicate through speech, writing, or signs.

astigmatism (GK. *stigma,* points or marks + -ism, condition) uneven curvature of the cornea or lens of the eye that prevents the sharp focus of an image on the retina.

bradykinesia (brady-, slow + -kinesia, movement) abnormal slowness of movement or sluggishness of mental and physical processes.

cephalalgia (cephal/o, head + -algia, pain) headache.

cerebral concussion (cerebr/o, brain + -al, pertaining to) loss of consciousness, either temporary or prolonged, as a result of a blow to the head.

cerebral contusion bruising of brain tissue as a result of head injury.

cerebral hemorrhage (hem/o, blood + -rrhage, excessive bleeding) result of the rupture of a sclerosed, diseased, or injured blood vessel in the brain.

cerebral palsy brain disorder characterized by paralysis and lack of muscle coordination; it results from developmental defects in the brain or trauma at birth.

coma state of unconsciousness from which the patient cannot be aroused, even by powerful stimulation.

diplegia (di-, two + -plegia, paralysis) paralysis affecting like parts on both sides of the body.

diplopia (dipl/o, double + -opia, vision) double vision, the perception of two images of a single object.

dyslexia (dys-, difficult + -lexia, words) inability to read, spell, and write words despite the ability to see and recognize letters.

dysphagia (-phagia, eating, swallowing) difficulty in swallowing, usually associated with obstruction or other disorder of the esophagus.

dysphasia (-phasia, speech) speech impairment caused by a lesion in the brain; characterized by lack of coordination and failure to arrange words properly.

electromyography (my/o, muscle) preparation, study, and interpretation of an electromyogram, a graphic record of the contraction of a muscle as a result of electrical stimulation.

encephalitis (encephal/o, brain + -itis, inflammation) inflammation of the brain.

encephalocele hernial protrusion of brain substance through a congenital or traumatic opening of the skull; craniocele.

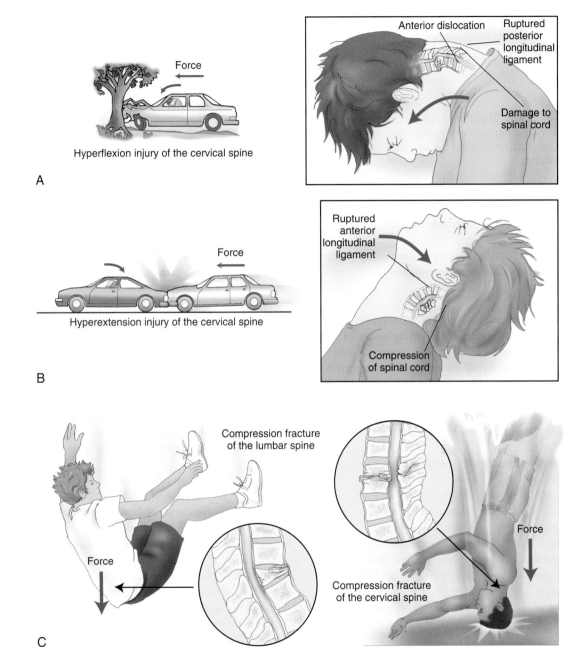

Figure 13-8 Closed spinal cord injuries. Fractures and dislocations to the vertebral column can result in injury to the spinal cord. These types of vertebral injuries occur most often at points where a relatively mobile portion of the spine meets a relatively fixed segment. **A,** Hyperflexion of the cervical vertebrae. **B,** Hyperextension of the cervical vertebrae. **C,** Vertical compression of the lumbar spine and the cervical spine.

-cele = herniation
mening/o = meninges

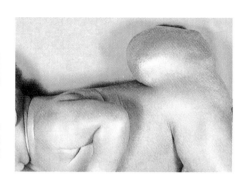

Figure 13-9 Meningocele. The spinal meninges have formed a hernial cyst that is filled with cerebrospinal fluid and is protruding through a defect in the vertebral column.

encephalomalacia (-malacia, softening) softening of the brain.

encephalomeningitis (mening/o, meninges) inflammation of the brain and meninges.

encephalopathy (-pathy, disease) any disease of the brain.

epilepsy (-lepsy, seizure) group of neurologic disorders characterized by recurrent episodes of convulsive seizures, sensory disturbances, loss of consciousness, or all of these. An uncontrolled electrical discharge from the nerve cells of the cerebral cortex is common to all types of epilepsy.

glaucoma abnormal condition of increased pressure within the eye.

hemiplegia (hemi-, half) paralysis of one side of the body.

hyperkinesia (hyper-, excessive + -kinesia, movement) abnormally increased activity or motor function.

hyperopia (-opia, vision) farsightedness, an error of refraction in which the rays of light entering the eye are brought to a focus behind the retina.

Meniere disease chronic disease of the inner ear characterized by recurrent episodes of dizziness.

meningitis (mening/o, meninges) inflammation of the meninges.

meningocele herniation of the meninges through a defect in the skull or vertebral column (Figure 13-9).

multiple sclerosis (scler/o, hard + -osis, condition) chronic CNS disease with progressive destruction of the myelin sheaths of the neurons.

The resulting scar tissue interferes with the normal transmission of nerve impulses.

myasthenia gravis (my/o, muscle + -asthenia, weakness) disease characterized by muscle weakness and abnormal fatigue.

myelitis (myel/o, bone marrow or spinal cord) inflammation of the bone marrow or spinal cord.

myelography radiographic examination of the spinal cord by injection of a radiopaque medium.

myopia nearsightedness, a defect in vision in which the rays of light entering the eye are brought to a focus in front of the retina.

narcolepsy (narc/o, sleep) chronic ailment involving sudden attacks of sleep that occur at intervals.

neuralgia (neur/o, nerve) pain along the course of a nerve.

neuritis inflammation of a nerve.

neuropathy any disease of the nerves.

paraplegia (para-, near or beside) paralysis of the legs and lower part of the body.

Parkinson disease chronic nervous disease characterized by a fine, slowly spreading tremor, muscular weakness, rigidity, and often a peculiar gait.

quadriplegia (quadri-, four) paralysis of all four extremities; also called tetraplegia.

retinal detachment separation of the retina from the back of the eye, usually resulting from a hole or tear in the retina (Figure 13-10).

retinopathy any disease of the retina.

shingles (herpes zoster) acute, infectious eruption of vesicles, usually on the trunk of the body along a peripheral nerve.

tinnitus (L. *tinnire*, to tinkle) subjective ringing of one or both ears.

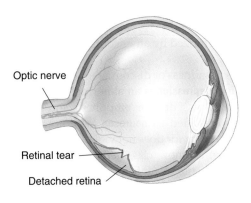

Optic nerve

Retinal tear

Detached retina

-al, -ic = pertaining to
ophthalm/o = eye
opt/o = vision
retin/o = retina
-scopy = visual examination

Figure 13-10 Retinal detachment. The onset of separation of the retina from the back of the eye is usually sudden and painless. The person may experience bright flashes of light or floating dark spots in the affected eye. Sometimes there is loss of visual field, as though a curtain is being pulled over part of the visual field. Retinal detachments are usually visible using ophthalmoscopy.

MATCH IT!

EXERCISE 9

Match the terms in the left column with the meanings in the right column.

_____ **1.** akinesia

_____ **2.** aphagia

_____ **3.** cephalgia

_____ **4.** diplegia

_____ **5.** dysphasia

_____ **6.** encephalocele

_____ **7.** hyperopia

_____ **8.** myopia

_____ **9.** narcolepsy

_____ **10.** paraplegia

A. farsightedness

B. headache

C. herniation of the brain through the skull

D. inability or refusal to swallow

E. loss of muscle movement

F. nearsightedness

G. paralysis affecting like parts on both sides of the body

H. paralysis of the legs and lower part of the body

I. speech impairment

J. sudden attacks of sleep

Psychologic Disorders

Psychologic disorders are unlike most diseases or disorders that confront health professionals because there often is no change in the body structure, and sometimes not even detectable changes in chemistry, thus making the abnormalities difficult to demonstrate and treat in the usual sense. **Psycho+somat+ic** means pertaining to the mind-body relationship or having physical symptoms of emotional origin.

psych/o = mind
somat/o = body
-ic = pertaining to

There are many classifications of psychologic disorders. The most serious form, a **psychosis**, refers to any major mental disorder characterized by a gross impairment in reality testing and often characterized by inappropriate mood and diminished impulse control. Symptoms may include hallucinations (false sensory perceptions), delusions (false beliefs), and strange behavior. Three examples of psychoses follow:

- **Schizo+phren+ia,** which involves gross distortion of reality, disorganization and fragmentation of thought and emotional reaction, and withdrawal from social interaction

schizo/o = split
phren/o = mind

bi- = two

pyr/o = fire
-mania = excessive
    preoccupation

🏃 **QUICK TIP**

Neuroses is plural of
neurosis.

WORD ORIGIN

agora (Gk.,
marketplace)
Ancient Greek
marketplaces were
large open spaces.

---

neur/o = nerve
-asthenia =
    weakness

🏃 **QUICK TIP**

Atrophy of the cerebral
cortex occurs in
Alzheimer disease.

- Bipolar disorders, characterized by manic episodes, major depression, or mixed moods
- **Pyro+mania,** an impulse control disorder characterized by an uncontrollable urge to set fires

Most persons experience occasional feelings of sadness or discouragement resulting from personal loss or tragedy. However, **clinical depression** is an abnormal emotional state characterized by exaggerated feelings of sadness, despair, emptiness, and hopelessness. Many disorders that were formerly classified as **neuroses** (symptoms are distressing to the person, reality testing is intact, behavior does not violate gross social norms, and there is no apparent organic cause) are now classified as disorders or combinations of disorders. These include anxiety disorders (anticipation of impending danger and dread, the source of which is largely unknown or unrecognized) and mood disorders.

Anxiety disorders sometimes include panic attacks, marked by intense apprehension or terror accompanied by difficult breathing, sweating, chest pain, or racing of the heart. An obsessive-compulsive disorder is a type of anxiety disorder characterized by recurrent and persistent thoughts, ideas, feelings (obsessions), or compulsions sufficiently severe to cause marked distress, repetitive acts (compulsions), or significant interference with the patient's functioning.

A **phobia** is a persistent, irrational, intense fear of something specific, such as fear of fire, an activity, meeting strangers, or leaving the familiar setting of home. One example is **agora+phobia,** an intense, irrational fear of open spaces, characterized by marked fear of venturing out alone or of being in public places, where escape would be difficult or help might be unavailable.

Anorexia nervosa is an eating disorder primarily seen in adolescent girls and usually associated with emotional stress or conflict, such as anxiety, irritation, anger, and fear. It is characterized by a prolonged refusal to eat, resulting in wasting, emotional disturbance concerning body image, and fear of becoming obese. **Neur+asthenia** is a nervous condition characterized by chronic weakness, fatigue, and sometimes exhaustion. It sometimes follows depression.

Signs of psychologic disorders can appear in a very young child, such as autism and attention deficit disorder (ADD). **Autism** is characterized by withdrawal and impaired development in social interaction and communication. ADD and attention deficit–hyperactivity disorder (ADHD) are characterized by short attention span, poor communication, and, in ADHD, hyperactivity.

Only a few psychologic disorders have observable pathologic conditions of the brain. An example of an observable pathologic condition is **Alzheimer disease,** which is progressive mental deterioration with several characteristics, including confusion, memory failure, disorientation, restlessness, and inability to carry out purposeful movement. The symptoms worsen with age.

MATCH IT!
EXERCISE 10

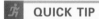

Match the psychologic terms in the left column with their descriptions.

___ **1.** Alzheimer disease   **A.** chronic weakness and fatigue, often following depression

___ **2.** anorexia nervosa   **B.** eating disorder that results in wasting of the body

___ **3.** neurasthenia   **C.** progressive mental deterioration

___ **4.** pyromania   **D.** uncontrollable urge to set fires

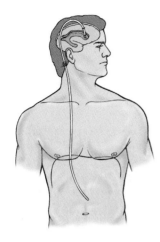

-al = pertaining to
cerebr/o = brain
peritone/o = peritoneum
spin/o = spine
ventricul/o = ventricle

Figure 13-11 Ventriculoperitoneal shunt. This type of shunt consists of plastic tubing between a cerebral ventricle and the peritoneum, to drain excess cerebrospinal fluid from the brain in hydrocephalus.

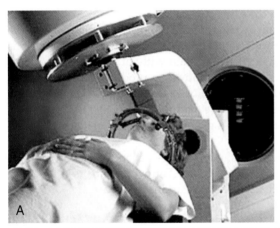

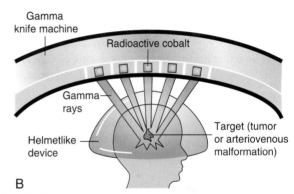

Figure 13-12 Gamma "knife" treatment assisted by stereotaxis. A, The stereotactic frame holds the patient's head in a fixed position. **B,** In a gamma knife treatment, beams are intense only at the targeted area.

Surgical and Therapeutic Interventions

Cranial surgery may be needed for vascular abnormalities, brain tumors, trauma, or removal of pus and necrotic products of infection. Any surgical opening into the skull is a **craniotomy. Cranioplasty** is surgical repair of the skull after surgery or injury to the skull. **Shunts** (passages or bypasses between two vessels) are used to redirect cerebrospinal fluid from one area to another using a tube or an implanted device (Figure 13-11).

Stereotactic radiosurgery involves closed-skull destruction of a target (e.g., tumor) using ionizing radiation. The patient's head is held in a frame. In a gamma knife procedure, a high dose of radiation is delivered to precisely targeted tumor tissue (Figure 13-12).

Neuroplasty is plastic surgery to repair a nerve or nerves. **Neuro+rrhaphy** is suturing of a cut nerve. **Neuro+lysis** has several meanings: release of a nerve sheath by cutting it longitudinally; surgery to break up adhesions surrounding a nerve; relief of tension on a nerve; and disintegration of nerve tissue.

QUICK TIP
Called gamma "knife" procedure because controlled radiation replaces surgical knife.

neur/o = nerve
-rrhaphy = suture
-lysis = destruction

cutane/o = skin
-ous = pertaining to
trans- = across

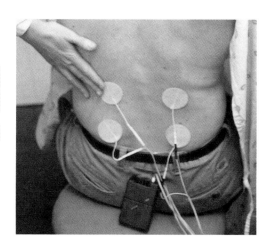

Figure 13-13 Transcutaneous electrical nerve stimulation (TENS). The TENS unit is being used in this example to control low back pain. Electrodes are placed on the skin and attached to a stimulator by flexible wires. The electrical impulses block transmission of pain signals to the brain. TENS is nonaddictive and has no known side effects, but it is contraindicated in patients with artificial cardiac pacemakers.

trans- = across *or* through
cutane/o = skin
-ous = pertaining to

Nerve blocks are used to reduce pain by temporarily blocking transmission of nerve impulses. Pain management may be for a short time (e.g., after surgery) or longer, as in chronic pain. **Analgesics** are agents that relieve pain without causing loss of consciousness. **Hypnotics** are drugs often used as sedatives to produce a calming effect. Trans+cutane+ous electrical nerve stimulation (TENS) is a method of pain control by the application of electrical impulses to the nerve endings (Figure 13-13). Pain signals to the brain are blocked by electrical impulses generated by a stimulator attached to electrodes on the skin.

In addition to analgesics and anesthetics, many drugs act on the central nervous system. **Anticonvulsants** relieve or prevent convulsions. Antipyretics are used to reduce fever, and antiparkinsonian drugs are used to treat Parkinson disease.

MATCH IT!
EXERCISE 11

Match the surgical terms in the left column with their descriptions.

_____ **1.** analgesics
_____ **2.** cranioplasty
_____ **3.** craniotomy
_____ **4.** hypnotics
_____ **5.** neurolysis
_____ **6.** neuroplasty
_____ **7.** neurorrhaphy

A. agents that are often used as sedatives
B. agents that relieve pain
C. incision of the skull
D. surgical relief of tension on a nerve
E. surgical repair of a nerve
F. surgical repair of the skull
G. suturing of a cut nerve

⚠ **Be Careful with These!**

-asthenia (weakness) versus *-esthesia* (sensation, perception)
-lexia (words, phrases) versus *-orexia* (appetite)
cerebell/o (cerebellum) versus *cerebr/o* (brain)

SELF-TEST Work the following exercises to test your understanding of the material in Chapter 13. Complete all the exercises before using Appendix VIII to check your answers.

A. WRITE IT! *Write a word in each blank to complete these sentences.*

1. The brain and spinal cord are part of the _____ nervous system.
2. The various nerves that connect the brain and the spinal cord with receptors, muscles, and glands make up the _____ nervous system.
3. The _____ nervous system is the control center of the body.
4. The main type of nerve cell is called a(n) _____.
5. Nerve cells that provide special support and protection are called _____ cells.
6. Protective membranes called _____ cover the brain and spinal cord.
7. The type of receptor stimulated by light is called a(n) _____.
8. The type of receptor stimulated by chemicals is called a(n) _____.
9. The sense organ that enables us to maintain a sense of balance is the _____.
10. Agents that relieve pain without causing loss of consciousness are called _____.

B. CIRCLE IT! *Choose the one correct response (a, b, c, or d) for each question.*

1. What is the term for protrusion of the brain through a defect in the skull?
   (a) cranioplasty   (b) encephalitis   (c) encephalocele   (d) encephalomyeloma
2. In which type of hematoma is blood found within the brain tissue itself?
   (a) epidural   (b) intracerebral   (c) subdural   (d) vascular
3. Which of the following diseases or disorders is characterized by sudden attacks of sleep?
   (a) astigmatism   (b) diplegia   (c) encephalomalacia   (d) narcolepsy
4. Which of the following is an infectious eruption that usually occurs on the trunk of the body?
   (a) Alzheimer disease   (b) multiple sclerosis   (c) myelitis   (d) shingles
5. Which of the following means recording of the electrical activity of the brain?
   (a) akinesia   (b) electroencephalography   (c) encephalopathy   (d) narcolepsy
6. Which term means inflammation of the brain?
   (a) adrenitis   (b) encephalitis   (c) meningitis   (d) myelitis
7. Which term means a headache?
   (a) cephalalgia   (b) cephalotomy   (c) dyslexia   (d) dysphagia
8. Which of the following is an abnormal emotional state characterized by exaggerated feelings of sadness and hopelessness?
   (a) clinical depression   (b) myopia   (c) psychosis   (d) psychosomatic disorder
9. Which of the following is an irrational fear of open spaces, characterized by marked fear of venturing out alone?
   (a) agoraphobia   (b) anorexia nervosa   (c) attention deficit disorder   (d) autism
10. Which term means complete loss of muscle movement?
   (a) akinesia   (b) aphasia   (c) aphonia   (d) dyskinesia

Continued

SELF-TEST (cont'd)

C. WRITE IT! *Write one-word terms for these meanings.*

1. abnormal preoccupation with fire _____
2. incision of the skull _____
3. any disease of the brain _____
4. destruction of nerve tissue _____
5. double vision _____
6. nearsightedness _____
7. persistent, irrational fear or dread _____
8. paralysis of the arms and legs _____
9. surgical repair of the skull _____
10. suturing of a cut nerve _____

D. SPELL IT! *Circle all incorrectly spelled terms, and write the correct spelling.*

1. glawcoma _____
2. periferal _____
3. retina _____
4. subdural _____
5. thalmus _____

E. FINDING THE CLUE! *Use a clue to write terms for these descriptions. Solve Question 1; each ending letter becomes the clue for the first letter of the next answer.*

1. the record obtained by electromyography _____
2. hernial protrusion of meninges _____
3. outside or above the dura mater _____
4. crying _____
5. pain of a nerve _____
6. refusal or loss of the ability to swallow _____
7. loss of speech, writing, or comprehending _____
8. agent that prevents or relieves convulsions _____
9. nerve ending sensitive to temperature change _____
10. any disease of the retina _____

F. READING HEALTH CARE REPORTS   *Read the health care report, then write terms from the report that match the descriptions.*

MEDICAL REPORT   **Mid-City Medical Center**

222 Medical Center Drive   **Main City, USA 63017-1000**   **Phone:** (555) 434-0000
                                                                            Fax: (555) 434-0001

HISTORY AND PHYSICAL

Patient's Name: Emma Lang   **Date of Admission:** 12/04/2009
Admitting Complaint: Multiple sclerosis
History of Admitting Complaint: Diagnosis of multiple sclerosis was made in 1999 by MRI scan. Family has noted progressive confusion over last 3-4 months, especially in the morning, and anorexia. She frequently chokes on liquids and has difficulty understanding speech, weakness in both arms and legs, and severe spasticity. She seldom speaks. She is catheterized 3-4 times per day due to urinary retention.
Allergies: None.
Physical Examination
  Cardiovascular, Pulmonary, and Gastrointestinal: No unusual findings.
  General: Disoriented to time, place, and person. Carries out simple commands.
  Neurologic: Eyes and ears appear normal except for possible diplopia. Muscle power is decreased in both arms. Tone is increased in right leg.
  Genitourinary: No unusual findings.
Family History: Mother had Alzheimer disease.
Impression: Progressive neurologic disorder with dementia, dysarthria, neurogenic bladder, and dysphasia.

Milton Freeberger
Milton Freeberger, M.D.

MEF: aba
Date: 12/6/2009

---

1. difficulty in language function   _____
2. double vision   _____
3. progressive, degenerative disease of the brain   _____
4. loss of appetite   _____
5. chronic disease characterized by progressive destruction of the myelin   _____
   sheaths of neurons

Q&E List

Use the Companion CD or audio CDs to review the terms presented in Chapter 13. Look closely at the spelling of each term as it is pronounced.

afferent (**af´ər-ənt**)
agoraphobia (**ag˝ə-rə-fo´be-ə**)
akinesia (**a˝kĭ-ne´zhə**)
Alzheimer disease (**awltz´hi-mər dĭ-zēz´**)
analgesic (**an˝əl-je´zik**)
anesthesia (**an˝es-the´zhə**)
anorexia nervosa (**an˝o-rek´se-ə nur-vo´sə**)
anticonvulsant (**an˝te-, an˝ti-kən-vul´sənt**)
aphagia (**ə-fa´jə**)
aphasia (**ə-fa´zhə**)
astigmatism (**ə-stig´mə-tiz-əm**)
autism (**aw´tiz-əm**)
autonomic nervous system (**aw˝tə-nom´ik
   nur´vəs sis´təm**)
axon (**ak´son**)
bradykinesia (**brad˝e-kĭ-ne´zhə**)
central nervous system (**sen´trəl nur´vəs sis´təm**)
cephalalgia (**səf˝ə-lal´jə**)
cerebellum (**ser˝ə-bel´əm**)
cerebral concussion (**ser´ə-brəl, sə-re´brəl
   kən-kush´ən**)
cerebral contusion (**ser´ə-brəl, sə-re´brəl
   kən-too´zhən**)
cerebral hemorrhage (**ser´ə-brəl, sə-re´brəl hem´ə-rəj**)
cerebral palsy (**ser´ə-brəl, sə-re´brəl pawl´ze**)
cerebrospinal fluid (**ser˝ə-bro-spi´nəl floo´id**)
cerebrovascular (**ser˝ə-bro-vas´ku-lər**)
cerebrum (**ser´ə-brəm, sə-re´brəm**)
cervical (**sur´vĭ-kəl**)
chemoreceptor (**ke˝mo-re-sep´tər**)
clinical depression (**klin´ĭ-kəl dĭ-presh´ən**)
coccygeal (**kok-sij´e-əl**)
cochlea (**kok´le-ə**)
coma (**ko´mə**)
cornea (**kor´ne-ə**)
cranioplasty (**kra´ne-o-plas˝te**)
craniotomy (**kra˝ne-ot´ə-me**)
cranium (**kra´ne-əm**)
cytoplasmic (**si˝to-plaz´mik**)
dendrite (**den´drīt**)
diencephalon (**di˝ən-sef´ə-lon**)
diplegia (**di-ple´je-ə**)

diplopia (**dĭ-plo´pe-ə**)
dyslexia (**dis-lek´se-ə**)
dysphagia (**dis-fa´je-ə**)
dysphasia (**dis-fa´zhə**)
efferent (**ef´ər-ənt**)
electroencephalogram (**e-lek˝tro-en-sef´ə-lo-gram˝**)
electroencephalography (**e-lek˝tro-ən-sef˝ə-log´rə-fe**)
electromyography (**e-lek˝tro-mi-og´rə-fe**)
encephalitis (**en-sef˝ə-li´tis**)
encephalocele (**en-sef´ə-lo-sēl˝**)
encephalomalacia (**en-sef˝ə-lo-mə-la´shə**)
encephalomeningitis (**en-sef˝ə-lo-men˝in-ji´tis**)
encephalopathy (**en-sef˝ə-lop´ə-the**)
epidural hematoma (**ep˝ĭ-doo´rəl he˝mə-to´mə**)
epilepsy (**ep´ĭ-lep˝se**)
equilibrium (**e˝kwĭ-lib´re-əm**)
glaucoma (**glaw-, glou-ko´mə**)
glia (**gli´ə**)
hemiplegia (**hem˝e-ple´jə**)
hydrocephalus (**hi˝dro-sef´ə-ləs**)
hyperkinesia (**hi˝pər-kĭ-ne´zhə**)
hyperopia (**hi˝pər-o´pe-ə**)
hypnotic (**hip-not´ik**)
hypothalamus (**hi˝po-thal´ə-məs**)
intracerebral hematoma (**in˝trə-ser´ə-brəl
   he˝mə-to´mə**)
lacrimal (**lak´rĭ-məl**)
lacrimation (**lak˝rĭ-ma´shən**)
lumbar (**lum´bər, lum´bahr**)
medulla oblongata (**mə-dul´ə ob˝long-gah´tə**)
Meniere disease (**mĕ-nyār´ dĭ-zēz´**)
meninges (**mə-nin´jēz**)
meningitis (**men˝in-ji´tis**)
meningocele (**mə-ning´go-sēl˝**)
multiple sclerosis (**mul´tĭ-pəl sklə-ro´sis**)
myasthenia gravis (**mi˝əs-the´ne-ə gră´vis**)
myelin sheath (**mi´ə-lin shēth**)
myelitis (**mi˝ə-li´tis**)
myelography (**mi´ə-log´rə-fe**)
myopia (**mi-o´pe-ə**)
narcolepsy (**nahr´ko-lep˝se**)
nasolacrimal (**na˝zo-lak´rĭ-məl**)

neuralgia (nŏŏ-ral´jə)
neurasthenia (noor˝əs-the´ne-ə)
neurilemma (noor˝ĭ-lem´ə)
neuritis (nŏŏ-ri´tis)
neuroglia (nŏŏ-rog´le-ə)
neurolysis (nŏŏ-rol´ĭ-sis)
neuron (noor´on)
neuropathy (nŏŏ-rop´ə-the)
neuroplasty (noor´o-plas˝te)
neurorrhaphy (nŏŏ-ror´ə-fe)
neuroses (nŏŏ-ro´sēz)
paraplegia (par˝ə-ple´jə)
Parkinson disease (pahr´kin-sən dĭ-zēz´)
peripheral nervous system (pə-rif´ər-əl nur´vəs sis´təm)
phobia (fo´be-ə)
photoreceptor (fo˝to-re-sep´tər)
pons (ponz)
psychosis (si-ko´sis)
psychosomatic (si˝ko-so-mat´ik)
pyromania (pi˝ro-ma´ne-ə)

quadriplegia (kwod˝rĭ-ple´jə)
retina (ret´ĭ-nə)
retinal detachment (ret´ĭ-nəl de-tach´mənt)
retinopathy (ret˝ĭ-nop´ə-the)
sacral (sa´krəl)
schizophrenia (skit˝so-, skiz˝o-fre´ne-ə)
semicircular canals (sem˝e-sər´kyə-lər kə-nals´)
shingles (shing´gəlz)
shunt (shunt)
somatic (so-mat´ik)
stereotactic radiosurgery (ster˝e-o-tak´tik
     ra´de-o-sur´jər-e)
subdural hematoma (səb-doo´rəl he˝mə-to´mə)
thalamus (thal´ə-məs)
thermoreceptor (thur˝mo-re-sep´tər)
thoracic (thə-ras´ik)
tinnitus (tin˝ĭ-təs, tĭ-ni´təs)
transient ischemic attack (tran´shent,
     tran´se-ənt is-ke´mik ə-tak´)

 evolve Don't forget the games on the Companion CD and http://evolve.elsevier.com/Leonard/quick/ for additional review activities, including questions on Spanish medical terms.

ESPAÑOL Enhancing Spanish Communication

English	Spanish (pronunciation)
anxiety	ansiedad (an-se-ay-DAHD)
concussion	concusión (con-coo-se-ON)
conscious	consciente (cons-se-EN-tay)
convulsion	convulsión (con-vool-se-ON)
cranium	cráneo (CRAH-nay-o)
fainting	desmayo (des-MAH-yo)
nervous	nervioso (ner-ve-O-so)
neurology	neurología (nay-oo-ro-lo-HEE-ah)
sleep	sueño (soo-AY-nyo)

CHAPTER 14

Endocrine System

CONTENTS

Function First
Structures of the Endocrine System
  Select Hormones
Diseases, Disorders, and Diagnostic Terms

Surgical and Therapeutic Interventions
Self-Test
Q&E List
Enhancing Spanish Communication

OBJECTIVES

After completing Chapter 14, you will be able to:

1. Recognize or write the functions of the endocrine system.
2. Recognize or write the meanings of Chapter 14 word parts and use them to build and analyze terms.
3. Write terms for selected structures of the endocrine system and their associated hormones and functions, or match them with their descriptions.

4. Write the names of the diagnostic terms and pathologies related to the endocrine system when given their descriptions, or match terms with their meanings.
5. Match surgical and therapeutic interventions for the endocrine system, or write the names of the interventions when given their descriptions.
6. Spell terms for the endocrine system correctly.

Function First

endo- = inside
-crine = secrete

dys- = "bad," impaired

The **endo+crine** system coordinates with the nervous system to regulate body activities. This is accomplished by endocrine hormones that affect various processes throughout the body, such as growth, metabolism, and secretions from other organs. Dysfunctional hormone production may involve either a deficiency (**hyposecretion**) or an excess (**hypersecretion**).

WRITE IT! / EXERCISE 1

Write answers to these questions.

1. What is the function of the endocrine gland? _____
2. What is the meaning of hyposecretion? _____
3. What is the meaning of hypersecretion? _____

Use Appendix VIII to check your answers to all the exercises in Chapter 14.

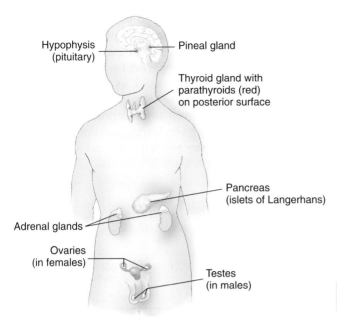

Hypophysis (pituitary) — Pineal gland

Thyroid gland with parathyroids (red) on posterior surface

Pancreas (islets of Langerhans)

Adrenal glands

Ovaries (in females)

Testes (in males)

hypo- = beneath (*or* below normal)
para- = near or beside (*also* abnormal)
-physis = growth

Figure 14-1 Location of major glands of the endocrine system.

Structures of the Endocrine System

The endocrine system, also called the "hormonal system," is composed of glands that have the ability to manufacture or release chemical substances (**hormones**) that are discharged into the bloodstream and used in other parts of the body. Glands are classified as endocrine or **exo+crine** on the basis of the presence or absence of ducts. Endocrine glands are ductless and secrete their hormones into the bloodstream. Exocrine glands open onto a body surface and discharge their secretions through ducts (e.g., sweat glands). Exocrine glands are not part of the endocrine system.

exo- = outside

The organ or structure toward which the effects of a hormone are primarily directed is called the **target organ**. Endocrine glands release hormones in one of two ways:

1. Hormones are released in response to the nervous system.
2. The pituitary produces hormones that act on endocrine glands, which then produce hormones.

Thus the pituitary gland is nicknamed the "master gland." Another way to understand pituitary function follows:

Pituitary produces stimulating hormones → Other endocrine glands → Other hormones

An example of the master gland acting on another gland involves gonado+tropic hormones (also called gonadotropins), which are produced by the pituitary gland and act on the gonads (ovaries or testicles).

The locations of the major glands of the endocrine system, including the pituitary, are shown in Figure 14-1. Observe that the **pituitary** gland is also called the **hypophysis**, so named because it is attached by a stalk at the base of the brain. Other endocrine glands include the pineal gland, the thyroid and parathyroid glands, islets of Langerhans within the **pancreas,** adrenal glands, the ovaries in females, and the testes in

QUICK TIP

Gonadotropins act on the ovaries or testicles, the target organs.

hypo- = below
-physis = growth

males. The **pineal gland,** also called the pineal body, is shaped like a pinecone and is attached to the posterior part of the brain. Its precise function has not been established, but it is believed to secrete the hormone melatonin. The **thyroid** gland, located at the front of the neck, consists of bilateral lobes that are connected by a narrow strip of thyroid tissue. **Parathyroid** glands are located near the thyroid, as the name implies, and are actually embedded in the posterior surface of the thyroid. The pancreas is an elongated structure that has digestive functions as well as endocrine functions. The **islets of Langerhans** are **pancreatic** cells that perform an endocrine function. An **adrenal** gland lies above each of the two kidneys. The ovaries and testes are endocrine glands as well as organs that produce ova or sperm, respectively.

QUICK TIP

Islets of Langerhans, named for their discoverer, Dr. Paul Langerhans, is an eponym.

WRITE IT!   **EXERCISE 2**

Write answers to these questions.

1. What is the general name for the structures that compose the endocrine system?
   _____

2. What is the term that means the chemical substances that are secreted by endocrine glands?
   _____

3. Describe the difference between endocrine and exocrine glands? _____
   _____

4. Which type of gland functions as part of the endocrine system? _____

5. What is the general term for the organ or structure toward which the effects of a hormone are directed?
   _____

6. Describe two ways in which endocrine glands are stimulated to release hormones.
   _____
   _____

7. Write the name of the master gland: _____.

8. In no particular order (a to g), list the names of seven endocrine glands, not including the master gland (*hint:* two are the male and female sex glands): (a) _____,
   (b) _____, (c) _____, (d) _____,
   (e) _____, (f) _____, and (g) _____

Commit the word parts in the following table to memory.

Word Parts: Endocrine System	
Combining Forms	**Meaning**
aden/o	gland
adren/o	adrenal glands
andr/o	male or masculine
gigant/o	giant
gonad/o	gonad
insulin/o	insulin
iod/o	iodine
myx/o	mucus

Word Parts: Endocrine System—cont'd

Combining Forms	Meaning
pancreat/o	pancreas
parathyroid/o	parathyroids
pituitar/o, hypophys/o	pituitary gland
ren/o	kidney
thyr/o, thyroid/o	thyroid gland
toxic/o	poison

Suffixes	
-gen	beginning, origin
-physis	growth
-tropic	stimulate
-tropin	that which stimulates
-uria	urine, urination

Use the electronic flashcards on the Evolve site or make your own set of flashcards using the above list. Select the word parts just presented, and study them until you know their meanings. Do this each time a set of word parts is presented.

MATCH IT!
EXERCISE 3

Match the meanings in the left column with the combining forms.

_____ **1.** adrenal gland   **A.** aden/o

_____ **2.** giant   **B.** adren/o

_____ **3.** gland   **C.** andr/o

_____ **4.** iodine   **D.** gigant/o

_____ **5.** kidney   **E.** iod/o

_____ **6.** male or masculine   **F.** myx/o

_____ **7.** mucus   **G.** ren/o

_____ **8.** poison   **H.** toxic/o

WRITE IT!
EXERCISE 4

Write suffixes for these meanings.

1. beginning   _____

2. growth   _____

3. origin   _____

4. stimulate   _____

5. that which stimulates   _____

6. urination   _____

Select Hormones

Some of the most discussed hormones include cortisone and steroids that are banned by most major sports organizations. Growth hormone injections are included in the list of athletic performance–enhancing drugs. You may also be familiar with cortisone injections to relieve pain and inflammation, or use of cortisone in topical creams and ointments to relieve skin inflammation. Female sex hormones are used in several birth control methods, including oral contraceptives (pills and patches).

Table 14-1   Select Hormones and Corresponding Endocrine Glands

Hormone	Endocrine Gland	Major Function(s)
adrenaline (also known as epinephrine)	adrenals	Potent stimulator of the "fight or flight" response, increasing blood pressure and cardiac output
androgen (major androgen is testosterone)	testicles	Development and maintenance of masculinizing characteristics
antidiuretic hormone (ADH)	pituitary*	Suppression of urine formation
cortisone	adrenals	Important in regulation of body metabolism
estrogen (female sex hormones; includes estradiol and estrone)	ovaries (primarily)	During menstrual cycle, estrogens act on the female genitalia to produce a suitable site for fertilization, implantation, and nutrition of the early embryo
growth hormone	pituitary	Stimulation of body growth, and maintenance of size once growth is obtained
insulin	pancreas	Regulation of blood glucose by coordinating with other hormones
thyroxine (iodine-containing hormone)	thyroid	Cell metabolism

*ADH is synthesized by the hypothalamus (a structure of the brain), which also controls its secretion by the pituitary.

Insufficient secretion or improper use of the hormone insulin leads to diabetes mellitus. Insulin and other important hormones are summarized in Table 14-1.

MATCH IT!   EXERCISE 5

Match the endocrine glands in the left column with the hormone they secrete.

_____ **1.** adrenals   **A.** androgen

_____ **2.** ovaries   **B.** antidiuretic hormone

_____ **3.** pancreas   **C.** epinephrine

_____ **4.** pituitary   **D.** estrogen

_____ **5.** testicles   **E.** insulin

Diseases, Disorders, and Diagnostic Terms

hyper- = above normal

ex- = outward
ophthalm/o = eye

Most endocrine glands are not accessible for examination in a routine physical examination; however, the testicles and thyroid gland are exceptions. The testicles are examined visually for masses or a difference in size. The thyroid gland can be observed and palpated for any unusual bulging over the thyroid area (Figure 14-2, *A*). Both enlargement and masses are abnormal findings and indicate additional testing is necessary. **Hyperthyroidism** is abnormally increased activity of the thyroid. A classic finding associated with hyperthyroidism is **ex+ophthalmos**, that is, protrusion of the eyeballs, but further tests are required with this condition because hyperthyroidism is not always the cause. The patient in Figure 14-2, *B*, has both exophthalmos and a **goiter,**

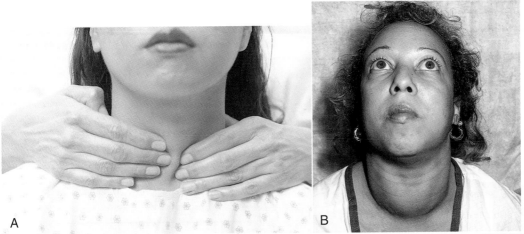

A   B

Figure 14-2 Physical examination of the thyroid gland. A, Using the hands to feel for thyroid enlargement or masses. **B,** Observing the patient for thyroid enlargement and exophthalmos, protrusion of the eyeballs. This patient shows both exophthalmos and a goiter, which is an enlarged thyroid gland, evidenced by the swelling in the neck.

> ex- = out
> ophthalm/o = eye

an enlarged thyroid gland that is usually evident as a pronounced swelling in the neck.

A person who is described as **eu+thyroid** has normal thyroid function.

Hypo+thyroid+ism is decreased activity of the thyroid. Several blood tests and radiologic studies are used to determine thyroid function. Thyroid scans consist of administering a radioactive substance, allowing time for the thyroid gland to absorb the radiation, scanning the thyroid, and imaging the radiation distribution.

> eu- = normal
> hypo- = below
>   normal

Physical indications of endocrine disorders also include unusually tall or short stature, coarsening of facial features, edema (accumulation of fluid in the interstitial tissues), hair loss, or excessive facial hair in women. Laboratory testing includes blood tests and urine tests, depending on the symptoms. Magnetic resonance imaging (MRI) is useful in identifying tumors involving the pituitary.

Diabetes insipidus is a disorder associated with a deficiency of antidiuretic hormone (ADH), one hormone produced by the pituitary gland, or inability of the kidneys to respond to ADH. Do not confuse diabetes insipidus with **diabetes mellitus** (DM), the well-known type of diabetes that produces hyperglycemia and is associated with insufficient or improper use of insulin. Type 1 diabetes mellitus is characterized by abrupt onset of symptoms and a dependence on insulin injections to sustain life. Type 2 diabetes mellitus is usually characterized by a gradual onset; dietary control, sometimes combined with oral hypoglycemic medications, may be effective in regulating the disorder. "Diabetics" are persons who have diabetes mellitus. Diabetes insipidus has some of the characteristics of diabetes mellitus: **poly+uria** and **poly+dipsia**. The two terms mean frequent urination and increased thirst, respectively. However, diabetes insipidus is not associated with insulin deficiency, **hyper+glyc+emia** (increased level of glucose in the blood), or **glycos+uria** (sugar in the urine). Table 14-2 compares the characteristics of these two types of diabetes.

> **QUICK TIP**
> *Diuretic* means promoting urine excretion. *Antidiuretic* has the opposite meaning.

> poly- = many
> -uria = urination
> -dipsia = thirst

> hyper- = increased
> glyc/o = sugar
> -emia = blood

Table 14-2 **Comparison of Diabetes Insipidus with Diabetes Mellitus**		
Characteristic	**Diabetes Insipidus**	**Diabetes Mellitus**
ADH deficiency	Yes	No
Polyuria	Yes	Yes
Polydipsia	Yes	Yes
Insufficient or improper use of insulin	No	Yes
Two types, I and II	No	Yes
Hyperglycemia	No	Yes
Glycosuria	No	Yes

WRITE IT!   EXERCISE 6

Write terms for these descriptions.

1. disorder associated with a deficiency of ADH _____

2. disorder associated with insufficient or improper use of insulin _____

3. decreased activity of the thyroid _____

4. frequent urination _____

5. increased level of blood glucose _____

6. increased thirst _____

7. protrusion of the eyeballs _____

8. sugar in the urine _____

The following list provides information about other disorders related to the endocrine system.

acromegaly (acr/o, extremity + -megaly, enlarged) disorder in which there is abnormal enlargement of the extremities of the skeleton—nose, jaws, fingers, and toes—caused by hypersecretion of growth hormone after maturity (Figure 14-3).

adenoma (-oma, tumor) tumor of a gland.

cretinism condition caused by congenital deficiency of thyroid secretion and marked by arrested physical and mental development (Figure 14-4).

acr/o = extremities
-megaly = enlargement

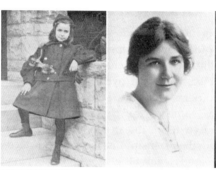
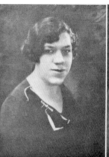
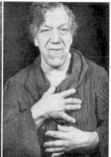

Figure 14-3 Progression of acromegaly. The patient is shown at age 9 years, age 16, age 33 with well-established acromegaly, and age 52 in the late stage of acromegaly.

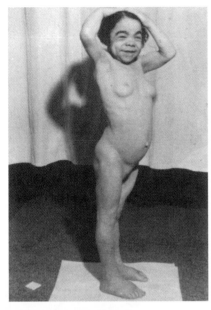

-al, -ary, -ic = pertaining to
axill/o = axilla
faci/o = facial
pub/o = pubis
umbilic/o = umbilicus (navel)

Figure 14-4 Cretinism. This 33-year-old untreated adult with cretinism exhibits characteristic features. She is only 44 inches tall, has underdeveloped breasts, protruding abdomen, umbilical hernia, widened facial features, and scant axillary and pubic hair.

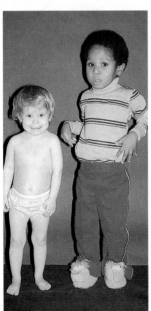

Figure 14-5 A growth hormone deficiency. A normal 3-year-old boy and a short 3-year-old girl who exhibits the characteristic "Kewpie doll" appearance, suggesting a diagnosis of growth hormone deficiency. This deficiency leads to dwarfism unless identified early and treated.

dwarfism disease caused by hyposecretion of growth hormone during childhood; it causes a person to be much smaller than normal size (Figure 14-5).

gigantism (gigant/o, large + -ism, condition) condition in which a person reaches an abnormal stature; it results from hypersecretion of growth hormone during childhood. Compare dwarfism and gigantism (Figure 14-6).

hyperinsulinism excessive secretion of insulin by the pancreas, which causes hypoglycemia.

hyperparathyroidism increased activity of the parathyroid glands.

hypoglycemia (hypo-, decreased) abnormally low blood sugar.

hypoparathyroidism decreased activity of the parathyroid glands.

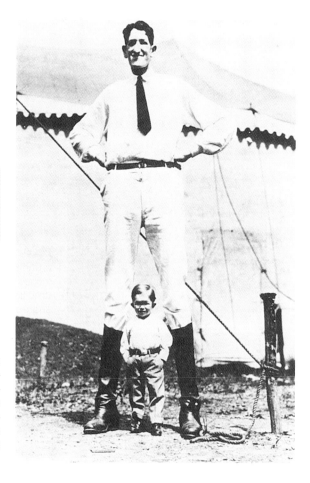

acr/o = extremities
gigant/o = large
hyper- = more than normal
-ism = condition
-megaly = enlargement

Figure 14-6 Gigantism and dwarfism. Both result from abnormal secretion of growth hormone (GH). Hypersecretion of GH during the early years results in gigantism. The person usually has normal body proportions and normal sexual development. The same hypersecretion in an adult causes acromegaly. Hyposecretion of GH during the early years produces a dwarf unless the child is treated with GH injections.

hypopituitarism diminished activity of the pituitary gland.

myxedema (myx/o, mucus + -edema, swelling) condition resulting from hypofunction of the thyroid gland, characterized by a dry, waxy swelling of the skin.

thyrotoxicosis (thyr/o, thyroid + toxic/o, poison + -osis, condition) morbid condition caused by excessive thyroid secretion.

MATCH IT!
EXERCISE 7

Match the diagnostic terms in the left column with their descriptions.

_____ **1.** acromegaly
_____ **2.** cretinism
_____ **3.** diabetes insipidus
_____ **4.** diabetes mellitus
_____ **5.** exophthalmos
_____ **6.** gigantism
_____ **7.** goiter

A. abnormal enlargement of the extremities
B. abnormally tall stature
C. condition caused by congenital deficiency of thyroid secretion
D. disorder associated with insufficient or improper use of insulin
E. disorder caused by insufficient ADH or inability of kidneys to respond to ADH
F. enlarged thyroid gland that results in swelling of the neck
G. outward protrusion of the eyeballs

WRITE IT!
EXERCISE 8

Write terms for these descriptions.
1. abnormally low blood sugar   _____
2. an iodine-containing thyroid hormone _____
3. excessive secretion of insulin   _____
4. normal thyroid function   _____
5. tumor of a gland   _____

Surgical and Therapeutic Interventions

Hormonal deficiencies are often treated by administration of the deficient hormone or substances that simulate hormonal effects. Because the most common cause of hypopituitarism is a pituitary tumor, treatment consists of surgery or radiation to remove the tumor, followed by administration of the deficient hormones. **Hypophysectomy** is surgical removal or destruction of the pituitary gland (Figure 14-7).

> hypophys/o = pituitary
> -ectomy = excision

Overproduction of hormones sometimes requires suppression or removal of all or part of the target organ responsible for the overproduction (e.g., overproduction of thyroid-stimulating hormone by the pituitary gland leads to hyperthyroidism and overproduction of thyroid hormones). The treatment of hyperthyroidism is destruction of large amounts of the thyroid tissue or the use of antithyroid drugs to block the production of thyroid hormones. **Adenectomy** means removal of a gland, but **thyroidectomy** specifically means removal of the thyroid gland.

The goal of treatment of diabetes mellitus is to maintain a balance of the body's insulin (a glucose-lowering agent) and glucose. Type 1 diabetes mellitus is controlled by administration of insulin, proper diet, and exercise. An insulin pump is a portable,

> **QUICK TIP**
> Type 1 diabetics are insulin dependent.

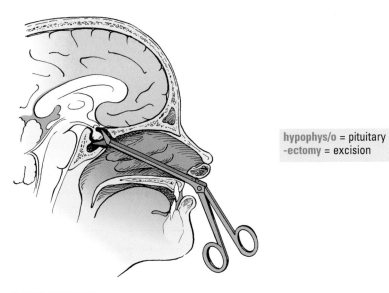

> hypophys/o = pituitary
> -ectomy = excision

Figure 14-7 Hypophysectomy. Surgical removal of the pituitary gland may be performed to excise a pituitary tumor or to slow the growth and spread of endocrine-dependent malignant tumors. Hypophysectomy is done only if other treatments fail to destroy all the pituitary tumor.

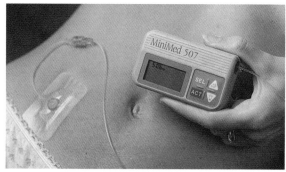

Figure 14-8 External insulin pump. This portable instrument delivers a measured amount of insulin through the abdominal wall at preset intervals. It can be programmed to deliver varied amounts of insulin according to the body's needs at different times of the day.

battery-operated instrument worn by many diabetics (Figure 14-8). Type 2 diabetes is controlled by diet, exercise, oral agents, and sometimes insulin. Oral agents are another type of glucose-lowering agent.

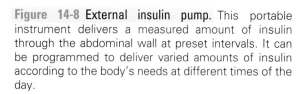

WRITE IT! **EXERCISE 9**

Write a one-word term in each blank to complete these sentences.

1. A term for surgical removal or destruction of the pituitary gland is _____.

2. Type 1 diabetes is controlled by administration of _____, proper diet, and exercise.

3. Type 2 diabetes is generally controlled by diet, exercise, and _____-lowering agents, if needed.

4. The term for removal of a gland is _____.

5. The term for removal of the thyroid gland is _____.

⚠ Be Careful with These!

aden/o (gland) versus *adren/o* (adrenal gland) versus *andr/o* (male)
-tropic (stimulate) versus *-tropin* (that which stimulates)

SELF-TEST   Work the following exercises to test your understanding of the material in Chapter 14. Complete all the exercises before using Appendix VIII to check your answers.

A. WRITE IT!   *Write answers to these questions.*

1. What is the function of the endocrine system? _____
_____

2. What is the difference between a gland and a hormone?
_____
_____

3. Which gland is the "master gland"? _____

4. What is a target organ? _____

5. What are two general types of dysfunctions in hormone production? _____
_____

SELF-TEST (cont'd)

B. WRITE IT! *List the names of seven endocrine glands, not including the master gland:*

1. _____
2. _____
3. _____
4. _____
5. _____
6. _____
7. _____

C. CIRCLE IT! *Choose the one correct response (a, b, c, or d) for each question.*

1. What is the general term for chemical substances that are discharged into the bloodstream and used in some other part of the body?
   (a) cortisones (b) estrogens (c) excretions (d) hormones
2. Which of the following is characterized by an abnormal enlargement of the extremities?
   (a) acromegaly (b) hyperparathyroidism (c) hypoglycemia (d) thyrotoxicosis
3. Which term means increased activity of the thyroid gland?
   (a) euthyroid (b) hyperthyroidism (c) hypothyroidism (d) thyroxine
4. The presence or absence of what determines whether a gland is classified as an endocrine gland or an exocrine gland?
   (a) blood vessels (b) ducts (c) fluids (d) islets
5. Which term means an enlargement of the thyroid gland, resulting in swelling at the front of the neck?
   (a) goiter (b) hyperparathyroidism (c) hyperthyroidism (d) hypothyroidism
6. Which of the following is associated with insufficient production or improper use of insulin?
   (a) diabetes insipidus (b) diabetes mellitus (c) myxedema (d) thyrotoxicosis
7. Which of the following is a disease caused by insufficient secretion of growth hormone during childhood?
   (a) acromegaly (b) cretinism (c) dwarfism (d) gigantism
8. Which term means excessive secretion of insulin?
   (a) diabetes (b) hyperinsulinism (c) hypoinsulinism (d) polydipsia
9. Which gland is responsible for the production of insulin?
   (a) adrenal (b) pancreas (c) parathyroid (d) thyroid
10. Which of the following disorders results from hypofunction of the thyroid gland?
   (a) acromegaly (b) exophthalmos (c) hypoparathyroidism (d) myxedema

D. WRITE IT! *Write a one-word term for each meaning.*

1. abnormally large stature _____
2. abnormally low blood sugar _____
3. decreased activity of the parathyroid gland _____
4. excision of the thyroid _____
5. increased thirst _____
6. frequent urination _____
7. tumor of a gland _____
8. removal of a gland _____
9. removal of the pituitary gland _____
10. toxic condition of the thyroid _____

SELF-TEST (cont'd)

E. FINDING THE CLUE! *Use a clue to write terms for these descriptions. Solve Question 1; each ending letter becomes the clue for the first letter of the next answer.*

1. gland believed to produce melatonin   _____
2. discoverer of insulin-producing cells   _____
3. meaning of the suffix -tropic   _____
4. type of gland that has ducts   _____
5. another term for hormonal   _____
6. normal thyroid   _____
7. person with diabetes mellitus   _____
8. congenital deficiency of thyroid secretion   _____
9. results from hypothyroidism   _____
10. suppressing the rate of urine formation   _____

F. READING HEALTH CARE REPORTS *Write the meanings of underlined terms in the following health care report.*

MEDICAL REPORT   **Mid-City Medical Center**

222 Medical Center Drive   **Main City, USA 63017-1000**   **Phone:** (555) 434-0000
                                                                     Fax: (555) 434-0001

Patient: W.A. Harter (62-year-old female)   **Date of Admission:** 6/10/09
Symptoms: Palpitations, hyperexcitability, weight loss, and exophthalmos.
History: Osteoporosis; currently in hospital with fractured hip after a fall.
Physical examination: Goiter present; pulse 120; blood pressure 170/96 mm Hg; appears anxious.
Diagnosis: Hyperthyroidism.
Plan: Conservative treatment with Tapazole for now. Consider possible thyroidectomy.

---

1. exophthalmos _____
2. goiter _____
3. hyperthyroidism _____
4. thyroidectomy _____

G. SPELL IT! *Circle all incorrectly spelled terms, and write the correct spelling.*

1. adrenalene   _____
2. cretenism   _____
3. homeostases   _____
4. hypersekretion   _____
5. mixedema   _____

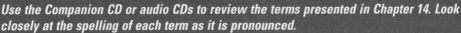

Q&E List

Use the Companion CD or audio CDs to review the terms presented in Chapter 14. Look closely at the spelling of each term as it is pronounced.

acromegaly (**ak˝ro-meg´ə-le**)
adenectomy (**ad˝ə-nek´tə-me**)
adenoma (**ad˝ə-no´mə**)
adrenal (**ə-dre´nəl**)
adrenaline (**ə-dren´ə-lin**)
androgen (**an´dro-jən**)
antidiuretic hormone (**an˝te-, an˝ti-di˝u-ret´ik hor´mōn**)
cortisone (**kor´tĭ-sōn**)
cretinism (**kre´tin-iz-əm**)
diabetes insipidus (**di˝ə-be´tēz in-sip´ĭ-dəs**)
diabetes mellitus (**di˝ə-be´tēz mel´lĕ-təs, mə-li´tis**)
dwarfism (**dworf´iz-əm**)
endocrine (**en´do-krīn, en´do-krin**)
estrogen (**es´trə-jən**)
euthyroid (**u-thi´roid**)
exocrine (**ek´so-krin**)
exophthalmos (**ek˝sof-thal´mos**)
gigantism (**ji-gan´tiz-əm, ji´gan-tiz-əm**)
glycosuria (**gli˝ko-su´re-ə**)
goiter (**goi´tər**)
growth hormone (**grōth hor´mōn**)
hormone (**hor´mōn**)
hyperglycemia (**hi˝pər-gli-se´me-ə**)
hyperinsulinism (**hi˝pər-in´sə-lin-iz˝əm**)

hyperparathyroidism (**hi˝pər-par´ə-thi´roid-iz-əm**)
hypersecretion (**hi˝pər-se-kre´shən**)
hyperthyroidism (**hi˝pər-thi´roĭd-iz-əm**)
hypoglycemia (**hi˝po-gli-se´me-ə**)
hypoparathyroidism (**hi˝po-par´ə-thi´roid-iz-əm**)
hypophysectomy (**hi poff˝ ə-sek´tə-me**)
hypophysis (**hi-pof´ə-sis**)
hypopituitarism (**hi˝po-pĭ-too´ĭ-tə-riz˝əm**)
hyposecretion (**hi˝po-sə-kre´shən**)
hypothyroidism (**hi˝po-thi´roid-iz-əm**)
insulin (**in´sə-lin**)
islets of Langerhans (**i´lets ov lahng´ər-hahnz**)
myxedema (**mik˝sə-de´mə**)
pancreas (**pan´kre-əs**)
pancreatic (**pan˝kre-at´ik**)
parathyroid (**par´ə-thi´roid**)
pineal gland (**pin´e-əl gland**)
pituitary (**pĭ-too´ĭ-tar˝e**)
polydipsia (**pol˝e-dip´se-ə**)
polyuria (**pol˝e-u´re-ə**)
target organ (**tahr´gət or´gən**)
thyroid (**thi´roid**)
thyroidectomy (**thi˝roid-ek´tə-me**)
thyrotoxicosis (**thi˝ro-tok˝sĭ-ko´sis**)
thyroxine (**thi-rok´sin**)

evolve Don't forget the games on the Companion CD and http://evolve.elsevier.com/Leonard/quick/ for additional review activities, including questions on Spanish medical terms.

ESPAñOL Enhancing Spanish Communication

English	Spanish (pronunciation)
adrenaline	adrenalina (**ah-dray-nah-LEE-nah**)
diabetes	diabetes (**de-ah-BAY-tes**)
feminine	femenina (**fay-may-NEE-na**)
giant	gigante (**he-GAHN-tay**)
hormone	hormona (**or-MOH-nah**)
insulin	insulina (**in-soo-LEE-nah**)
masculine	masculino (**mas-coo-LEE-no**)
pituitary	pituitario (**pe-too-e-TAH-re-o**)
thyroid	tiroides (**te-RO-e-des**)

Review of Chapters 1 Through 14

CONTENTS

Answering Multiple-Choice Questions
Writing Medical Terms

OBJECTIVES

After completing the material in Quick & Easy Medical Terminology, *you will be able to:*

1. Analyze medical terms and recognize their correct meanings.
2. Demonstrate understanding of the rules for using word parts by combining them correctly to write medical terms.
3. Correctly spell medical terms.

This section is included to help you test yourself on how well you remember the material in this book. Work all questions in this review if you have completed Chapters 1 through 14. If you did not complete all chapters in the book, do not work the questions relating to chapters that you did not cover.

The following two types of questions are included in this review chapter:

I. Answering multiple-choice questions

II. Writing medical terms

It is better to do all the questions in a set before checking the answers against those in Appendix VIII. As you work through the exercises, prepare a study sheet of terms that you do not remember. When you have completed the exercises, grade your answers as though it were an actual test. Look through the chapter material and find the correct answers for all multiple-choice questions that you missed. Analyze the component parts of these terms.

The following review is a representative sample of chapter material and does not include every term. Refer to your study sheet several times before taking the test that your instructor prepares, and study the list of terms at the end of each chapter, being sure you remember the meaning of each term.

I. Answering Multiple-Choice Questions

Circle the correct response (a, b, c, or d) to each question.

Chapter 2

1. What is the term for the presence of abnormally large amounts of fluid in the tissues?
   (a) dilatation   (b) edema   (c) emesis   (d) ptosis
2. Which term means excessive preoccupation with fire?
   (a) hydrophobia   (b) kleptomania   (c) paranoia   (d) pyromania
3. What is the meaning of carcinoma?
   (a) an abnormal fear of something   (b) another term for cancer
   (c) any disease of a body structure   (d) excessive preoccupation with illness
4. What does prolapse mean?
   (a) cramping   (b) discharge   (c) sagging   (d) rupture
5. Which term means inflammation of the eye?
   (a) ophthalmalgia   (b) ophthalmitis   (c) ophthalmopathy   (d) ophthalmorrhexis
6. Which term means suture of a blood vessel?
   (a) angiectomy   (b) angioplasty   (c) angiorrhaphy   (d) angiotomy
7. What is the term for surgical puncture of the thin membrane that surrounds the fetus?
   (a) adenectomy   (b) amniocentesis   (c) angiorrhexis   (d) glycolysis
8. Which of the following terms means pain along the course of a nerve?
   (a) neuralgia   (b) neurocele   (c) neuroplasty   (d) neurosis
9. What is the correct term for protrusion of all or part of an organ through the wall of the cavity that contains it?
   (a) hernia   (b) dilatation   (c) edema   (d) emesis
10. Which term means stretching of a structure?
    (a) dilatation   (b) ptosis   (c) prolapse   (d) spasm

Chapter 3

11. Which term means pertaining to the skin?
    (a) dermal   (b) dermatology   (c) dermatopathy   (d) dermatosis
12. Which of the following means a record or tracing of the electrical impulses of the heart?
    (a) electrocardiograph   (b) electrocardiogram   (c) electrocardiography   (d) electrocardiopathy
13. A disease caused by defective nutrition or metabolism is:
    (a) dystrophy   (b) necrosis   (c) oncology   (d) rachischisis
14. Which of the following conditions is caused by a deficiency of oxygen and results in a slightly bluish, slatelike color of the skin?
    (a) cyanosis   (b) erythrocytosis   (c) melancholy   (d) xanthosis
15. Pyoderma is:
    (a) an inflammatory disease of the skin in which pus is produced
    (b) any inflamed condition of the skin
    (c) the structure, function, and composition of the skin
    (d) an abnormal fear of touching dead tissue
16. A condition characterized by a yellowish discoloration of the skin and mucous membranes is:
    (a) albinism   (b) chloropia   (c) jaundice   (d) necrosis
17. A chronic ailment that consists of recurrent attacks of drowsiness and sleep is:
    (a) epilepsy   (b) narcolepsy   (c) photophobia   (d) polydipsia
18. Aphonia is:
    (a) absence of speech   (b) difficult speech   (c) rapid speech   (d) absence or loss of voice

19. A serious condition in which the body temperature is greatly elevated due to retention of body heat is:
   (a) cryptorchidism   (b) hyperthermia   (c) hypothermia   (d) orthopnea

20. Which term means a muscle that draws a body part away from the midline of the body?
   (a) abductor   (b) adductor   (c) aerosol   (d) antepartum

Chapter 4

21. Which term means a procedure that introduces a hollow flexible tube into a body cavity?
   (a) cannula   (b) catheter   (c) catheterization   (d) catheterize

22. Which of the following describes a procedure in which the image data are digitized and immediately displayed on a monitor or recorded?
   (a) computed radiography   (b) radiation oncology   (c) radiograph   (d) sonogram

23. Which term describes a procedure that involves entry into a body cavity?
   (a) invasive   (b) palpation   (c) therapeutic   (d) systolic

24. Which of the following terms means the branch of medicine concerned with the diagnosis and treatment of disease using any of the various sources of radiant energy?
   (a) radiogram   (b) radiograph   (c) radiography   (d) radiology

25. Which term describes a technique that offers continuous imaging of the motion of internal structures?
   (a) computed tomography   (b) fluoroscopy   (c) magnetic resonance imaging
   (d) positron emission tomography

26. Which term specifically means an antimicrobial agent that is derived from cultures of a microorganism or is produced semisynthetically and used to treat infections?
   (a) analgesic   (b) antibiotic   (c) chemotherapy   (d) therapeutic

27. What is the term for the rhythmic expansion of an artery that occurs as the heart beats?
   (a) blood pressure   (b) diastolic pressure   (c) pulse   (d) systolic pressure

28. What is the term for a small sample taken from the body for testing?
   (a) sign   (b) specimen   (c) symptom   (d) tomogram

29. Which of the following is not strictly a vital sign?
   (a) blood pressure   (b) body temperature   (c) pulse rate   (d) respiration rate

30. Which term means placing radioactive materials into body organs for the purpose of imaging?
   (a) computed tomography   (b) magnetic resonance   (c) nuclear scan   (d) sonography

Chapter 5

31. Which term means softening of the nails?
   (a) onychectomy   (b) onychoma   (c) onychomalacia   (d) onychomycosis

32. Which term means the presence of lacrimal stones?
   (a) allergic rhinitis   (b) dacryocystitis   (c) dacryolithiasis   (d) sialitis

33. Which term means a sticking together of two structures that are normally separated?
   (a) abdominocentesis   (b) adhesion   (c) laparogastrotomy   (d) mucosa

34. Which term means examination of the abdominal cavity using an endoscope?
   (a) anaphylaxis   (b) dactylography   (c) diaphoresis   (d) laparoscopy

35. Which term means formation and excretion of sweat?
   (a) adrenal   (b) ascites   (c) hidradenoma   (d) hidrosis

36. Which term describes a person who is able to walk?
   (a) ambulant   (b) lateral   (c) superior   (d) supine

37. Which term means the opposite of distal?
   (a) proximal   (b) inferior   (c) superior   (d) ventral

38. Which body cavity is divided into the cranial and spinal cavities?
   (a) dorsal (b) pericardial (c) thoracic (d) ventral
39. What structure lines the abdominopelvic cavity and enfolds the internal organs?
   (a) lymph (b) pericardium (c) peritoneum (d) visceral
40. Which term means inflammation of the navel?
   (a) dactylitis (b) dermatitis (c) omphalitis (d) sialitis

Chapter 6

41. What does rachialgia mean?
   (a) fused spine (b) painful spine (c) opposite of rachiodynia (d) same as spondylitis
42. Which of the following means excision of a wrist bone?
   (a) carpectomy (b) carposclerosis (c) tarsectomy (d) tarsosclerosis
43. Which term means inflammation of the vertebrae?
   (a) carpitis (b) phalangitis (c) spondylitis (d) tarsitis
44. Which term means between the ribs?
   (a) costovertebral (b) intercostal (c) intracostal (d) subcostal
45. Which word means pertaining to the wrist and fingers?
   (a) carpophalangeal (b) metacarpal (c) metatarsal (d) tarsophalangeal
46. Which term means excision of a portion of the skull?
   (a) angiectomy (b) coccygectomy (c) craniectomy (d) craniotomy
47. Which adjective does *not* pertain to a bone of the arm?
   (a) costal (b) humeral (c) radial (d) ulnar
48. Which term means lateral curvature of the spine?
   (a) kyphosis (b) rickets (c) scoliosis (d) spina bifida
49. What is the common name of the sternum?
   (a) breastbone (b) collarbone (c) shoulder blade (d) skull
50. What is the meaning of a myocele?
   (a) fascial hernia (b) fibrous muscle (c) hardened muscle (d) painful muscle

Chapter 7

51. Which term means enlarged spleen?
   (a) hyperchondria (b) hypochondria (c) spleenomegaly (d) splenomegaly
52. A general term that designates primary myocardial disease is:
   (a) cardiomyopathy (b) congenital heart defect (c) heart block (d) ischemia
53. Which term means swelling that results from obstruction of a lymphatic vessel?
   (a) lymphangiography (b) lymphangitis (c) lymphedema (d) lymphography
54. Which of the following is a mass of undissolved matter brought by the circulating blood to a vessel?
   (a) embolus (b) ischemia (c) occlusion (d) thrombosis
55. What is another name for stroke or stroke syndrome?
   (a) aneurysm (b) cerebrovascular accident (c) myocardial infarction (d) necrosis
56. Which term means a thickening and loss of elasticity of the arterial walls?
   (a) arteriography (b) arteritis (c) arteriosclerosis (d) polyarteritis
57. Radiography of the heart and great vessels using contrast media is:
   (a) angiocardiography (b) angiography (c) angiology (d) cardiology
58. Which term means passage of a long flexible tube into the heart chamber through a vein?
   (a) catheterization (b) echocardiography (c) electrocardiogram (d) electrocardiography

59. Which term indicates severe chest pain caused by insufficient blood supply?
(a) angina pectoris (b) hypertension (c) hypotension (d) infarction

60. Which word means equilibrium of the internal environment of the body?
(a) homeostasis (b) necrosis (c) pallor (d) plasma

Chapter 8

61. What is the appropriate term for absence of breathing?
(a) apnea (b) dyspnea (c) hypopnea (d) hyperpnea

62. Which of the following is a respiratory condition in which there is breathing discomfort in any position except sitting erect or standing?
(a) apnea (b) bradypnea (c) orthopnea (d) tachypnea

63. What is the term for material raised from inflamed membranes of the respiratory tract?
(a) emphysema (b) saliva (c) sputum (d) tussive

64. What structure is inflamed in rhinitis?
(a) chest (b) nose (c) throat (d) voice box

65. Which term means labored or difficult breathing?
(a) bradypnea (b) dyspnea (c) hyperpnea (d) tachypnea

66. Which term means pertaining to the windpipe and the bronchi?
(a) bronchiectasis (b) laryngobronchial (c) pharyngobronchial (d) tracheobronchial

67. Which of the following is a respiratory condition characterized by paroxysmal dyspnea and wheezing?
(a) asthma (b) bronchitis (c) emphysema (d) influenza

68. To what does pneumocardial pertain?
(a) chest and lungs (b) heart and kidneys (c) heart and lungs (d) kidneys and lungs

69. What is the name of the membrane that surrounds each lung?
(a) diaphragm (b) esophagus (c) pleura (d) trachea

70. Which term means the inability to communicate through speech, writing, or signs and is caused by improper functioning of the brain?
(a) aphasia (b) aphonia (c) dysphasia (d) dysphonia

Chapter 9

71. Which of the following is a lesion of the mucous membrane of the stomach?
(a) biliary (b) gastric ulcer (c) gastrocele (d) hiatus

72. Which term means a type of duodenal anastomosis?
(a) colostomy (b) gastroduodenostomy (c) laparoscopy (d) vagotomy

73. To what does biliary refer?
(a) bile (b) gallbladder (c) gallstones (d) saliva

74. Which condition results when the output of body fluid exceeds fluid intake?
(a) achlorhydria (b) dehydration (c) enterostasis (d) peristalsis

75. Cirrhosis is a disease of which organ?
(a) gallbladder (b) liver (c) pancreas (d) stomach

76. Which structure is herniated when a gastrocele exists?
(a) gallbladder (b) intestine (c) liver (d) stomach

77. What is meant by eupepsia?
(a) deficient appetite (b) excessive appetite (c) normal digestion
(d) sluggish intestinal action

78. Which term means under the tongue?
(a) hypoglossal (b) infrajejunal (c) subcecal (d) subgingival

79. Which of these physicians specializes in diseases of the anus, rectum, and colon?
(a) gastroenterologist   (b) gerontologist   (c) otolaryngologist   (d) proctologist

80. Which term means inflammation of the bile ducts?
(a) cholangiogram   (b) cholangiography   (c) cholangitis   (d) cholitis

Chapter 10

81. Diminished capacity to form urine, excreting less than 500 mL of urine per day, is:
(a) anuria   (b) dysuria   (c) oliguria   (d) polyuria

82. An agent that increases urination is called a:
(a) dialysis   (b) diuresis   (c) diuretic   (d) glomerulus

83. The name of the functional unit of the kidney is:
(a) glomerulus   (b) nephron   (c) tubule   (d) ureter

84. A bladder hernia that protrudes into the vagina is a:
(a) bladder polyp   (b) cystocele   (c) pyelolith   (d) vaginal fissure

85. Which of the following is a toxic condition of the body associated with failure of the kidneys to function properly?
(a) hematuria   (b) incontinence   (c) pyuria   (d) uremia

86. Which of the following conditions is marked by degenerative, but not inflammatory, changes in the kidney?
(a) cystitis   (b) nephritis   (c) nephrosis   (d) pyelolithiasis

87. Which of the following is a surgical procedure to remove a renal calculus?
(a) nephrectomy   (b) nephrolithotomy   (c) nephrosclerosis   (d) nephrotomy

88. What is the name of the instrument used in cystoscopy?
(a) cystogram   (b) cystograph   (c) cystoscope   (d) cystotome

89. X-ray images of the urinary tract are taken after injection of contrast medium in which procedure?
(a) nephroscopy   (b) nephrosonography   (c) urogram   (d) urography

90. Which of the following is a major waste product found in the urine of a normal individual?
(a) blood   (b) protein   (c) sugar   (d) urea

Chapter 11

91. What is the name of the transparent sac that encloses the fetus in utero?
(a) amniocentesis sac   (b) amniotic sac   (c) congenital membrane   (d) trisomic membrane

92. Which term means the same as menopause?
(a) amenorrhea   (b) climacteric   (c) dysmenorrhea   (d) fistula

93. Which term means an abnormal tubelike passage?
(a) adhesion   (b) colposcopy   (c) fistula   (d) polyp

94. Which of the following means childbirth?
(a) gestation   (b) neonatality   (c) obstetrics   (d) parturition

95. Which term means excision of any part of the body or removal of a growth?
(a) ablation   (b) dilation and curretage   (c) circumcision   (d) orchiotomy

96. Which branch of medicine specializes in the care of females during pregnancy and childbirth?
(a) gynecology   (b) internal medicine   (c) obstetrics   (d) pediatrics

97. Which hormone has the primary responsibility of developing and maintaining female sexual characteristics?
(a) amnion   (b) estrogen   (c) testosterone   (d) uterine

98. Which term means a woman who has had one pregnancy that resulted in viable offspring?
(a) nullipara   (b) secundipara   (c) tripara   (d) unipara

99. What are reproductive organs called?
(a) genitalia (b) gonadotropin (c) uteri (d) vulva

100. Which of the following is characterized by cauliflower-like genital and anal lesions?
(a) AIDS (b) condyloma acuminatum (c) genital herpes (d) syphilis

Chapter 12

101. Which of the following is characterized by thinning of the skin and loss of characteristic markings?
(a) atrophy (b) cellulitis (c) hypopigmentation (d) psoriasis

102. Which of the following is also called a boil?
(a) furuncle (b) pediculosis (c) scabies (d) urticaria

103. Which of the following cause erection of the hairs of the skin?
(a) pilomotor muscles (b) sebaceous glands (c) sudoriferous glands (d) sweat glands

104. Which type of skin lesion is the result of skin being scraped or rubbed away by friction?
(a) abrasion (b) contusion (c) incision (d) laceration

105. Which of the following terms means a piercing wound?
(a) melanoma (b) nodule (c) plaque (d) puncture

106. Which term means removal of foreign material and dead or damaged tissue from a wound?
(a) debridement (b) cryosurgery (c) dermabrasion (d) necrosis

107. Which term means ulceration of tissue?
(a) erosion (b) macule (c) vesicle (d) wheal

108. Which term means a cavity that contains pus?
(a) abscess (b) cellulitis (c) cyanosis (d) petechiae

109. Which of the following is an inflammatory skin disease that begins on the scalp but may involve other areas, particularly the eyebrows?
(a) acne vulgaris (b) carcinoma (c) mycodermatitis (d) seborrheic dermatitis

110. To what does the term adipose pertain?
(a) fat (b) perspiration (c) sebum (d) skin

Chapter 13

111. Which of the following is characterized by gross distortion of reality and disorganization of thought and emotional reaction?
(a) anorexia nervosa (b) clinical depression (c) neurasthenia (d) schizophrenia

112. Which term means complete loss of muscle movement?
(a) akinesia (b) aphasia (c) aphonia (d) dyskinesia

113. Which of the following means recording and analysis of the electrical activity of the brain?
(a) akinesia (b) electroencephalography (c) encephalopathy (d) narcolepsy

114. Which of the following is an irrational fear of open spaces, characterized by marked fear of venturing out alone?
(a) agoraphobia (b) anorexia nervosa (c) attention deficit disorder (d) autism

115. Protrusion of the brain through a defect in the skull is:
(a) craniocele (b) cranioplasty (c) encephalitis (d) encephalomyeloma

116. In which type of hematoma is blood found within the brain tissue itself?
(a) epidural (b) intracerebral (c) subdural (d) vascular

117. Which of the following diseases or disorders is characterized by sudden attacks of sleep?
(a) astigmatism (b) diplegia (c) encephalomalacia (d) narcolepsy

118. Which of the following is an infectious eruption that usually occurs on the trunk of the body?
(a) Alzheimer disease (b) multiple sclerosis (c) myelitis (d) shingles

119. Which term means inflammation of the brain?
   (a) adrenitis   (b) encephalitis   (c) meningitis   (d) myelitis
120. Which term means a headache?
   (a) cephalalgia   (b) cephalotomy   (c) dyslexia   (d) dysphagia

Chapter 14

121. Which of the following is a disease caused by insufficient secretion of growth hormone during childhood?
   (a) acromegaly   (b) cretinism   (c) dwarfism   (d) gigantism
122. Which term means excessive secretion of insulin?
   (a) diabetes   (b) hyperinsulinism   (c) hypoinsulinism   (d) polydipsia
123. What is the general term for chemical substances that are discharged into the bloodstream and used in some other part of the body?
   (a) cortisones   (b) estrogens   (c) excretions   (d) hormones
124. Which of the following is the master gland?
   (a) adrenal   (b) parathyroid   (c) pineal   (d) pituitary
125. Which term means increased activity of the thyroid gland?
   (a) euthyroid   (b) hyperthyroidism   (c) hypothyroidism   (d) thyroxine
126. The presence or absence of what in particular determines whether a gland is classified as an endocrine gland or an exocrine gland?
   (a) blood vessels   (b) ducts   (c) fluids   (d) islets
127. Which of the following disorders results from hypofunction of the thyroid gland?
   (a) acromegaly   (b) exophthalmos   (c) hypoparathyroidism   (d) myxedema
128. Which term means an enlargement of the thyroid gland?
   (a) goiter   (b) hyperparathyroidism   (c) hyperthyroidism   (d) hypothyroidism
129. Which gland is responsible for the production of insulin?
   (a) adrenal   (b) pancreas   (c) parathyroid   (d) thyroid
130. Which of the following is associated with insufficient production or improper use of insulin?
   (a) diabetes insipidus   (b) diabetes mellitus   (c) myxedema   (d) thyrotoxicosis

Use Appendix VIII to check your answers.

II. Writing Medical Terms

Write the correct term for each meaning. When checking your answers, carefully look at how words are spelled.

Chapter 2

1. heart specialist   _____
2. surgical removal of a gland   _____
3. surgical repair of the ear   _____
4. crushing of a stone   _____
5. specialty of a geriatrician   _____
6. pertaining to the heart   _____
7. cramping of the hand   _____
8. resembling mucus   _____
9. specialist who cares for newborns   _____
10. inflammation of a vein   _____

Chapter 3

11. under the skin _____

12. viewing things with the microscope _____

13. another term for stones _____

14. without symptoms _____

15. benign fatty tumor _____

16. red blood cell _____

17. study of fungi _____

18. condition characterized by excessive thirst _____

19. capable of surviving without oxygen _____

20. decreased pulse rate _____

Chapter 4

21. objective evidence of an illness or disorder _____

22. existing over a long period _____

23. using a stethoscope to listen for sounds within the body _____

24. illuminated instrument for viewing inside a body cavity _____

25. not permitting the passage of x-rays _____

26. treatment using heat _____

27. drug that relieves pain _____

28. predicted outcome _____

29. tapping the body with the fingertips to evaluate internal organs _____

30. drug that produces insensibility or stupor _____

Chapter 5

31. lying down _____

32. paralysis of the eyelid _____

33. pertaining to the extremities _____

34. plastic surgery of the hand _____

35. blood in the urine _____

36. capable of breaking up mucus _____

37. behind and above _____

38. large organs in the ventral cavity _____

39. pertaining to the abdomen and thorax _____

40. pertaining to the head and pelvis _____

Chapter 6

41. muscular weakness   _____

42. slight or partial paralysis   _____

43. inflammation of a joint   _____

44. loss of calcium from bone   _____

45. pertaining to the tailbone   _____

46. below the cartilage   _____

47. pertaining to the shoulder blade   _____

48. infection of the bone and bone marrow   _____

49. instrument used to view a joint   _____

50. pertaining to the ilium and the pubis   _____

Chapter 7

51. excision of a vein   _____

52. acting against elevated blood pressure   _____

53. enlarged heart   _____

54. any disease of the lymph nodes   _____

55. inflammation of the myocardium   _____

56. elevated blood pressure   _____

57. any disease of the arteries   _____

58. inflammation of the aorta   _____

59. increased pulse rate   _____

60. tumor consisting of lymph vessels   _____

Chapter 8

61. plastic surgery of the nose   _____

62. incision of the windpipe   _____

63. pertaining to the voice box   _____

64. loss of voice   _____

65. inflammation of the lungs and bronchi   _____

66. pertaining to the air sacs of the lung   _____

67. inflammation of a sinus   _____

68. agents used to prevent coughing   _____

69. chronic dilation of the bronchi   _____

70. pertaining to the diaphragm   _____

Chapter 9

71. enzyme that breaks down starch _____

72. excision of a pancreatic stone _____

73. loss of appetite for food _____

74. x-ray examination of the gallbladder _____

75. decreased blood sugar _____

76. pertaining to the duodenum _____

77. excessive vomiting _____

78. pertaining to the common bile duct _____

79. pertaining to the stomach _____

80. enlarged liver _____

Chapter 10

81. inflammation of the renal pelvis _____

82. pertaining to the urethra _____

83. softening of the kidney _____

84. pertaining to the kidney _____

85. surgical repair of a ureter _____

86. absence of urination _____

87. instrument used to surgically crush a stone _____

88. presence of kidney stones _____

89. forming a new opening into the bladder _____

90. visual examination of the bladder _____

Chapter 11

91. excision of the prostate _____

92. prolapse of the uterus _____

93. most common type of fetal presentation _____

94. disease caused by gonococci _____

95. pertaining to the prostate _____

96. absence of menstrual flow, when normally expected _____

97. newborn infant _____

98. removal of an ovary _____

99. inflammation of a uterine tube _____

100. pertaining to the ovaries _____

Chapter 12

101. inhibiting the growth of bacteria   _____

102. pertaining to the armpit   _____

103. sac filled with clear fluid   _____

104. tumor consisting of fat cells   _____

105. using a needle to withdraw fluid   _____

106. any disease of the nail   _____

107. blisters larger than 1 cm   _____

108. deep splits through the epidermis   _____

109. excessive dryness of the skin   _____

110. inflammation of a sweat gland   _____

Chapter 13

111. incision of the skull   _____

112. inability or refusal to swallow   _____

113. paralysis of one side of the body   _____

114. persistent, irrational fear or dread   _____

115. suturing of a cut nerve   _____

116. double vision   _____

117. ringing of the ears   _____

118. softening of the brain   _____

119. loss of sensation   _____

120. sedatives used to produce a calming effect   _____

Chapter 14

121. increased thirst   _____

122. normal thyroid function   _____

123. excision of the pituitary   _____

124. excision of a gland   _____

125. tumor of a gland   _____

126. abnormal enlargement of the extremities   _____

127. abnormally tall stature   _____

128. enlarged thyroid gland that results in swelling of the neck   _____

129. excision of the thyroid gland   _____

130. frequent urination   _____

Use Appendix VIII to check your answers.

APPENDIX I
Medical Abbreviations

PART ONE

Chapter 2

ED	emergency department
ENT	ear, nose, and throat
ER	emergency room
GP	general practitioner
GYN, Gyn, gyn	gynecology
ICU	intensive care unit
OB	obstetrics
PA	physician assistant; posteroanterior

Chapter 3

ECG, EKG	electrocardiogram
EEG	electroencephalogram
IM	intramuscular
IV	intravenous

Chapter 4

BP	blood pressure
CT, CAT	computed tomography, computerized (computed) axial tomography
Dx	diagnosis
MRI	magnetic resonance imaging

OTC	over-the-counter (drug)
PET	positron emission tomography
Sx	symptoms
WNL	within normal limits

Chapter 5

AIDS	acquired immunodeficiency syndrome
CA	cancer, carcinoma
CBC, cbc	complete blood count
CDC	Centers for Disease Control and Prevention
CSF	cerebrospinal fluid
FEMA	Federal Emergency Management Agency
HIV	human immunodeficiency virus
LLQ	left lower quadrant
LUQ	left upper quadrant
RBC	red blood cell, red blood cell count
RLQ	right lower quadrant
RUQ	right upper quadrant
WBC	white blood cell, white blood cell count
WMD	weapons of mass destruction

PART TWO

Chapter 6

C1 ... C7	first cervical vertebra ... seventh cervical vertebra
DJD	degenerative joint disease
DMARD	disease-modifying antirheumatic drug
fx	fracture
L1 ... L5	first lumbar vertebra ... fifth lumbar vertebra

LE	lupus erythematosus
NSAID	nonsteroidal antiinflammatory drug
RA	rheumatoid arthritis; right atrium
T1 ... T12	first thoracic vertebra ... twelfth thoracic vertebra

Chapter 7

ASD	atrial septal defect
AV, A-V	atrioventricular (also arteriovenous)
CABG	coronary artery bypass graft
CAD	coronary artery disease
CHF	congestive heart failure
CPR	cardiopulmonary resuscitation
ECHO, echo	echocardiography
MI, AMI	myocardial infarction (acute MI)
T&A	tonsillectomy and adenoidectomy
VSD	ventricular septal defect

Chapter 8

ARDS	adult respiratory distress syndrome; acute respiratory distress syndrome
COLD	chronic obstructive lung disease
COPD	chronic obstructive pulmonary disease
LRT	lower respiratory tract
SARS	severe acute respiratory syndrome
SIDS	sudden infant death syndrome
SOB	shortness of breath
TB	tuberculosis
URT	upper respiratory tract
VC	vital capacity

Chapter 9

DM	diabetes mellitus
ERCP	endoscopic retrograde cholangiopancreatography
GERD	gastroesophageal reflux disease
GI	gastrointestinal
IBS	inflammatory bowel syndrome
LGI	lower gastrointestinal tract

Chapter 10

ADH	antidiuretic hormone
ARF	acute renal failure
BUN	blood urea nitrogen
CRF	chronic renal failure
ESWL	extracorporeal shock wave lithotripsy
IVP	intravenous pyelogram
pH	hydrogen ion concentration, "potential" hydrogen
TUR	transurethral resection
TURP	transurethral resection of the prostate
U/A, UA	urinalysis
UTI	urinary tract infection

Chapter 11

AIDS	acquired immunodeficiency syndrome
BBT	basal body temperature

BPH	benign prostatic hyperplasia
CS, C-section	cesarean section
D&C	dilation and curettage
EDD	expected delivery date
GC	gonococcus
GU	genitourinary
HBV	hepatitis B virus
HCV	hepatitis C virus
HDV	hepatitis D virus
HCG, hCG	human chorionic gonadotropin
HIV	human immunodeficiency virus
HPV	human papillomavirus
HRT	hormone replacement therapy
HSV-2	herpes simplex virus type 2 (genital herpes)
IUD	intrauterine device
IUS	intrauterine system
IVF	in vitro fertilization
LMP	last menstrual period
Pap	Papanicolaou smear, stain, or test
PID	pelvic inflammatory disease
PMS	premenstrual syndrome
PSA	prostate-specific antigen
STD	sexually transmitted disease
TUMT	transurethral microwave thermotherapy
TUNA	transurethral needle ablation
TURP	transurethral resection of the prostate

Chapter 12

Bx, bx	biopsy
DLE	discoid lupus erythematosus
TBSA	total body surface area

Chapter 13

ADD	attention deficit disorder
ADHD	attention deficit–hyperactivity disorder
CNS	central nervous system
CSF	cerebrospinal fluid
CVA	cerebrovascular accident; costovertebral angle
PNS	peripheral nervous system
TENS	transcutaneous electrical nerve stimulation
TIA	transient ischemic attack

Chapter 14

ADH	antidiuretic hormone
DM	diabetes mellitus

APPENDIX II
Finding Medical Abbreviations

acquired immunodeficiency syndrome	AIDS	degenerative joint disease	DJD
acute myocardial infarction	AMI	diabetes mellitus	DM
acute renal failure	ARF	diagnosis	Dx
adult respiratory distress syndrome	ARDS	dilation and curettage	D&C
antidiuretic hormone	ADH	discoid lupus erythematosus	DLE
atrial septal defect	ASD	disease-modifying antirheumatic drug	DMARD
atrioventricular	AV, A-V	ear, nose, and throat	ENT
attention deficit disorder	ADD	echocardiography	ECHO, echo
attention deficit–hyperactivity disorder	ADHD	electrocardiogram	ECG, EKG
basal body temperature	BBT	electroencephalogram	EEG
benign prostatic hyperplasia	BPH	emergency department	ED
biopsy	Bx, bx	emergency room	ER
blood pressure	BP	endoscopic retrograde cholangiopancreatography	ERCP
blood urea nitrogen	BUN		
cancer	CA	expected delivery date	EDD
carcinoma	CA	extracorporeal shock wave lithotripsy	ESWL
cardiopulmonary resuscitation	CPR	Federal Emergency Management Agency	FEMA
Centers for Disease Control and Prevention	CDC	fracture	fx
central nervous system	CNS	gastroesophageal reflux disease	GERD
cerebrospinal fluid	CSF	gastrointestinal	GI
cerebrovascular accident	CVA	general practitioner	GP
cervical vertebrae	C1-C7	genitourinary	GU
cesarean section	CS, C-section	gonococcus	GC
chronic obstructive lung disease	COLD	gynecology	Gyn
chronic obstructive pulmonary disease	COPD	hepatitis B virus	HBV
chronic renal failure	CRF	hepatitis C virus	HCV
complete blood count	CBC, cbc	hepatitis D virus	HDV
computed tomography, computerized (computed) axial tomography	CT, CAT	herpes simplex virus	HSV
		herpes simplex virus type 2 (genital herpes)	HSV-2
congestive heart failure	CHF	hormone replacement therapy	HRT
coronary artery bypass graft	CABG	human chorionic gonadotropin	HCG, hCG
coronary artery disease	CAD	human immunodeficiency virus	HIV
costovertebral angle	CVA	human papillomavirus	HPV

in vitro fertilization	IVF	prostate-specific antigen	PSA
inflammatory bowel syndrome	IBS	red blood cell, red blood cell count	RBC
intensive care unit	ICU	rheumatoid arthritis	RA
intramuscular	IM	right atrium	RA
intrauterine device	IUD	right lower quadrant	RLQ
intrauterine system	IUS	right upper quadrant	RUQ
intravenous	IV	severe acute respiratory syndrome	SARS
intravenous pyelogram	IVP	sexually transmitted disease	STD
last menstrual period	LMP	shortness of breath	SOB
left atrium	LA	sudden infant death syndrome	SIDS
left lower quadrant	LLQ	symptoms	Sx
left upper quadrant	LUQ	thoracic vertebrae	T1-T12
lower gastrointestinal tract	LGI	tonsillectomy and adenoidectomy	T&A
lower respiratory tract	LRT	total body surface area	TBSA
lumbar vertebrae	L1-L5	transcutaneous electrical nerve stimulation	TENS
lupus erythematosus	LE	transient ischemic attack	TIA
magnetic resonance imaging	MRI	transurethral microwave thermotherapy	TUMT
myocardial infarction	MI	transurethral needle ablation	TUNA
nonsteroidal antiinflammatory drug	NSAID	transurethral resection	TUR
obstetrics	OB	transurethral resection of the prostate	TURP
over the counter (drug)	OTC	tuberculosis	TB
Papanicolaou smear, stain, or test	Pap	upper respiratory tract	URT
pelvic inflammatory disease	PID	urinalysis	UA, U/A
peripheral nervous system	PNS	urinary tract infection	UTI
physician assistant	PA	ventricular septal defect	VSD
positron emission tomography	PET	vital capacity	VC
"potential" hydrogen, hydrogen ion concentration	pH	weapons of mass destruction	WMD
		white blood cell, white blood cell count	WBC
premenstrual syndrome	PMS	within normal limits	WNL

APPENDIX III
Pharmacology Overview

Erinn Kao, PharmD

Pharmacology is the science that deals with the origin, nature, chemistry, effects, and uses of drugs. A drug may modify one or more of the body's functions. Drugs are used in medicine to prevent, diagnose, or treat a disease or abnormal condition. Another term for drugs is *pharmaceuticals.* Drugs used specifically to treat a condition are also referred to as *therapeutics.* Radioactive drugs that are used for medicinal diagnosis or treatment are called *radiopharmaceuticals.*

Giving a drug to a patient is called *drug administration.* The various ways a drug may be administered are called the *routes of administration.* Although most drugs are administered orally or by injection, some can be administered via the skin (transdermal patches) or mucous membranes (e.g., nasal spray). *Parenteral administration* includes all the routes a drug may be administered except via the digestive tract.

How the drug is utilized in the body after administration is referred to as *pharmacokinetics* and involves the drug's absorption, distribution, metabolism, and elimination. Once administered, a drug may remain at the site of administration, or it may enter the blood. The movement of the drug from the administration site into the blood is called *absorption* of the drug. The transportation of the drug to other body tissues is called the *distribution* of the drug. Many drugs are chemically changed within the body by a process called *metabolism.* Where and how a drug interacts with a site in the body is called the *action* of the drug. If the effect is confined to the site of administration, the drug has a *local* effect. If it acts on many sites away from the administration site, the effect is said to be *systemic.* The drug eventually is removed from the body in a process called *elimination.*

A measured amount of a drug is called a *dose.* The greater the effect with a single dose, the more potent a drug is. A *placebo* is an inactive mimic of another drug, usually given as a control in a clinical drug study.

A *prescription* is an order for a drug made by authorized medical personnel (usually a physician) for a specific patient. An over-the-counter (OTC) drug is available without a prescription and, as with prescription drugs, is approved for safety and efficacy by the U.S. Food and Drug Administration (FDA). Herbal and dietary supplements are also available without a prescription but are not regulated by the FDA and are not classified as "drugs."

Drug abuse is the use of any drug in a way that deviates from its prescribed use. *Drug addiction* is caused by excessive or continued use of habit-forming drugs. Any pharmaceutical with a potential for abuse or addiction is classified as a *controlled substance.*

The *generic name* (e.g., acetaminophen) of a drug is the common name for the drug and is used by every company for identification, whereas the *trade name* or *brand name* (e.g., Tylenol) is the property of only one company and cannot be used by other companies. The first letter of the trade name is capitalized, whereas a generic name's first letter is not capitalized.

Drugs are generally grouped into several *classes* based on their major effects. Actions, reactions, and interactions with other drugs are often shared by drugs of the same class. Pharmacists provide information regarding a medication's possible *side effects,* which are reactions to or the consequences of taking the particular medication. *Adverse drug reactions* are harmful, unexpected reactions to a drug. Pharmacists also provide information about potential interactions with other drugs, supplements, and food.

Chapters 2 Through 5

Major drug classes and their general functions are listed. The information that is provided serves only as an introduction to the various drug classes and is not meant to be a comprehensive list of drugs. Each drug class has a few example drugs listed below the heading. The generic name of the drug is followed by the trade name in parentheses. Some generic drugs may be marketed under multiple trade names, but only one will be noted here. The "General Pharmacology" list of drugs pertains to the whole body rather than to any one particular body system and corresponds to The Basics (Chapters 2 through 5) of *Quick and Easy Medical Terminology*, Sixth Edition.

General Pharmacology

Drug Class	Effects and Uses
Minerals calcium iodine iron magnesium potassium sodium zinc	Essential inorganic substances for proper growth and function
Vitamins	Essential organic substances for proper growth and function

A: Beta-carotene, retinol
B: B_1 (thiamine), B_2 (riboflavin), B_3 (niacin), B_5 (pantothenic acid), B_6 (pyridoxine), B_7 (biotin), B_9 (folic acid), B_{12} (cyanocobalamin)
C: Ascorbic acid
D: D_2 (ergocalciferol), D_3 (cholecalciferol)
E: Alpha-tocopherol
K: K_1 (phylloquinone), K_2 (menaquinone), K_3 (menadione)

Drug Class	Effects and Uses
Analgesics	Relieve pain
Narcotic Analgesics codeine (in many combination products) fentanyl (Duragesic) morphine (MS Contin) oxycodone (OxyContin) propoxyphene (Darvocet) tramadol (Ultram)	Potential for addiction or abuse
Non-Narcotic Analgesics acetaminophen (Tylenol) aspirin (Bayer) ibuprofen (Motrin)	No potential for addiction or abuse
Anesthetics	Reduce physical sensations
Local Anesthetics benzocaine (Orajel) lidocaine (Xylocaine) procaine (Novocain)	Local numbing effect at site of administration
General Anesthetics halothane (Fluothane) nitrous oxide ("laughing gas") propofol (Diprivan)	Loss of all body sensation, and some induce loss of consciousness
Antiinfectives/Antimicrobials	Kill or stop growth of microorganisms
Antibiotics	Target various microorganisms (bacteria, fungi, protozoa, or helminths)
Anthelmintics ivermectin (Stromectol) mebendazole (Vermox)	Destroy or expel parasitic worms
Antibacterials amoxicillin (Amoxil) ampicillin (Principen) azithromycin (Zithromax) ceftazidime (Fortaz) cephalexin (Keflex) ciprofloxacin (Cipro) erythromycin (E-Mycin) sulfamethoxazole/trimethoprim (Septra) tetracycline (Sumycin) vancomycin (Vancocin)	Treat bacterial infections; antibacterials are grouped in many subclasses such as aminoglycosides, cephalosporins, fluoroquinolones, macrolides, penicillins, sulfonamides, and tetracyclines based on the drug's chemical structure, method of action, and type of bacteria it is effective against
Antifungals amphotericin B (Fungizone) fluconazole (Diflucan) ketoconazole (Nizoral) nystatin (Mycostatin)	Treat fungal infections

Drug Class	Effects and Uses
Antiprotozoals atovaquone (Mepron) hydroxychloroquine (Plaquenil) metronidazole (Flagyl)	Treat protozoal infections; antimalarials are antiprotozoals that specifically treat malaria
Antitubercular Agents ethambutol (Myambutol) isoniazid (Nydrazid) pyrazinamide rifampin (Rifadin)	Antibacterials that specifically treat tuberculosis
Antivirals acyclovir (Zovirax) amantadine (Symmetrel) efavirenz (Sustiva) famciclovir (Famvir) oseltamivir (Tamiflu) zidovudine (Retrovir)	Treat viral infections; antiretrovirals specifically treat HIV
Antineoplastic/Cytotoxic/ Chemotherapeutic Agents cisplatin (Platinol) cyclophosphamide (Cytoxan) doxorubicin (Adriamycin) fluorouracil (Adrucil) methotrexate (Trexall) paclitaxel (Taxol) rituximab (Rituxan) tamoxifen (Nolvadex) vincristine (Oncovin)	Treat various cancers. Some are useful in treating other diseases such as arthritis. Subclasses include alkylating agents, anthracyclines, antimetabolites, mitotic inhibitors (plant alkaloids), topoisomerase inhibitors, and monoclonal antibodies. Differentiating agents target cancerous cells to mature them into normal cells.
Antiinflammatory Drugs	Reduce inflammation
Corticosteroids cortisone dexamethasone (Decadron) hydrocortisone (Cortef) methylprednisolone (Medrol) prednisone (Deltasone) triamcinolone (Aristocort)	The chemical structure of each drug determines the degree of glucocorticoid and mineralocorticoid properties exhibited
Nonsteroidal Antiinflammatory Drugs (NSAIDs) aspirin (Bayer) celecoxib (Celebrex) ibuprofen (Motrin) indomethacin (Indocin) ketorolac (Toradol) naproxen (Aleve) oxaprozin (Daypro)	Often used for antiinflammatory effects, but also have mild pain reducing effects

Drug Class	Effects and Uses
Antipyretics acetaminophen (Tylenol) aspirin (Bayer) ibuprofen (Motrin)	Reduce fever; these drugs often have other actions such as pain relief or to reduce inflammation
Antihistamines cetirizine (Zyrtec) diphenhydramine (Benadryl) hydroxyzine (Atarax) loratadine (Claritin)	Block histamine-1 receptors to relieve allergy symptoms
Immunosuppressants azathioprine (Imuran) cyclosporine (Neoral) mycophenolate (CellCept) tacrolimus (Prograf)	Inhibit immune system to treat autoimmune disease or to prevent transplant rejection
Opioid Antagonists naloxone (Narcan) naltrexone (ReVia)	Block opioid receptors to treat dependence or overdose to alcohol or narcotics
Radiopharmaceuticals iodine-131 strontium-89 (Metastron) technetium-99m tetrofosmin (Myoview) thallium-201	Assess various internal functions (diagnostic) or treat certain cancers or tissue hyperfunction (therapeutic)
Vaccines diphtheria, tetanus toxoids, acellular pertussis vaccine (DTaP) hepatitis vaccine (A or B) human papillomavirus quadrivalent vaccine (Gardasil) inactivated poliovirus (IPV) influenza vaccine (Fluzone) measles, mumps, rubella vaccine (MMR) pneumococcal conjugate vaccine (Prevnar)	Induce resistance to a specific disease by providing the body with a modified version of the disease that stimulates the immune system's formation of defenses

 Material for chapters 6 through 14 includes pharmaceutical classes specific to each chapter's body system, and is on the companion CD.

Spanish Pronunciation of Select Terms

English/Inglés	Spanish/Español (pronunciation)	English/Inglés	Spanish/Español (pronunciation)
abdomen	abdomen (**ab-DOH-men**), vientre (**ve-EN-tray**)	breathe	alentar (**ah-len-TAR**), respirar (**res-pe-RAR**)
acidity	acidez (**ah-se-DES**)	breathing	respiración (**res-pe-rah-se-ON**)
acute	agudo (**ah-GOO-do**)	bruise	contusión (**con-too-se-ON**), moretón (**mo-ray-TON**)
adrenaline	adrenalina (**ah-dray-nah-LEE-nah**)	burn	quemadura (**kay-mah-DOO-rah**)
aged	envejecido (**en-vay-hay-SEE-do**)	calcium	calcio (**CAHL-se-o**)
allergy	alergia (**ah-LEHR-he-ah**)	calculus	cálculo (**CAHL-coo-lo**)
anemia	anemia (**ah-NAY-me-ah**)	cancer	cáncer (**CAHN-ser**)
anesthesia	anestesia (**ah-nes-TAY-se-ah**)	capillary	capilar (**cah-pe-LAR**)
anesthetic	anestésico (**ah-nes-TAY-se-co**)	cartilage	cartílago (**car-TEE-lah-go**)
ankle	tobillo (**to-BEEL-lyo**)	catheter	catéter (**cah-TAY-ter**)
antibiotic	antibiótico (**an-te-be-O-te-co**)	cheek	mejilla (**may-HEEL-lyah**)
anxiety	ansiedad (**an-se-ay-DAHD**)	chest	pecho (**PAY-cho**)
appendix	apéndice (**ah-PEN-de-say**)	chew	masticar (**mas-te-CAR**)
appetite	apetito (**ah-pay-TEE-to**)	child	niña (**NEE-nya**), niño (**NEE-nyo**)
arm	brazo (**BRAH-so**)	childbirth	parto (**PAR-to**)
armpit	sobaco (**so-BAH-co**)	cholesterol	colesterol (**co-les-tay-ROL**)
artery	arteria (**ar-TAY-re-ah**)	chronic	crónico (**CRO-ne-co**)
asphyxia	asfixia (**as-FEEC-se-ah**)	circumcision	circuncisión (**ser-coon-se-se-ON**)
asthma	asma (**AHS-mah**)	clot	coágulo (**co-AH-goo-lo**)
augmentation	aumento (**ah-oo-MEN-to**)	collarbone	clavícula (**clah-VEE-coo-lah**)
axilla	sobaco (**so-BAH-co**)	conception	concepción (**con-sep-se-ON**)
back	espalda (**es-PAHL-dah**)	concussion	concusión (**con-coo-se-ON**)
belly	barriga (**bar-REE-gah**)	condom	condón (**con-DON**)
benign	benigno (**bay-NEEG-no**)	conscious	consciente (**cons-se-EN-tay**)
biopsy	biopsia (**be-OP-see-ah**)	consciousness	conciencia (**con-se-EN-se-ah**)
birth	nacimiento (**nah-se-me-EN-to**)	contraception	contracepción (**con-trah-cep-se-ON**)
black	negro (**NAY-gro**)	convulsion	convulsión (**con-vool-se-ON**)
bladder	vejiga (**vay-HEE-gah**)	cough	tos (**tos**)
blood	sangre (**SAHN-gray**)	cranium	cráneo (**CRAH-nay-o**)
blood pressure	presión sanguínea (**pray-se-ON san-GEE-nay-ah**)	cream	crema (**CRAY-mah**)
blood sample	muestra de sangre (**moo-AYS-trah day SAHN-gray**)	cry	llorar (**lyo-RAR**)
		defecate	evacuar (**ay-vah-coo-AR**)
blue	azul (**ah-SOOL**)	dentist	dentista (**den-TEES-tah**)
body	cuerpo (**coo-ERR-po**)	dermatology	dermatología (**der-mah-to-lo-HEE-ah**)
bone	hueso (**oo-AY-so**)	destruction	destrucción (**des-trooc-se-ON**)
brain	cerebro (**say-RAY-bro**)	diabetes	diabetes (**de-ah-BAY-tes**)
breasts	senos (**SAY-nos**)	diagnosis	diagnóstico (**de-ag-NOS-te-co**)

English/Inglés	Spanish/Español (pronunciation)
dialysis	diálisis (de-AH-le-sis)
diaphragm	diafragma (de-ah-FRAHG-mah)
digestion	digestión (de-hes-te-ON)
disease	enfermedad (en-fer-may-DAHD)
dizziness	vértigo (VERR-te-go)
ear	oreja (o-RAY-hah)
edema	hidropesía (e-dro-pay-SEE-ah)
elbow	codo (CO-do)
electricity	electricidad (ay-lec-tre-se-DAHD)
enzyme	enzima (en-SEE-mah)
epilepsy	epilepsia (ay-pe-LEP-se-ah)
erect, straight	derecho (day-RAY-cho)
erection	erección (ay-rec-se-ON)
esophagus	esófago (ay-SO-fah-go)
excretion	excreción (ex-cray-se-ON)
extremity	extremidad (ex-tray-me-DAHD)
eye	ojo (O-ho)
eyeball	globo del ojo (GLO-bo del O-ho)
eyebrow	ceja (SAY-hah)
eyelash	pestaña (pes-TAH-nyah)
eyelid	párpado (PAR-pah-do)
face	cara (CAH-rah)
fainting	languidez (lan-gee-DES), desmayo (des-MAH-yo)
fatigue	fatiga (fah-TEE-gah)
fear	miedo (me-AY-do)
feces	excremento (ex-cray-MEN-to)
feminine	femenina (fay-may-NEE-na)
fetus	feto (FAY-to)
fever	fiebre (fe-AY-bray)
fiber	fibra (FEE-brah)
finger	dedo (DAY-do)
fingerprint	impresión digital (im-pray-se-ON de-he-TAHL)
fire	fuego (foo-AY-go)
fluid	fluido (floo-EE-do)
foam	espuma (es-POO-mah)
foot, feet	pie (pe-AY), pies (pe-AYS)
forearm	antebrazo (an-tay-BRAH-so)
fracture	fractura (frac-TOO-rah)
gallbladder	vesícula biliar (vay-SEE-coo-la be-le-AR)
gallstone	cálculo biliar (CAHL-coo-lo be-le-AR)
giant	gigante (he-GAHN-tay)
gland	glándula (GLAN-doo-lah)
glucose	glucosa (gloo-CO-sah)
gray	gris (grees)
green	verde (VERR-day)
gum, gingiva	encía (en-SEE-ah)
gynecology	ginecología (he-nay-co-lo-HEE-ah)
hair	pelo (PAY-lo)
hand	mano (MAH-no)
head	cabeza (cah-BAY-sah)
headache	dolor de cabeza (do-LOR day cah-BAY-sa)

English/Inglés	Spanish/Español (pronunciation)
heart	corazón (co-rah-SON)
heat	calor (cah-LOR)
heel	talón (tah-LON)
hemorrhage	hemorragia (ay-mor-RAH-he-ah)
hernia	hernia (AYR-ne-ah), quebradura (kay-brah-DOO-rah)
high blood pressure	hipertensión (e-per-ten-se-ON), presión alta (pray-se-ON AHL-tah)
hip	cadera (cah-DAY-rah)
hives	roncha (RON-chah)
hormone	hormona (or-MOH-nah)
hunger	hambre (AHM-bray)
hypodermic	hipodérmico (e-po-DER-me-co)
imperfect	imperfecto (im-per-FEC-to)
impotency	impotencia (im-po-TEN-se-ah)
incision	incisión (in-se-se-ON), corte (COR-tay)
influenza	gripe (GREE-pay)
injection	inyección (in-yec-se-ON)
injury	daño (DAH-nyo)
instrument	instrumento (ins-troo-MEN-to)
insulin	insulina (in-soo-LEE-nah)
intercourse, sexual	cópula (CO-poo-lah)
intestine	intestino (in-tes-TEE-no)
jaw	mandíbula (man-DEE-boo-lah)
joint	articulación (ar-te-coo-lah-se-ON), coyuntura (co-yoon-TOO-rah)
kidney	riñón (ree-NYOHN)
knee	rodilla (ro-DEEL-lyah)
kneecap	rótula (RO-too-lah)
laboratory	laboratorio (lah-bo-rah-TO-re-o)
leg	pierna (pe-ERR-nah)
leukemia	leucemia (lay-oo-SAY-me-ah)
life	vida (VEE-dah)
ligament	ligamento (le-gah-MEN-to)
light	luz (loos)
lips	labios (LAH-be-os)
liver	hígado (EE-ga-do)
lobe	lóbulo (LO-boo-lo)
lung	pulmón (pool-MON)
lymph	linfa (LEEN-fa)
lymphatic	linfático (lin-FAH-te-co)
malignant	maligno (mah-LEEG-no)
masculine	masculino (mas-coo-LEE-no)
membrane	membrana (mem-BRAH-nah)
menopause	menopausia (may-no-PAH-oo-se-ah)
menstruation	menstruación (mens-troo-ah-se-ON)
microscope	microscopio (me-cros-CO-pe-o)
milk	leche (LAY-chay)
mind	mente (MEN-te)
mouth	boca (BO-cah)
movement	movimiento (mo-ve-me-EN-to)
mucus	moco (MO-co)
murmur	murmullo (moor-MOOL-lyo)
muscle	músculo (MOOS-coo-lo)

English/Inglés	Spanish/Español (pronunciation)	English/Inglés	Spanish/Español (pronunciation)
nails	uñas (**OO-nyahs**)	renal calculus	cálculo renal (**CAHL-coo-lo ray-NAHL**)
narcotic	narcótico (**nar-CO-te-co**)	reproduction	reproducción (**ray-pro-dooc-se-ON**)
narrow	estrecho (**es-TRAY-cho**)	respiration	respiración (**res-pe-rah-se-ON**)
navel	ombligo (**om-BLEE-go**)	rhythm	ritmo (**REET-mo**)
neck	cuello (**coo-EL-lyo**)	rhythm method	método de ritmo (**MAY-to-do day REET-mo**)
nerve	nervio (**NERR-ve-o**)	rib	costilla (**cos-TEEL-lyah**)
nervous	nervioso (**ner-ve-O-so**)	rupture	ruptura (**roop-TOO-rah**)
neurology	neurología (**nay-oo-ro-lo-HEE-ah**)	sacrum	hueso sacro (**oo-AY-so SAH-cro**)
newborn	recién nacida (**ray-se-EN nah-SEE-dah**)	saliva	saliva (**sah-LEE-vah**)
nipple	pezón (**pay-SON**)	same	mismo (**MEES-mo**)
nose	nariz (**nah-REES**)	seizure	ataque (**ah-TAH-kay**)
nostril	orificio de la nariz (**or-e-FEE-se-o day lah nah-REES**)	sexual	sexual (**sex-soo-AHL**)
nutrition	nutrición (**noo-tre-se-ON**)	shoulder	hombro (**OM-bro**)
obstruction	obstrucción (**obs-trooc-se-ON**)	shoulder blade	espaldilla (**es-pal-DEEL-lyah**)
optician	óptico (**OP-te-co**)	skeleton	esqueleto (**es-kay-LAY-to**)
orange (color)	anaranjado (**ah-nah-ran-HAH-do**), naranjado (**nah-ran-HAH-do**)	skin	piel (**pe-EL**)
orthodontist	ortodóntico (**or-to-DON-te-co**)	skull	cráneo (**CRAH-nay-o**)
ovarian	ovárico (**o-VAH-re-co**)	sleep	sueño (**soo-AY-nyo**)
ovary	ovario (**o-VAH-re-o**)	sole	planta (**PLAHN-tah**)
oxygen	oxígeno (**ok-SEE-hay-no**)	sound	sonido (**so-NEE-do**)
pain	dolor (**do-LOR**)	spasm	espasmo (**es-PAHS-mo**)
painful	doloroso (**do-lo-RO-so**)	speech (language)	habla (**AH-blah**), lenguaje (**len-goo-AH-hay**)
palm	palma (**PAHL-mah**)	spinal column	columna vertebral (**co-LOOM-nah ver-tay-BRAHL**)
pancreas	páncreas (**PAHN-cray-as**)	spine	espinazo (**es-pe-NAH-so**)
paralysis	parálisis (**pah-RAH-le-sis**)	spiral	espiral (**es-pe-RAHL**)
parturition	parto (**PAR-to**)	spleen	bazo (**BAH-so**)
pathology	pathología (**pah-to-lo-HEE-ah**)	sprain, to	torcer (**tor-SERR**)
penis	pene (**PAY-nay**)	starch	almidón (**al-me-DON**)
perspiration	sudor (**soo-DOR**)	sterile	estéril (**es-TAY-reel**)
phalanges	falanges (**fah-LAHN-hays**)	sternum	esternón (**es-ter-NON**)
phosphorus	fósforo (**FOS-fo-ro**)	stiff	tieso (**te-AY-so**)
physical examination	examen físico (**ek-SAH-men FEE-se-co**)	stomach	estómago (**es-TOH-mah-go**)
pink	rosa (**RO-sah**)	stone	cálculo (**CAHL-coo-lo**)
pituitary	pituitario (**pe-too-e-TAH-re-o**)	surgeon	cirujano(a) (**se-roo-HAH-no (-na)**)
pneumonia	neumonía (**nay-oo-mo-NEE-ah**), pulmonía (**pool-mo-NEE-ah**)	surgery	cirugía (**se-roo-HEE-ah**)
pregnancy	embarazo (**em-bah-RAH-so**)	suture	sutura (**soo-TOO-rah**)
pregnant	embarazada (**em-bah-rah-SAH-dah**)	swallow	tragar (**trah-GAR**)
prolapse	prolapso (**pro-LAHP-so**)	sweat	sudor (**soo-DOR**)
prostate	próstata (**PROS-ta-tah**)	swelling (to swell)	hinchar (**in-CHAR**)
prostatic	prostático (**pros-TAH-te-co**)	symptom	síntoma (**SEEN-to-mah**)
prostatitis	prostatitis (**pros-ta-TEE-tis**)	tears	lágrimas (**LAH-gre-mahs**)
psychiatry	psiquiatría (**se-ke-ah-TREE-ah**)	temperature	temperatura (**tem-pay-rah-TOO-rah**)
psychology	psicología (**se-co-lo-HEE-ah**)	temple	sien (**se-AYN**)
pulse	pulso (**POOL-so**)	tendon	tendón (**ten-DON**)
radiation	radiación (**rah-de-ah-se-ON**)	testicle	testículo (**tes-TEE-coo-lo**)
radiograph	radiografía (**rah-de-o-grah-FEE-ah**)	therapy	terapia (**ter-ah-PEE-ah**)
radiology	radiología (**rah-de-o-lo-HEE-ah**)	thermometer	termómetro (**ter-MO-may-tro**)
rectum	recto (**REK-to**)	thigh	muslo (**MOOS-lo**)
red	rojo (**RO-ho**)	thirst	sed (**sayd**)
reduction	reducción (**ray-dooc-se-ON**)	throat	garganta (**gar-GAHN-tah**)
renal artery	arteria renal (**ar-TAY-re-ah ray-NAHL**)	thumb	pulgar (**pool-GAR**)
		thyroid	tiroides (**te-RO-e-des**)

English/Inglés	Spanish/Español (pronunciation)	English/Inglés	Spanish/Español (pronunciation)
toe	dedo del pie (**DAY-do del PE-ay**)	uterus	útero (**OO-tay-ro**)
tongue	lengua (**LEN-goo-ah**)	vagina	vagina (**vah-HEE-nah**)
tonsil	tonsila (**ton-SEE-lah**), amígdala (**ah-MEEG-dah-lah**)	varicose veins	venas varicosas (**VAY-nahs vah-re-CO-sas**)
tooth, teeth	diente (**de-AYN-tay**), dientes (**de-AYN-tays**)	vein	vena (**VAY-nah**)
trachea	tráquea (**TRAH-kay-ah**)	vertebral column	columna vertebral (**co-LOOM-nah ver-tay-BRAHL**)
trauma	daño (**DAH-nyo**), herida (**ay-REE-dah**)	vessel	vaso (**VAH-so**)
treatment	tratamiento (**trah-tah-me-EN-to**)	vision	visión (**ve-se-ON**)
ulcer	ulcera (**OOL-say-rah**)	voice	voz (**vos**)
urea	urea (**oo-RAY-ah**)	voiding	orinar (**o-re-NAR**)
urinalysis	urinálisis (**oo-re-NAH-le-sis**)	vomiting	vómito (**VO-me-to**)
urinary	urinario (**oo-re-NAH-re-o**)	water	agua (**AH-goo-ah**)
urinary system	sistema urinario (**sis-TAY-mah oo-re-NAH-re-o**)	weakness	debilidad (**day-be-le-DAHD**)
urinate	orinar (**o-re-NAR**)	white	blanco (**BLAHN-co**)
urination	urinación (**oo-re-nah-se-ON**)	wound	lesión (**lay-se-ON**)
urine	orina (**o-REE-nah**)	wrist	muñeca (**moo-NYAY-cah**)
urology	urología (**oo-ro-lo-HEE-ah**)	x-ray (image)	radiografía (**rah-de-o-grah-FEE-ah**)
		yellow	amarillo (**ah-mah-REEL-lyo**)

Translation of Select Spanish Terms

Spanish/Español	English/Inglés	Spanish/Español	English/Inglés
acidez	acidity	capilar	capillary
adrenalina	adrenaline	cara	face
agua	water	cartílago	cartilage
agudo	acute	catéter	catheter
alentar	breathe	ceja	eyebrow
alergia	allergy	cerebro	brain
almidón	starch	circuncisión	circumcision
amarillo	yellow	cirugía	surgery
amígdala	tonsil	cirujano(a)	surgeon
anaranjado	orange (color)	clavícula	collarbone
anemia	anemia	coágulo	clot
anestesia	anesthesia	codo	elbow
anestésico	anesthetic	colesterol	cholesterol
ansiedad	anxiety	columna vertebral	spinal column, vertebral column
antebrazo	forearm	concepción	conception
antibiótico	antibiotic	conciencia	consciousness
apéndice	appendix	concusión	concussion
apetito	appetite	condón	condom
arteria	artery	consciente	conscious
articulación	joint	contracepción	contraception
asfixia	asphyxia	contusión	bruise
asma	asthma	convulsión	convulsion
ataque	seizure	cópula	sexual intercourse
aumento	augmentation	corazón	heart
azul	blue	corte	incision
barriga	belly	costilla	rib
bazo	spleen	coyuntura	joint
benigno	benign	cráneo	cranium, skull
biopsia	biopsy	crema	cream
blanco	white	crónico	chronic
boca	mouth	cuello	neck
brazo	arm	cuerpo	body
cabeza	head	daño	trauma, injury
cadera	hip	debilidad	weakness
calcio	calcium	dedo	finger
cálculo	calculus, stone	dedo del pie	toe
cálculo biliar	gallstone	dentista	dentist
cálculo renal	renal calculus	derecho	erect, straight
calor	heat	dermatología	dermatology
cáncer	cancer	desmayo	fainting

Spanish/Español	English/Inglés	Spanish/Español	English/Inglés
destrucción	destruction	hinchar	swelling, to swell
diafragma	diaphragm	hipertensión	high blood pressure
diagnóstico	diagnosis	hipodérmico	hypodermic
diálisis	dialysis	hombro	shoulder
diente, dientes	tooth, teeth	hormona	hormone
dolor	pain	hueso	bone
dolor de cabeza	headache	hueso sacro	sacrum
doloroso	painful	imperfecto	imperfect
electricidad	electricity	impotencia	impotency
embarazada	pregnant	impresión digital	fingerprint
embarazo	pregnancy	incisión	incision
encía	gum, gingival	instrumento	instrument
envejecido	aged	insulina	insulin
enzima	enzyme	intestino	intestine
epilepsia	epilepsy	inyección	injection
erección	erection	labios	lips
esófago	esophagus	laboratorio	laboratory
espalda	back	lágrimas	tears
espaldilla	shoulder blade	languidez	fainting
espasmo	spasm	leche	milk
espinazo	spine	lengua	tongue
espiral	spiral	lenguaje	speech (language)
espuma	foam	lesión	wound
esqueleto	skeleton	leucemia	leukemia
estéril	sterile	ligamento	ligament
esternón	sternum	linfa	lymph
estómago	stomach	linfático	lymphatic
estrecho	narrow	llorar	to cry
evacuar	defecate	lóbulo	lobe
examen físico	physical examination	luz	light
excreción	excretion	maligno	malignant
excremento	feces	mandíbula	jaw
extremidad	extremity	mano	hand
falanges	phalanges	masculino	masculine
fatiga	fatigue	masticar	to chew
femenina	feminine	mejilla	cheek
feto	fetus	membrana	membrane
fibra	fiber	menopausia	menopause
fiebre	fever	menstruación	menstruation
fluido	fluid	mente	mind
fósforo	phosphorus	método de ritmo	rhythm method
fractura	fracture	microscopio	microscope
fuego	fire	miedo	fear
garganta	throat	mismo	same
gigante	giant	moco	mucus
ginecología	gynecology	movimiento	movement
glándula	gland	muestra de sangre	blood sample
globo del ojo	eyeball	muñeca	wrist
glucosa	glucose	murmullo	murmur
gripe	influenza	músculo	muscle
gris	gray	muslo	thigh
habla	talk, speech	nacimiento	birth
hambre	hunger	naranjado	orange (color)
hemorragia	hemorrhage	narcótico	narcotic
hidropesía	edema	nariz	nose
hígado	liver	negro	black

Spanish/Español	English/Inglés	Spanish/Español	English/Inglés
nervio	nerve	respiración	breathing, respiration
nervioso	nervous	respirar	breathe
neumonía	pneumonia	riñón	kidney
neurología	neurology	ritmo	rhythm
niño, niña	child	rodilla	knee
nutrición	nutrition	rojo	red
obstrucción	obstruction	roncha	hives
ojo	eye	rosa	pink
ombligo	navel	rótula	kneecap
óptico	optician	ruptura	rupture
oreja	ear	sangre	blood
orificio de la nariz	nostril	sed	thirst
orina	urine	senos	breasts
orinar	urinate	sien	temple
ortodóntico	orthodontist	síntoma	symptom
ovárico	ovarian	sistema urinario	urinary system
ovario	ovary	sobaco	armpit, axilla
oxígeno	oxygen	sonido	sound
palma	palm	sudor	sweat, perspiration
páncreas	pancreas	sueño	sleep
parálisis	paralysis	sutura	suture
párpado	eyelid	talón	heel
parto	childbirth, parturition	temperatura	temperature
patología	pathology	tendón	tendon
pecho	chest	terapia	therapy
pelo	hair	termómetro	thermometer
pene	penis	testículo	testicle
pestaña	eyelash	tieso	stiff
pezón	nipple	tiroides	thyroid
pie, pies	foot, feet	tobillo	ankle
piel	skin	tonsila	tonsil
pierna	leg	torcer	to sprain
pituitario	pituitary	tos	cough
planta	sole	tragar	swallow
presión alta	high blood pressure	tráquea	trachea
presión sanguínea	blood pressure	tratamiento	treatment
prolapso	prolapse	ulcera	ulcer
próstata	prostate	uñas	nails
prostático	prostatic	urinación	urination
prostatitis	prostatitis	urinálisis	urinalysis
psicología	psychology	urinario	urinary
psiquiatría	psychiatry	urología	urology
pulgar	thumb	útero	uterus
pulmón	lung	vaso	vessel
pulmonía	pneumonia	vejiga	bladder
pulso	pulse	vena	vein
quebradura	hernia	venas varicosas	varicose veins
quemadura	burn	verde	green
radiación	radiation	vértigo	dizziness
radiografía	radiograph, x-ray (image)	vesícula biliar	gallbladder
radiología	radiology	vida	life
recién nacida	newborn	vientre	abdomen
recto	rectum	visión	vision
reducción	reduction	vómito	vomiting
reproducción	reproduction	voz	voice

Word Parts and Their Meanings

Word Part	Meaning	Word Part	Meaning
a-	no, not, without	axill/o	axilla (armpit)
ab-	away from	bacter/i, bacteri/o	bacteria
abdomin/o	abdomen	bi-	two
-able, -ible	capable of, able to	bil/i	bile
-ac, -al, -an, -ar, -ary	pertaining to	bi/o	life or living
acr/o	extremities (arms and legs)	blast/o	embryonic form
ad-	toward	blephar/o	eyelid
aden/o	gland	brady-	slow
adenoid/o	adenoids	bronch/o, bronchi/o	bronchi
adip/o	fat	bronchiol/o	bronchiole
adren/o	adrenal glands	burs/o	bursa
aer/o	air	calcane/o	calcaneus (heel bone)
agora-	open marketplace	calc/i	calcium
alb/o, albin/o	white	cancer/o, carcin/o	cancer
albumin/o	albumin	cardi/o	heart
algesi/o	sensitivity to pain	carp/o	carpus (wrist)
-algia	pain	caud/o	tail, in a posterior direction
alveol/o	alveolus	cec/o	cecum
amni/o	amnion	-cele	hernia
amyl/o	starch	cellul/o	little cell or compartment
an-	no, not, without	-centesis	surgical puncture
an/o	anus	centi-	one hundred or one-hundredth
andr/o	male, masculine	cephal/o	head, toward the head
angi/o, vascul/o	vessel	cerebell/o	cerebellum
ankyl/o	stiff	cerebr/o	brain, cerebrum
ante-	before	cervic/o	neck, uterine cervix
anter/o	anterior, toward the front	cheil/o	lips
anti-	against	chem/o	chemical
aort/o	aorta	chir/o	hand
append/o, appendic/o	appendix	chlor/o	green
arter/o, arteri/o	artery	chol/e	bile
arteriol/o	articulation, joint	cholecyst/o	gallbladder
arthr/o	joint	choledoch/o	common bile duct
-ase	enzyme	chondr/o	cartilage
-asthenia	weakness	-cidal	killing
atel/o	imperfect	circum-	around
ather/o	yellow fatty plaque	cirrh/o	orange-yellow
-ation	action or process	clavicul/o	clavicle (collarbone)
audi/o	hearing	coccyg/o	coccyx
aut/o	self	col/o, colon/o	colon or large intestine

Word Part	Meaning	Word Part	Meaning
colp/o	vagina	eu-	normal, good
coni/o	dust	-eum, -ium	membrane
contra-	against	ex-, exo-	out, without, away from
corpor/o	body	extra-	outside
cost/o	rib	faci/o	face
crani/o	cranium, skull	femor/o	femur (thigh bone)
crin/o, -crine	secrete	fet/o	fetus
cry/o	cold	fibr/o	fiber
crypt/o	hidden	fibul/o	fibula
cutane/o	skin	fluor/o	emitting or reflecting light
cyan/o	blue	follicul/o	follicle
cyst/o	cyst, bladder, sac	gastr/o	stomach
cyt/o, -cyte	cell	gen/o, -gen	beginning, origin
dacry/o	tear, tearing, crying	-genesis	producing, forming
dactyl/o	digit (toe, finger, or both)	-genic	produced by or in
de-	down, from, removing, reversing	genit/o	genitals
		ger/a, ger/o, geront/o	aged, elderly
dendr/o	tree	gigant/o	giant
dent/i, dent/o	teeth	gingiv/o	gums
derm/a, dermat/o, derm/o, -derm	skin	gli/o	neuroglia or sticky substance
		glomerul/o	glomerulus
di-	two	gloss/o	tongue
dia-	through	glyc/o, glycos/o	sugar
diplo-	double	gon/o	genitals, reproduction
dips/o	thirst	gonad/o	gonad
dist/o	far or distant from the origin or point of attachment	gram/o	to record
		-gram	a record
dors/o	directed toward or situated on the back side	-graph	recording instrument
		-graphy	process of recording
duoden/o	duodenum	gynec/o	female
dur/o	dura mater	hem/a, hem/o, hemat/o	blood
-dynia	pain	hemi-	half, partly
dys-	"bad," difficult	hepat/o	liver
-eal	pertaining to	herni/o	hernia
ech/o	sound	hidr/o	perspiration
-ectasia, -ectasis	dilation, stretching	hist/o	tissue
ecto-	out, without, away from	home/o	sameness
-ectomy	excision	humer/o	humerus
-edema	swelling	hydr/o	water
electr/o	electricity	hyper-	excessive, more than normal
embol/o	embolus	hypo-	beneath or below normal
-emesis	vomiting	hypophys/o	pituitary (hypophysis)
-emia	blood	hyster/o	uterus
en-	inside	-ia, -iasis	condition
encephal/o	brain	-iac	one who suffers
end-, endo-	inside	-iatrician	practitioner
enter/o	intestines, small intestine	-iatrics, -iatric, -iatry	medicine
epi-	above or upon (on)	-ic	pertaining to
epiglott/o	epiglottis	ichthy/o	fish
-er	one who	ile/o	ileum
erythemat/o	erythema or redness	ili/o	ilium
erythr/o	red	immun/o	immune
-esis	action, process, or result of	in-	not, inside, in
esophag/o	esophagus	infer/o	lowermost, below
-esthesia	sensation, perception	infra-	below
esthesi/o	feeling	insulin/o	insulin

Word Part	Meaning	Word Part	Meaning
inter-	between	-meter	instrument used to measure
intestin/o	intestines	metr/i	uterine tissue
intra-	within	metr/o	measure, uterine tissue
iod/o	iodine	-metry	process of measuring
ischi/o	ischium	micro-	small
-ism	condition, theory	mid-	middle
-ist	one who	milli-	one thousand or one-thousandth
-itis	inflammation		
-ium	membrane	mono-	one or single
-ive	pertaining to	muc/o	mucus
jejun/o	jejunum	multi-	many
kerat/o	hard or horny tissue, cornea	muscul/o	muscle
kinesi/o, -kinesia, -kinesis	movement, motion	my/o	muscle
lacrim/o	tear, tearing, crying	myc/o	fungus
lact/o	milk	myel/o	bone marrow, spinal cord
lapar/o	abdominal wall	myx/o	mucus
laryng/o	larynx	narc/o	stupor
later/o	toward the side, farther from the midline of the body or a structure	nas/o	nose
		nat/i, nat/o	birth
		ne/o	new
leps/o, -lepsy	seizure	necr/o	dead, death
leuc/o, leuk/o	white	nephr/o	kidney
-lexia	words, phrases	nerv/o, neur/o	nerve
lingu/o	tongue	nulli-	none
lip/o	fat, lipid	obstetr/o	midwife
lith/o, -lith	stone, calculus	ocul/o	vision
lob/o	lobe	odont/o	teeth
log/o	knowledge, words	-oid	resembling
-logic, -logical	pertaining to the science or study of	-ole	little
		olig/o	few
-logist	one who studies, specialist	-oma	tumor (occasionally, swelling)
-logy	study or science of	omphal/o	umbilicus (navel)
lumb/o	lower back	-on	body
lymph/o	lymph, lymphatics	onc/o	tumor
lymphat/o	lymphatics	onych/o	nail
lys/o	destruction, dissolving	oophor/o	ovary
-lysin	that which destroys	ophthalm/o	eye
-lysis	dissolving, destruction, freeing	-opia	vision
-lytic	capable of destroying	optic/o, opt/o	vision
macro-	large	or/o	mouth
mal-	"bad," poor, abnormal	orchi/o, orchid/o	testes
malac/o	soft, softening	-orexia	appetite
-malacia	softening	orth/o	straight
mamm/o, mast/o	breast	-ose	sugar
-mania	excessive preoccupation	-osis	condition
medio-	middle or nearer the middle	oste/o	bone
megal/o, mega-	enlargement	ot/o	ear
-megaly	large, enlarged	-ous	pertaining to, characterized by
melan/o	black	ovar/o	ovary
men/o	month	ox/o	oxygen
mening/o	meninges	pan-	all
ment/o	mind, chin	pancreat/o	pancreas
meso-	middle	par/o	to bear offspring
meta-	change or next in a series	para-	near, beside, abnormal
metacarp/o	metacarpals	-para	female who has given birth
metatars/o	metatarsals	parathyroid/o	parathyroids

Word Part	Meaning	Word Part	Meaning
patell/o	patella (kneecap)	py/o	pus
path/o	disease	pyel/o	renal pelvis
-pathy	disease	pyr/o	fire
ped/o	child, foot	quad-, quadri-	four
pelv/i	pelvis	rach/i, rachi/o	spine
pen/o	penis (occasionally, punishment)	radi/o	radius, radiant energy
		rect/o	rectum
-penia	deficiency	ren/o	kidney
-pepsia	digestion	retin/o	retina
per-	through, by	retro-	behind, backward
peri-	around	rheumat/o	rheumatism
periton/o	peritoneum	rhin/o	nose
-pexy	surgical fixation	roentgen/o	x-ray
phag/o, -phagia, -phagic, -phagy	eating, swallowing, ingesting	-rrhage	excessive bleeding
		-rrhagia	hemorrhage
phalang/o	phalanges (bones of fingers or toes)	-rrhaphy	suture
		-rrhea	flow, discharge
pharmac/o, pharmaceut/i	drugs, medicine	-rrhexis	rupture
pharyng/o	pharynx	sacr/o	sacrum
phas/o, -phasia	speech	salping/o	uterine tube
phleb/o	vein	-sarcoma	malignant tumor arising from connective tissue
-phobia	abnormal fear		
phon/o	voice	scapul/o	scapula (shoulder blade)
phot/o	light	schis/o, schiz/o, schist/o, -schisis	split, cleft
phren/o	mind, diaphragm		
physi/o	nature	scler/o, -sclerosis	hard, hardening
-physis	growth	scop/o	to examine, to view
pil/o	hair	-scope	instrument used for viewing
pituitar/o	pituitary	-scopy	process of visually examining
-plasia	development	scrot/o	scrotum
plast/o	repair	seb/o	sebum
-plasty	surgical repair	semi-	half, partly
pleg/o, -plegia	paralysis	semin/o	semen
pleur/o	pleura	seps/o	infection
-poiesis	production	sept/o	infection or septum
-poietin	substance that causes production	ser/o	serum
		sial/o	saliva, salivary gland
poly-	many	sigmoid/o	sigmoid colon
post-	after, behind	silic/o	silica
poster/o	posterior, toward the back, situated behind	som/a, somat/o	body
		son/o	sound
-pnea	breathing	-spasm	twitching, cramp
pneum/o	lung, air	spermat/o	sperm
pneumon/o	lung	spin/o	spine
pre-	before	spir/o	spiral, to breathe
primi-	first	splen/o	spleen
pro-	before	spondyl/o	vertebra
proct/o	anus, rectum	-stasis	stopping, controlling
prostat/o	prostate	-static	keeping stationary
prote/o, protein/o	protein	stern/o	sternum (breastbone)
proxim/o	nearer the origin or point of attachment	stomat/o	mouth
		-stomy	formation of an opening
psych/o	mind	sub-	under
-ptosis	sagging, prolapse	super-	excessive or above
pub/o	pubis	supra-	above, beyond
pulm/o, pulmon/o	lung	super/o	uppermost, above

Word Part	Meaning	Word Part	Meaning
sym-, syn-	joined, together	-tropin	that which stimulates
tachy-	fast	uln/o	ulna
tars/o	tarsals (ankle bones)	ultra-	beyond, excess
ten/o, tend/o, tendin/o	tendon	ungu/o	nail
test/o, testicul/o	testicle, testis	uni-	one, single
tetra-	four	ur/o	urine, urinary tract
therapeut/o, -therapy	treatment	ureter/o	ureter
therm/o	heat	urethr/o	urethra
thorac/o	thorax, chest	-uria	urine, urination
thromb/o	thrombus, clot	urin/o	urine or urination
thyr/o, thyroid/o	thyroid gland	uter/o	uterus
tibi/o	tibia	vag/o	vagus nerve
-tic	pertaining to	vagin/o	vagina
tom/o	to cut	vas/o	vessel, ductus deferens
-tome	instrument used for cutting	vascul/o	vessel
-tomy	incision	ven/o	vein
tonsill/o	tonsil	ventr/o	ventral or belly side
top/o	place, position	venul/o	venule
tox/o, toxic/o	poison	vertebr/o	vertebra
trache/o	trachea (windpipe)	vesic/o	bladder or vesicle
trans-	across, through	viscer/o	viscera
tri-	three	vulv/o	vulva
trich/o	hair	xanth/o	yellow
-tripsy	surgical crushing	xer/o	dry
troph/o, -trophic, -trophy	nutrition	-y	state, condition
-tropic	stimulate		

English Terms and Corresponding Word Parts

English Term(s)	Word Parts
abdomen	abdomin/o
abdominal wall	lapar/o
abnormal	para-
above	epi-, super-, supra-
across	trans-
action	-ation, -esis
adenoids	adenoid/o
adrenal glands	adren/o
after	post-
against	anti-, contra-
aged	ger/a, ger/o, geront/o
air	aer/o, pneum/o
air sac	alveol/o
all	pan-
alveolus	alveol/o
amnion	amni/o
ankle bone	tars/o
anus	an/o
anus and rectum	proct/o
aorta	aort/o
appendix	append/o, appendic/o
armpit	axill/o
arms and legs	acr/o
around	circum-, peri-
arteriole	arteriol/o
artery	arter/o, arteri/o
articulation	arthr/o
away from	ab-, ex-
back	dors/o
backward	retr/o
bacteria	bacter/i, bacteri/o
"bad" (difficult, poor)	dys-, mal-
before	ante-, pre-, pro-
beginning	gen/o, -gen, -genic, -genesis, -genous
behind	poster/o, post-, retro-
belly side	ventr/o
below or beneath	hypo-, sub-, infra-
below normal	hypo-
beside	par-, para-

English Term(s)	Word Parts
between	inter-
beyond	supra-
bile	bil/i, chol/e
birth	nat/i, nat/o
birth (give birth)	par/o
woman who has given birth	-para
black	melan/o
bladder	cyst/o
blood	hem/a, hem/o, hemat/o, -emia
blue	cyan/o
body	corpor/o, som/a, somat/o
bone	oste/o
bone marrow	myel/o
brain	cerebr/o, encephal/o
breast	mamm/o, mast/o
breastbone	stern/o
breathing	-pnea
bronchi	bronch/o, bronchi/o
bronchiole	bronchiol/o
bursa	burs/o
calcaneus	calcane/o
calcium	calc/i
calculus	lith/o, -lith
cancer	cancer/o, carcin/o
carpus	carp/o
cartilage	chondr/o
cecum	cec/o
cell	cyt/o, -cyte
compartment or little cell	cellul/o
cerebellum	cerebell/o
cerebrum	cerebr/o
cervix uteri	cervic/o
chemical	chem/o
chest	thorac/o
child	ped/o
chin	ment/o
clavicle	clavicul/o
clot (thrombus)	thromb/o

English Term(s)	Word Parts
coccyx	coccyg/o
cold	cry/o
collarbone	clavicul/o
colon	col/o, colon/o
color	chrom/o
common bile duct	choledoch/o
condition	-ia, iasis, -osis, -y
constant	home/o
controlling	-stasis
cornea	kerat/o
cramp	-spasm
cranium	crani/o
cut (to cut)	tom/o
incision or cutting	-tomy
instrument used to cut	-tome
cyst	cyst/o
death	necr/o
decreased or deficient	-penia
destruction	lys/o
that which destroys	-lysin
process of destroying	-lysis
capable of destroying	-lytic
development	-plasia
diaphragm	phren/o
difficult	dys-
digestion	-pepsia
digit	dactyl/o
dilation	-ectasia, -ectasis
discharge	-rrhea
disease	path/o, -osis, -pathy
dissolving	lys/o
distant	dist/o
double	diplo-
down	de-
drooping	-ptosis
drugs	pharmac/o, pharmaceut/i
dry	xer/o
duct	vas/o
ductus deferens	vas/o
duodenum	duoden/o
dura mater	dur/o
dust	coni/o
ear	ot/o
eat	phag/o
elderly	ger/a, ger/o, geront/o
electricity	electr/o
embolus	embol/o
embryonic form	-blast, blast/o
emitting or reflecting light	fluor/o
enzyme	-ase
epiglottis	epiglott/o
esophagus	esophag/o

English Term(s)	Word Parts
examine	scop/o
instrument used	-scope
process of examining	-scopy
excessive	hyper-, super-
excision	-ectomy
extremities	acr/o
eye	ophthalm/o
eyelid	blephar/o
face	faci/o
far	dist/o
fast	tachy-
fat	adip/o, lip/o
fear (abnormal)	-phobia
feeling	esthesi/o
female	gynec/o
femur	femor/o
fetus	fet/o
few	olig/o
fiber, fibrous	fibr/o
fibula	fibul/o
fingers or toes	dactyl/o
fire	pyr/o
first	primi-
fish	ichthy/o
flow	-rrhea
follicle	follicul/o
for	pro-
formation of an opening	-stomy
four	quadri-, tetra-
from	de-
front	anter/o
fungus	myc/o
gall	chol/e
gallbladder	cholecyst/o
giant	gigant/o
gland	aden/o
glomerulus	glomerul/o
gonad	gonad/o
good	eu-
green	chlor/o
growth	-physis
gums	gingiv/o
hair	pil/o, trich/o
half	hemi-, semi
hand	chir/o
hard, hardening	scler/o, kerat/o
head	cephal/o
hearing	audi/o
heart	cardi/o
heat	therm/o
hemorrhage	-rrhagia
hernia	-cele, herni/o
hidden	crypt/o
horny tissue	kerat/o
humerus	humer/o

English Term(s)	Word Parts	English Term(s)	Word Parts
ileum	ile/o	nail	onych/o, ungu/o
ilium	ili/o	narrowing	-stenosis
immune	immun/o	nature	physi/o
incision	tom/o, -tomy	near	par-, para-, proxim/o
instrument used	-tome	neck	cervic/o
increase	-osis	nerve	nerv/o, neur/o
infection	seps/o, sept/o	neuroglia	gli/o
inferior	infer/o	new	ne/o
inflammation	-itis	new opening	-stomy
ingest	phag/o, -phagia, -phagic, -phagy	no	a-, an-
inside	in-, en-, end-, endo-	none	nulli-
insulin	insulin/o	normal	norm/o, eu-
intestine	enter/o, intestin/o	nose	nas/o, rhin/o
iodine	iod/o	not	a-, an-, in-
ischium	ischi/o	nutrition	troph/o, -trophy
jejunum	jejun/o	obsessive	-mania
joined or together	sym-, syn-	preoccupation	
joint	arthr/o	old, elderly	ger/o, geront/o
keeping stationary	-static	one	uni-, mono-
kidney	nephr/o, ren/o	one hundred,	centi-
killing	-cidal	one-hundredth	
kneecap	patell/o	one-thousandth	milli-
large	gigant/o, macro-, megalo-,	one who	-er, -ist
	-megaly	one who studies	-logist
large intestine	col/o	orange-yellow	cirrh/o
larynx	laryng/o	organs of reproduction	genit/o, gon/o
life or living	bi/o	origin	gen/o, -gen, -genic, -genesis
light	phot/o	out	ex-, exo-
lip	cheil/o	outside	ecto-, exo-, extra-
liver	hepat/o	ovary	oophor/o
location	top/o	oxygen	ox/o
lower back	lumb/o	pain	-algia, -dynia
lung	pneum/o, pneumon/o, pulm/o,	painful	dys-
	pulmon/o	pancreas	pancreat/o
lymph	lymph/o	paralysis	pleg/o, -plegia
lymphatics	lymph/o, lymphat/o	parathyroids	parathyroid/o
male, masculine	andr/o	patella (kneecap)	patell/o
malignant tumor	-sarcoma	pelvis	pelv/i
many	multi-, poly-	perception	-esthesi/o, -esthesia
marketplace	agora-	peritoneum	periton/o
measure	metr/o	perspiration	hidr/o
instrument used	-meter	pertaining to	-ac, -al, -eal, -ic, -ous
process	-metry	pertaining to the	-logic, -logical
medicine	-iatrics, -iatric, -iatry, pharmac/o	science or study of	
membrane	-eum, -ium	phalanges	phalang/o
meninges	mening/o	pharynx	pharyng/o
middle	medi/o, meso-, mid-	phrases	-lexia
midwife	obstetr/o	pituitary	pituitar/o, hypophys/o
milk	lact/o	place (position)	top/o
mind	ment/o, phren/o, psych/o	pleura	pleur/o
month	men/o	poison	tox/o, toxic/o
more than normal	hyper-	practitioner	-iatrician
mouth	or/o, stomat/o	preoccupation	-mania
movement	kinesi/o	(excessive)	
mucus	muc/o, myx/o	process	-ation, -esis
muscle	muscul/o, my/o	production	-poiesis

English Term(s)	Word Parts	English Term(s)	Word Parts
prolapse	-ptosis	sperm, spermatozoa	spermat/o
prostate gland	prostat/o	spinal cord	myel/o
protein	prote/o, protein/o	spine	rach/i, rachi/o, spin/o, spondyl/o
pubis	pub/o	spleen	splen/o
pus	py/o	split	schis/o, schiz/o, -schisis, schist/o
radiant energy	radi/o	starch	amyl/o
radius	radi/o	sternum (breastbone)	stern/o
record (to record)	gram/o	sticky substance	gli/o
process of recording	-graphy	stimulate	-tropic
the record	-gram	stomach	gastr/o
recording instrument	-graph	stone	lith/o, -lith
rectum	rect/o	stopping	-stasis
red	erythr/o	straight	orth/o
redness	erythemat/o	stretching	-ectasia, -ectasis
removal	-ectomy	study or science of	-logy
renal pelvis	pyel/o	stupor	narc/o
repair	plast/o	substance that causes	-poietin
reproduction	gon/o	production	
resembling	-oid	sugar	glyc/o, glycos/o, -ose
result of	-esis	surgical crushing	-tripsy
retina	retin/o	surgical fixation	pex/o, -pexy
reversing	de-	surgical puncture	-centesis
rheumatism	rheumat/o	surgical repair	-plasty
ribs	cost/o	suture	-rrhaphy
rupture	-rrhexis	sweat	hidr/o
sac	cyst/o	swelling	-edema
sacrum	sacr/o	tail	caud/o
sag	-ptosis	tailbone	coccyg/o
saliva, salivary glands	sial/o	tarsals (ankle bones)	tars/o
sameness	home/o	tear (crying)	dacry/o, lacrim/o
scapula (shoulder	scapul/o	teeth	dent/i, dent/o, odont/o
blade)		tendon	ten/o, tend/o
sebum	seb/o	testis, testicle	orchi/o, orchid/o, test/o, testicul/o
secrete	crin/o, -crine	that which stimulates	-tropin
seizure	-lepsy	thirst	dips/o
self	aut/o	thorax	thorac/o
semen	semin/o	three	tri-
sensation	esthesi/o, -esthesia	throat	pharyng/o
sensitivity to pain	algesi/o	thrombus	thromb/o
septum	sept/o	through	dia-, trans-
shoulder blade	scapul/o	thyroid gland	thyr/o, thyroid/o
side	later/o	tibia	tibi/o
sigmoid colon	sigmoid/o	tissue	hist/o
single	mono-	to cut	tom/o
situated above	super/o, super-, supra-	tongue	gloss/o, lingu/o
situated below	infer/o, infra-	tonsil	tonsill/o
skin	cutane/o, derm/a, dermat/o,	toward	ad-
	derm/o, -derm	trachea	trache/o
skull	crani/o	treatment	therapeut/o, -therapy
slow	brady-	tree	dendr/o
small	micro-, -ole	tumor	onc/o, -oma
small intestine	enter/o	twice	di-
soft, softening	malac/o, -malacia	twitching	-spasm
sound	ech/o, son/o	two	bi-, di-
specialist	-ist	ulna	uln/o
speech	phas/o	umbilicus	omphal/o

English Term(s)	Word Parts	English Term(s)	Word Parts
under	sub-	vessel	angi/o, vas/o, vascul/o
upon (on)	epi-	viscera	viscer/o
uppermost	super/o	vision	opt/o, optic/o, -opia, ocul/o
ureter	ureter/o	voice	phon/o
urethra	urethr/o	vomiting	-emesis
urinary tract	ur/o	vulva	vulv/o
urination	urin/o	water	hydr/o
urine	ur/o, urin/o	weakness	-asthenia
uterine tissue	metr/o	white	alb/o, albin/o, leuk/o
uterine tube	salping/o	windpipe	trache/o
uterus	hyster/o, uter/o	within	intra-
vagina	colp/o, vagin/o	without	a-, an-, ex-
vagus nerve	vag/o	words	-lexia
vein	phleb/o, ven/o	wrist bone	carp/o
ventral	ventr/o	x-ray	roentgen/o
venule	venul/o	yellow	xanth/o
vertebra	spondyl/o, vertebr/o	yellow fatty plaque	ather/o

APPENDIX VIII
Answers to Exercises

PART ONE

Chapter 1
Exercises

1.
1. CF
2. CF
3. CF
4. WR
5. CF
6. WR

2.
1. A
2. C
3. C
4. A
5. B
6. C
7. B
8. A
9. B
10. C

3.
1. dyspnea
2. enteric
3. eupepsia
4. tonsillitis
5. uremia
6. antianxiety
7. leukocyte
8. appendicitis
9. hyperemia
10. endocardial

4.
1. A
2. A
3. B
4. A
5. B

5.
1. atria
2. bacilli
3. diagnoses
4. larynges
5. varices

6.
1. three
2. ek
3. kos
4. sen
5. net

Self-Test

A.
1. C
2. C
3. B
4. C
5. B
6. A
7. A
8. B
9. B
10. C

B.
1. C
2. B
3. A
4. B
5. A

C.
1. hypodermic
2. leukemia
3. melanoid
4. myocardial
5. thrombosis

D.
1. appendixes or appendices
2. bronchi
3. ilea
4. pharynges
5. prognoses

Chapter 2
Exercises

1.
1. E
2. B
3. D
4. A
5. E
6. B
7. C
8. F

2.
1. cardi/o; heart
2. dermat/o; skin
3. gynec/o; female
4. immun/o; immune
5. neur/o; nerve
6. onc/o; tumor
7. ophthalm/o; eye
8. path/o; disease
9. psych/o; mind
10. radi/o; radiation
11. rhin/o; nose
12. ur/o; urinary tract

3.
1. to secrete
2. intestines or small intestine
3. feeling or sensation
4. stomach
5. elderly
6. larynx
7. birth
8. new
9. midwife
10. straight
11. ear
12. child or foot

4.
1. cardiac
2. gynecologic
3. obstetrics
4. neonatology
5. ophthalmic
6. otolaryngology
7. rheumatologist
8. endocrine
9. oncologist
10. gastroenterologist

5.
1. D
2. I
3. H
4. E
5. G
6. F
7. J
8. C
9. B
10. A

6.
1. cardiology
2. radiology
3. immunology
4. endocrinology
5. rhinology
6. obstetrics
7. gastroenterology
8. urology
9. orthopedics
10. rheumatology

7.
1. J
2. G
3. B
4. I
5. K
6. C

391

7. L
8. D
9. A
10. E
11. F
12. H

8.
1. angi/o
2. oste/o
3. encephal/o
4. mast/o
5. derm/a

9.
1. col/o, colon; -pexy, surgical fixation
2. aden/o, gland; -ectomy, excision
3. col/o, large intestine; -stomy, formation of an opening
4. col/o, large intestine; -scopy, visual examination
5. mast/o, breast; -ectomy, excision
6. mast/o, breast; -itis, inflammation
7. mast/o, breast; -pexy, surgical fixation
8. neur/o, nerve; -ectomy, excision
9. neur/o, nerve; -lysis, loosening, freeing, or destroying
10. neur/o, nerve; -plasty, surgical repair

10.
1. angioplasty
2. mammoplasty
3. otoplasty
4. ophthalmoplasty
5. dermatoplasty

11.
1. appendectomy
2. encephalotome
3. ophthalmoscope
4. otic
5. tonsillectomy
6. colopexy

7. angiorrhaphy
8. otoscopy

12.
1. E
2. J
3. C
4. I
5. H
6. B
7. F
8. A
9. G
10. D

13.
1. deficiency
2. rupture
3. resembling
4. abnormal fear
5. prolapse
6. -oma
7. -pathy
8. -rrhea
9. spasm
10. -rrhage

14.
1. phlebitis
2. appendicitis
3. otitis
4. ophthalmitis
5. dermatitis

15.
1. chirospasm
2. angiectasis
3. pyromania
4. ophthalmorrhagia
5. encephalocele
6. gastrocele
7. dermatosis
8. neuralgia
9. ophthalmalgia
10. blepharoptosis
11. cardiorrhexis
12. hematemesis

16.
1. capable of, able to
2. pertaining to
3. sugar
4. enzyme
5. specialist; one who studies
6. pertaining to
7. membrane
8. condition or theory

9. one who
10. pertaining to

17.
1. lipids
2. stone
3. encephalitis
4. starch
5. hematemesis
6. small
7. lith/o

Self-Test

A.
1. amyl/o (starch) + -lysis (destruction)
2. appendic/o (appendix) + -itis (inflammation)
3. blephar/o (eyelid) + -ptosis (drooping)
4. dermat/o (skin) + -logist (specialist)
5. lip/o (lipid) + -ase (enzyme)
6. muc/o (mucus) + -oid (resembling)
7. neur/o (nerve) + -plasty (repair)
8. ophthalm/o (eye) + -rrhagia (hemorrhage)
9. ot/o (ear) + -ic (pertaining to)
10. tonsill/o (tonsil) + -ectomy (excision)

B.
1. gland
2. skin
3. study of
4. hand
5. surgical fixation
6. sugar
7. breast
8. nerve
9. eye
10. abnormal softening

C.
1. ophthalmic
2. cardiologists
3. spasm
4. malignant
5. triage
6. encephalitis
7. suture

8. excision
9. neoplasm
10. myelopathy

D.
1. B
2. K
3. F
4. J
5. E
6. H
7. L
8. D
9. C
10. A
11. G
12. I

E.
1. b
2. b
3. c
4. d
5. b
6. c
7. a
8. b
9. a
10. a
11. a
12. b
13. d
14. c
15. a
16. d
17. b
18. a

F.
1. amylase
2. ophthalmoscopy
3. tracheotomy
4. appendicitis
5. otitis
6. neural
7. tonsillectomy
8. dermatologist
9. lithotripsy
10. mastectomy

G.
1. (correct)
2. chirospasm
3. incision
4. (correct)
5. (correct)

Chapter 3
Exercises

1.
1. B
2. B
3. E
4. F
5. A
6. D
7. C
8. A

2.
1. di-, two
2. hyper-, excessive, more than normal
3. hemi-, half
4. hypo-, beneath
5. pan-, all
6. poly-, many
7. primi-, first
8. quadri-, four
9. semi-, partly
10. super-, excessive
11. tetra-, four
12. ultra-, excessive

3.
1. away from, toward
2. behind
3. inside, out
4. between, within
5. above

4.
1. circum-, around
2. dia-, through
3. exo-, out
4. endo-, inside
5. epi-, on
6. hypo-, beneath (below)
7. meso-, middle
8. peri-, around
9. per-, through
10. pre-, in front of (before)
11. retro-, back or backward
12. sub-, beneath or below
13. super-, beyond
14. syn-, together
15. trans-, across (through)

5.
1. B
2. E
3. F
4. D
5. C
6. B
7. C
8. D
9. A
10. C

6.
1. brady-, slow
2. tachy-, fast
3. hypo-, less than normal
4. hyper-, more than normal
5. in-, not
6. mal-, bad (poor)
7. anti-, against
8. in-, not
9. dys-, difficult
10. contra-, against
11. anti-, against
12. para-, near
13. para-, near

14. hypo-, less than normal
15. hyper-, more than normal
16. eu-, normal
17. hypo-, less than normal
18. hyper-, more than normal

7.
1. one
2. first
3. part (or half)
4. three
5. two
6. no (or zero)
7. partly (or partially)
8. many
9. many
10. four
11. one
12. below normal
13. large
14. excessive
15. many
16. small

8.
1. three
2. toward
3. transdermal
4. difficulty
5. bradykinesia
6. oxygen
7. anesthesia
8. without
9. water
10. without

9.
1. red; condition
2. yellow; condition
3. black; tumor
4. white; skin
5. green; vision
6. white; condition
7. blue; pertaining to

10.
1. process; instrument
2. process
3. hemolysin

4. cephalometer
5. carcinogenesis; cancer
6. disease
7. nutrition
8. eat
9. movement (or motion)

11.
1. movement
2. softening
3. eating
4. enlarged
5. hardening
6. eat
7. speech
8. paralysis
9. split
10. movement
11. large
12. split

12.
1. aer/o, air
2. phon/o, voice
3. carcin/o, cancer
4. cry/o, cold
5. electr/o, electricity
6. erythr/o, red
7. lith/o, stone
8. myc/o, fungus; dermat/o, skin
9. necr/o, dead
10. pharmac/o, drugs
11. psych/o, mind
12. py/o, pus; gen/o, origin

Self-Test
A.
1. F
2. D
3. H
4. J
5. E
6. I
7. B
8. A
9. C
10. G

B.
1. E
2. C
3. B
4. D
5. A
6. F

C.
1. aerobic
2. calculus
3. semiconscious
4. subcutaneous
5. suprarenal
6. lipid
7. diplopia
8. aerosol
9. lithiasis
10. symptomatic

D.
1. c
2. c
3. b
4. d
5. b
6. c
7. b
8. b
9. d
10. c

E.
1. dysphonia
2. melanoma
3. hyperlipemia (hyperlipidemia)
4. multicellular
5. polydipsia
6. tachycardia
7. endotracheal
8. cephalometry
9. hemiplegia
10. bradykinesia

F.
1. (correct)
2. dystrophy
3. (correct)
4. oncolytic
5. syndrome

Chapter 4
Exercises

1.
1. acute
2. chronic
3. diagnosis
4. prognosis

2.
1. A
2. A
3. B
4. B
5. A

3.
1. pulse
2. respiration
3. thermometer
4. systolic
5. palpation
6. percussion
7. auscultation

4.
1. electrocardiograph
2. electrocardiography
3. electrocardiogram
4. cephalometry

5. ophthalmoscope
6. ophthalmoscopy
7. microscope
8. otoscopy

5.
1. endoscopy
2. catheterization
3. catheterize
4. cannula

6.
1. ech/o; sound
2. fluor/o; emitting or reflecting light

3. radi/o; radiant energy
4. tom/o; to cut
5. son/o; sound

7.
1. E
2. D
3. A
4. B
5. C

8.
1. algesi/o; sensitivity to pain

2. chem/o; chemical
3. pharmaceut/i; drugs or medicine
4. therapeut/o; treatment
5. tox/o; poison

9. 1. analgesic
2. antineoplastic
3. chemotherapy
4. cryotherapy
5. cytotoxic
6. pharmacotherapy
7. radiotherapy
8. thermotherapy

Self-Test
A. 1. B
2. A
3. A
4. A
5. B
6. C
7. D
8. A
9. B

B. (no particular order)
1. pulse rate
2. respiration rate
3. body temperature

C. 1. b
2. a
3. b
4. b

5. d
D. 1. acute
2. echogram
3. malignant
4. therapeutic
5. cytotoxic
6. computed
7. diagnosis
8. stethoscope
9. electrocardiogram
10. magnetic

E. 1. narcotic
2. analgesic
3. sign
4. therapeutic
5. chemotherapy

6. acute
7. radiolucent
8. radiopaque
9. chronic
10. percussion

F. 1. fluoroscopy
2. neoplasm
3. symptom
4. stethoscope
5. (correct)

Chapter 5
Exercises

1. 1. cell
2. tissue
3. organ
4. body system
5. chemical

2. 1. D
2. C
3. B
4. A

3. 1. front, anterior
2. tail or inferior, caudal (caudad)
3. head, cephalad
4. far or distant, distal
5. back side, dorsal
6. lowermost or below, inferior
7. side, lateral
8. middle, medial, or median
9. back, posterior
10. nearer the origin, proximal
11. uppermost or above, superior
12. belly, ventral

4. 1. posterior
2. superior
3. distal
4. dorsal

5. 1. anter/o, front; medi/o, middle
2. poster/o, back
3. poster/o, back; medi/o, middle
4. dors/o, back; later/o, side

5. poster/o, back; later/o, side
6. anter/o, front; later/o, side
7. medi/o, middle; later/o, side
8. anter/o, front; super/o, above
9. poster/o, behind; super/o, above
10. infer/o, under; medi/o, middle

6. 1. C
2. A
3. B
4. F
5. E
6. D

7. 1. B
2. A
3. A
4. B

8. (any order)
1. head
2. neck
3. torso (or trunk)
4. extremities

9. 1. lapar/o
2. som/a, somat/o
3. dactyl/o
4. acr/o
5. blephar/o
6. onych/o
7. thorac/o
8. omphal/o

10. 1. acrocyanosis
2. laparoscopy
3. peritonitis
4. cephalometry

5. abdominothoracic
6. acral
7. blepharoplasty
8. omphalorrhexis
9. thoracentesis
10. thoracotomy

11. 1. blephar/o, eyelid; -itis, inflammation
2. blephar/o, eyelid; -edema, swelling
3. blephar/o, eyelid; -ptosis, sagging (prolapse)
4. onych/o, nail; -malacia, softening
5. thorac/o, chest; -dynia, pain
6. thorac/o, chest; -tomy, incision
7. thorac/o, chest; -plasty, surgical repair
8. thorac/o, chest; -scopy, visual examination

12. 1. E
2. G
3. A
4. H
5. B
6. F
7. C
8. D

13. 1. cyt/o (sometimes cellul/o)
2. thromb/o
3. coagul/o
4. erythr/o
5. leuk/o

14. 1. B
2. A
3. D
4. C
5. E

15. 1. thrombocytes
2. erythrocytes
3. leukocytes

16. 1. B
2. C
3. B
4. C
5. A

17. 1. plasma
2. hematoma
3. hemolysis
4. hemodialysis
5. coagulation
6. anticoagulant
7. thrombosis
8. thrombopenia
9. anemia
10. phagocytes
11. hematopoiesis
12. leukocytosis
13. leukopenia
14. erythrocytosis

18. 1. A
2. B
3. B
4. A
5. B

19. 1. A
2. A
3. B
4. B

20. 1. antigen
2. susceptible
3. nonspecific

4. specific
5. Active
6. immunodeficiency
21. 1. weapons
  2. Disease
  3. bioterrorism
  4. disseminated

Self-Test
A. 1. G
  2. J
  3. H
  4. C
  5. F
  6. B
  7. I
  8. D
  9. E
  10. A
B. 1. cell

2. tissue
3. organ
4. dysplasia
5. hyperplasia
6. eyelid
7. extremities
8. chest
9. nail
10. dorsal
11. quadrants
12. abdominal
13. intracellular
14. tears
15. platelets
C. 1. a
  2. c
  3. c
  4. c
  5. b

6. a
7. d
8. d
9. c
10. a
D. (no particular order)
  1. connective
  2. epithelial
  3. muscle
  4. nervous
E. 1. acrocyanosis
  2. sagittal
  3. laparoscope
  4. edema
  5. ambulant
  6. telecardiogram
  7. metastasize
  8. erythrocyte
  9. extracellular

10. recumbent
F. 1. antigen
  2. anticoagulant
  3. hematopoiesis
  4. anterolateral
  5. aplasia
  6. abdominothoracic
  7. thrombosis
  8. bioterrorism
  9. leukocytes
     (leucocytes)
  10. intracellular
G. 1. anaphylaxis
  2. fibrin
  3. hypertrophy
  4. immunosuppressant
  5. (correct)

PART TWO

Chapter 6
Exercises
1. 1. protection
  2. support
  3. movement
  4. formation
  5. fat
  6. minerals
2. 1. J
  2. D
  3. H
  4. I
  5. E
  6. E
  7. F
  8. B
  9. E
  10. G
  11. C
  12. A
3. 1. C
  2. E
  3. B
  4. A
  5. B
  6. D
4. 1. carpal
  2. cranial
  3. femoral
  4. humeral
  5. vertebral
  6. lumbar
  7. pelvic
  8. spinal
  9. costal

10. thoracic
11. radial
12. ulnar
5. 1. E
  2. D
  3. F
  4. A
  5. C
  6. B
6. 1. chondr/o
  2. vertebr/o;
     chondr/o
  3. cost/o;
     chondr/o
7. 1. fascia
  2. destruction
  3. disease
  4. muscle
  5. pain
8. 1. myofibrosis
  2. myasthenia
  3. paraplegia
  4. quadriplegia
  5. myocele
9. 1. B
  2. D
  3. A
  4. C
10. 1. cellulitis
  2. osteomyelitis
  3. osteochondritis
  4. chondrosarcoma
  5. fibrosarcoma
  6. leukemia
  7. osteoporosis

8. osteomalacia
11. 1. bifida
  2. scoliosis
  3. dystrophy
  4. arthritis
  5. osteoarthritis
  6. rheumatoid
  7. arthrodynia
  8. erythematosus
  9. gout
  10. hyperuricemia
12. 1. spondylarthritis
  2. polyarthritis
  3. ankylosis
  4. bursitis
  5. arthroscopy
13. 1. C
  2. D
  3. B
  4. A
14. 1. diskectomy
  2. myelosuppression
  3. antiinflammatories
  4. arthrocentesis
  5. myoplasty

Self-Test
A. 1. N
  2. F
  3. J
  4. L
  5. C
  6. M
  7. G
  8. G
  9. H

10. D
11. G
12. B
13. I
14. E
15. A
16. B
17. K
B. 1. G
  2. B
  3. E
  4. D
  5. A
  6. C
  7. F
C. 1. extension
  2. arthroscopy
  3. vertebroplasty
  4. scoliosis
  5. wrist
D. 1. b
  2. a
  3. c
  4. b
  5. c
  6. c
  7. d
  8. b
  9. c
  10. c
E. 1. degenerative joint
     disease;
     degenerative
     changes in the
     joints

2. chronic, systemic disease that often results in deformities of the joints
3. osteoarthritis (noninflammatory, degenerative arthritis) of the left knee

4. right knee replacement
5. right leg
F. 1. ankylosed
2. dislocation
3. nonarticular
4. radial
5. lumbar
6. rheumatism
7. myelitis

8. sternal
9. lateral
10. ligament
G. 1. myolysis
2. osteochondritis
3. myelosuppression
4. antiinflammatories
5. anti-osteoporotics
6. clavicular
7. cervical

8. humeral
9. tarsoptosis
10. reduction
H. 1. ankylosis
2. circumduction
3. femoral
4. flexion
5. laminectomy

Chapter 7
Exercises
1. 1. oxygen
   2. nutrients (nourishment)
   3. vitamins
   4. antibodies
   5. waste
   6. carbon dioxide
   7. acid-base
   8. hemorrhage
   9. temperature
2. (no particular order)
   1. arteries
   2. arterioles
   3. capillaries
   4. veins
   5. venules
3. 1. B
   2. A
   3. C
4. 1. C
   2. B
   3. A
   4. F
   5. D
   6. C
   7. C
   8. E
5. 1. F
   2. J
   3. I
   4. B

5. G
6. D
7. C
8. A
9. H
10. E
6. 1. arteriosclerosis
   2. aortitis
   3. cerebrovascular
   4. thrombophlebitis
   5. polyarteritis
7. 1. A
   2. F
   3. C
   4. E
8. 1. antiarrhythmic
   2. open
   3. cardiopulmonary
   4. beta
   5. pacemaker
9. 1. E
   2. C
   3. D
   4. B
   5. A
10. 1. CABG
    2. aortoplasty
    3. angioplasty
    4. phlebectomy
    5. antihypertensives
    6. antilipidemics
11. 1. G
    2. H

3. F
4. D
5. C
Self-Test
A. 1. lymphangi/o
   2. arter/o or arteri/o
   3. arteriol/o
   4. phleb/o or ven/o
   5. venul/o
B. 1. aorta
   2. arterioles
   3. oxygen
   4. veins
   5. atrium
   6. lymphatic
   7. coronary
   8. endocardium
   9. myocardium
   10. epicardium
C. 1. b
   2. b
   3. b
   4. d
   5. c
   6. a
   7. a
   8. c
   9. a
   10. d
D. 1. necrosis of a portion of cardiac muscle
   2. increased blood pressure

3. increased levels of lipids in the blood
4. introduction of a catheter into the heart
5. chest pain caused by insufficient oxygen to the heart
E. 1. hypotension
   2. antihypertensive
   3. splenomegaly
   4. lymphadenopathy
   5. tonsillectomy
   6. tachycardia
   7. lipids
   8. angiocardiography
   9. endocardium
   10. capillaries
F. 1. adenoidectomy
   2. cholesterol
   3. (correct)
   4. defibrillator
   5. infarction
G. 1. thrombolysis
   2. sinoatrial
   3. lymphadenitis
   4. stenosis
   5. septal
   6. lipid
   7. diastolic
   8. cardiac
   9. cholesterol
   10. lymphangiography

Chapter 8
Exercises
1. 1. homeostasis
   2. inspiration
   3. expiration
   4. oxygen
2. 1. A
   2. B
   3. G

4. E
5. C
6. F
7. D
8. D
9. E
10. H
3. 1. E
   2. D

3. B
4. A
5. F
6. C
4. 1. bronchi/o, bronchus
   2. pharyng/o, pharynx
   3. pneum/o, lung or air
   4. pneum/o, lungs; cardi/o, heart

5. pulmon/o, lungs; -ary or -ic, pertaining to
5. 1. polyp
   2. pharyngeal
   3. laryngeal
   4. laryngalgia
   5. aphonia
   6. aphasia

7. alveolar
8. rhinitis
9. sinusitis
10. sputum
6. 1. pneumonitis
2. bronchopneumonia
3. atelectasis
4. aphasia
5. syndrome
6. emphysema
7. asthma
8. pneumoconiosis
7. 1. C
2. B
3. E
4. D
5. A
8. 1. rhinoplasty
2. thoracocentesis
3. tracheotomy

4. pneumectomy
5. bronchodilator
6. mucolytic

Self-Test
A. 1. G
2. A
3. B
4. F
5. E
6. C
7. D
B. 1. mucolytic
2. antitussive
3. dysphonia
4. bronchoscopy
5. tracheotomy
6. pharyngitis
7. alveolar
8. bronchogram
9. rhinoplasty

10. endotracheal
C. 1. b
2. a
3. b
4. d
5. c
6. a
7. c
8. c
9. d
10. a
D. 1. endoscope
2. eupnea
3. aphasia
4. antihistamine
5. epiglottis
6. silicosis
7. sputum
8. mucolytic
9. cannula

10. alveolus
E. 1. pleural effusion
2. bronchiectasis
3. emphysema
4. bronchitis
5. pneumonia
6. dyspnea
7. sputum
8. pulmonary embolism
9. pneumothorax
10. bronchodilator
F. 1. asphyxiation
2. endoscopic
3. intubation
4. polyp
5. pulmonic

Chapter 9
Exercises
1. 1. ingestion
2. digestion
3. absorption
4. elimination
2. (no particular order)
1. carbohydrates
2. proteins
3. lipids (fats)
3. 1. B
2. B
3. D
4. E
5. F
6. A
7. C
8. G
4. 1. D
2. C
3. E
4. B
5. G
6. G
7. F
8. A
5. 1. an/o, anus
2. duoden/o, duodenum
3. gastr/o, stomach
4. enter/o, small intestine
5. esophag/o, esophagus
6. gastr/o, stomach
7. gloss/o, tongue

8. intestin/o, intestine
9. lingu/o, tongue
10. rect/o, rectum
6. 1. choledoch/o
2. pancreat/o
3. hepat/o
4. cholecyst/o
5. sial/o
7. 1. esophagogram
2. cholelithiasis
3. choledocholithiasis
4. pancreatolithiasis
5. sialography
6. esophagoscopy
7. colonoscopy
8. sigmoidoscopy
8. 1. mellitus
2. hyperglycemia
3. polyuria
4. polydipsia
5. glycosuria
6. gestational
7. hypoglycemia
8. lipids (fats)
9. hyperemesis
10. emaciation
11. anorexia
12. bulimia
9. 1. cholelithiasis
2. cirrhosis
3. an ulcer
4. gastrocele
5. glossitis
6. hemorrhoids
10. 1. esophagitis
2. gastroenteritis

3. enterostasis
4. gastroscopy
5. cholecystitis
6. cirrhosis
11. 1. F
2. C
3. A
4. D
5. H
6. G
7. E
8. B
Self-Test
A. 1. A
2. B
3. E
4. C
5. D
B. 1. C
2. A
3. D
4. B
C. 1. b
2. d
3. a
4. c
5. d
6. b
7. b
8. b
9. b
10. c
D. 1. jejunostomy
2. anorexiant
3. amylase
4. hyperemesis

5. pancreatolithectomy
6. vagotomy
7. gastritis
8. esophageal
9. dyspepsia
10. cholelithiasis
E. 1. cholangiography
2. enteral
3. hepatic
4. lithotriptor
5. diabetes mellitus
F. (no particular order)
1. carbohydrates
2. proteins
3. lipids (fats)
G. 1. stoma
2. anastomosis
3. sigmoid
4. diverticulum
5. mandible
6. eupepsia
7. alimentation
8. nasogastric
9. canker
10. rectum
H. 1. b
2. a
3. b
4. a
5. a
6. a
7. b
8. b

Chapter 10
Exercises
1.
1. water
2. blood
3. hydrogen
4. waste
5. pressure
6. erythropoietin
2.
1. C
2. A
3. D
4. B
5. F
6. E
3.
1. A
2. B
3. C
4. B
5. D
6. E
4.
1. B
2. A
3. C
4. D
5.
1. glomerular filtration
2. tubular reabsorption
3. tubular secretion

6.
1. albuminuria
2. hematuria
3. ketonuria
4. pyuria
5. glycosuria
6. nephrotomography
7. catheterization
8. urinalysis
7.
1. cystoscopy
2. polyuria
3. anuria
4. oliguria
5. nephromegaly
6. glomerulonephritis
7. pyelitis
8. nephroptosis
9. nephromalacia
10. nephrolithiasis
11. uremia
12. nephrosonography
8.
1. a
2. d
3. b
4. c
5. a
9.
1. a
2. a

3. d
4. b
5. b
Self-Test
A.
1. E
2. D
3. A
4. C
5. B
B.
1. voiding
2. glomerulus
3. stenosis
4. suprapubic
5. cystocele
6. excretion
7. nephroscope
8. erythropoietin
9. nephron
10. nephrolithotomy
C.
1. B
2. B
3. B
4. B
5. A
D.
1. c
2. b
3. a

4. c
5. a
6. a
7. b
8. b
9. c
10. b
E.
1. hematuria
2. nephron
3. cystoscopy
4. pyelitis
5. hemodialysis
6. pyelostomy
7. urethral
8. nephrolithiasis
9. nephropexy
10. ureteroplasty
F.
1. c
2. b
3. a
4. c
5. d
G.
1. catheterized
2. nephrectomy
3. (correct)
4. suprapubic
5. urinary

Chapter 11
Exercises
1.
1. genitalia
2. gonads
3. ovum
4. spermatozoon
5. ovary
6. testis or testicle
7. reproduction
2.
1. B
2. H
3. G
4. C
5. E
6. D
7. F
8. A
3.
1. D
2. B
3. E
4. C
5. A
4.
1. A
2. D
3. E
4. B
5. C

5.
1. cervical
2. ovarian
3. uterine
4. vaginal
5. vulval or vulvar
6. endometrium
7. perimetrium
8. myometrium
9. intrauterine
10. extrauterine
11. ovulation
12. menstruation
13. climacteric
14. fetus
15. progesterone
6.
1. speculum
2. Pap
3. dysplasia
4. colposcopy
5. hysteroscopy
6. hysterosalpingogram
7.
1. B
2. C
3. A
4. D
8.
1. B
2. A

3. D
4. C
9.
1. colpitis
2. endometriosis
3. colposcopy
4. hysteroptosis
5. endometritis
10.
1. abstinence
2. intrauterine
3. spermicides
4. coitus
5. rhythm
11.
1. hysterectomy
2. colpoplasty
3. colporrhaphy
4. oophorectomy
   (ovariectomy)
5. salpingorrhaphy
6. ligation
7. laparoscopy
8. curettage
9. laparotomy
10. conization
12.
1. amni/o
2. nat/i
3. fet/o
4. par/o

13.
1. C
2. A
3. B
4. D
14.
1. secundipara
2. fetus
3. ectopic pregnancy
4. neonatal
5. cephalic
6. amnion
7. Down syndrome
8. amniotomy
9. placenta
10. abruptio placentae
15.
1. A
2. D
3. B
4. C
16.
1. gon/o
2. pen/o
3. prostat/o
4. scrot/o
5. semin/o
6. spermat/o
7. orchi/o, orchid/o,
   test/o, testicul/o
8. vas/o

17.
1. penis
2. prostate
3. scrotum
4. semen
5. testis (testicle)

18.
1. cryptorchidism
2. hyperplasia
3. prostatitis
4. orchitis
5. hydrocele

19.
1. orchiopexy (orchidopexy)
2. circumcision
3. vasectomy
4. orchiectomy (orchidectomy)
5. prostatectomy
6. ablation

20.
1. gonorrhea
2. within
3. chancre
4. chlamydial
5. immunodeficiency
6. Kaposi
7. herpes
8. warts
9. hepatitis
10. trichomoniasis
11. candidiasis
12. lice

21.
1. D
2. B
3. A
4. D
5. D
6. A
7. D
8. A
9. C

Self-Test

A.
1. oophor/o
2. salping/o
3. hyster/o
4. cervic/o
5. colp/o
6. vas/o
7. urethr/o
8. pen/o
9. prostat/o
10. orchi/o
11. scrot/o

B.
1. D
2. A
3. B

4. E
5. C
6. F

C.
1. zygote
2. extrauterine
3. endometriosis
4. seminal
5. lactiferous
6. spermatogenesis
7. spirochete
8. ectopic
9. cryptorchidism
10. mastoptosis

D.
1. b
2. c
3. a
4. d
5. b
6. d
7. c
8. c
9. a
10. a
11. b
12. d
13. c
14. d
15. c
16. c
17. b
18. c
19. b
20. b

E.
1. neonate
2. implantation
3. amniotomy
4. episiotomy
5. climacteric
6. dysmenorrhea
7. cervical
8. hysteroptosis
9. amniocentesis
10. ovulation

F.
1. spherical bacteria in pairs located both within and outside cells
2. gonorrhea
3. gonococcus

G.
1. cervicocolpitis
2. (correct)
3. chorionic
4. cystocele
5. syphilis

Chapter 12
Exercises

1.
1. integument
2. microbes (microorganisms)
3. receptors
4. salts

2.
1. B
2. C
3. A

3.
1. xer/o
2. erythemat/o
3. adip/o or lip/o
4. ichthy/o
5. follicul/o
6. pil/o or trich/o
7. kerat/o
8. seps/o or sept/o
9. onych/o or ungu/o
10. seb/o

4.
1. accessory
2. axillary
3. sudoriferous
4. perspiration
5. sebaceous
6. ungual

5.
1. A
2. C
3. D
4. E
5. B

6.
1. B
2. A
3. C
4. D
5. E

7.
1. superficial
2. dermis
3. deep

8.
1. D
2. E
3. C
4. A
5. F
6. B
7. I
8. H
9. J
10. G

9.
1. D
2. C
3. A

4. B

Self-Test

A. (no particular order)
1. covers and protects the body
2. helps control body temperature
3. has receptors that receive stimuli
4. has sweat glands that excrete water and salt

B. (no particular order)
1. epidermis: protection from microorganisms
2. dermis: contains blood vessels, nerves, and glands
3. subcutaneous adipose tissue: insulation and cushion against shock

C.
1. petechia
2. abrasion
3. nodule
4. erythema
5. abscess
6. sudoriferous
7. seborrhea
8. acne
9. electrolysis
10. scabies

D.
1. A
2. F
3. C
4. D
5. G
6. E
7. B

E.
1. a
2. d
3. a
4. a
5. b
6. a
7. c
8. c
9. d
10. b

F.
1. furuncle
2. laceration
3. albinism
4. contusion
5. onychopathy
6. lipoma

7. scleroderma
8. xerosis or xeroderma
9. hidradenitis
10. ungual

G.
1. keloid

2. skin graft
3. sepsis
4. full- and partial-thickness
5. onychomycosis

H.
1. antiperspirant

2. axillary
3. follicle
4. integument
5. petechia or petechiae

Chapter 13
Exercises
1.
1. information (data)
2. movement
3. changes
4. homeostasis
5. afferent
6. efferent
7. somatic
8. autonomic

2. (no particular order)
1. central nervous system
2. peripheral nervous system

3.
1. central
2. peripheral
3. neuron
4. glial or neuroglial

4.
1. F
2. A
3. E
4. G
5. I
6. B
7. C
8. H
9. D
10. J

5.
1. open marketplace
2. weakness
3. cerebellum
4. coccyx

5. dura mater
6. brain
7. neuroglia or sticky substance
8. words, phrases
9. mind
10. nature

6.
1. C
2. A
3. B

7.
1. A
2. B
3. B
4. B
5. A

8.
1. stroke
2. hydrocephalus
3. electroencephalography
4. subdural
5. epidural
6. intracerebral

9.
1. E
2. D
3. B
4. G
5. I
6. C
7. A
8. F
9. J
10. H

10.
1. C
2. B
3. A
4. D

11.
1. B
2. F
3. C
4. A
5. D
6. E
7. G

Self-Test
A.
1. central
2. peripheral
3. central
4. neuron
5. glial or neuroglial
6. meninges
7. photoreceptor
8. chemoreceptor
9. ear
10. analgesics

B.
1. c
2. b
3. d
4. d
5. b
6. b
7. a
8. a
9. a
10. a

C.
1. pyromania
2. craniotomy
3. encephalopathy
4. neurolysis
5. diplopia
6. myopia
7. phobia
8. quadriplegia
9. cranioplasty
10. neurorrhaphy

D.
1. glaucoma
2. peripheral
3. (correct)
4. (correct)
5. thalamus

E.
1. electromyogram
2. meningocele
3. epidural
4. lacrimation
5. neuralgia
6. aphagia
7. aphasia
8. anticonvulsant
9. thermoreceptor
10. retinopathy

F.
1. dysphasia
2. diplopia
3. Alzheimer disease
4. anorexia
5. multiple sclerosis

Chapter 14
Exercises
1.
1. coordinates with the nervous system to regulate the body's activities
2. insufficient secretion
3. excessive secretion

2.
1. glands (endocrine glands)
2. hormones

3. Endocrine glands are ductless and secrete their hormones into the bloodstream. Exocrine glands open onto a body surface and discharge their hormones through ducts.
4. endocrine

5. target organ
6. Hormones are released in response to nervous system; or, endocrine glands respond to hormones produced by the pituitary gland.
7. pituitary (hypophysis)

8. (no particular order) pancreas, pineal gland, thyroid, parathyroid, adrenal, ovaries, testes

3.
1. B
2. D
3. A
4. E
5. G
6. C

7. F
8. H

4. 1. -gen
2. -physis
3. -gen
4. -tropic
5. -tropin
6. -uria

5. 1. C
2. D
3. E
4. B
5. A

6. 1. diabetes insipidus
2. diabetes mellitus
3. hypothyroidism
4. polyuria
5. hyperglycemia
6. polydipsia
7. exophthalmos
8. glycosuria

7. 1. A
2. C
3. E
4. D
5. G
6. B
7. F

8. 1. hypoglycemia
2. thyroxine
3. hyperinsulinism
4. euthyroid
5. adenoma

9. 1. hypophysectomy
2. insulin
3. glucose
4. adenectomy
5. thyroidectomy

Self-Test

A. 1. coordinates with the nervous system to regulate body activities
2. A gland is a structure that is specialized to secrete or excrete hormones. Hormones are chemical substances that have a specific effect on cells or organs.
3. pituitary (hypophysis)
4. organ or structure toward which a hormone is directed
5. deficiency (hyposecretion) or excess (hypersecretion)

B. (no particular order) pineal gland, thyroid, parathyroids, adrenals, pancreas, ovaries, testes

C. 1. d
2. a
3. b
4. b
5. a
6. b
7. c
8. b
9. b
10. d

D. 1. gigantism
2. hypoglycemia
3. hypoparathyroidism
4. thyroidectomy
5. polydipsia
6. polyuria

7. adenoma
8. adenectomy
9. hypophysectomy
10. thyrotoxicosis

E. 1. pineal
2. Langerhans
3. stimulate
4. exocrine
5. endocrine
6. euthyroid
7. diabetic
8. cretinism
9. myxedema
10. antidiuretic

F. 1. bulging outward of the eyes
2. enlarged thyroid
3. increased activity of the thyroid
4. excision of the thyroid

G. 1. adrenaline
2. cretinism
3. homeostasis
4. hypersecretion
5. myxedema

PART THREE

Review of Book
I. Chapter 2
1. b
2. d
3. b
4. c
5. b
6. c
7. b
8. a
9. a
10. a
Chapter 3
11. a
12. b
13. a
14. a
15. a
16. c
17. b
18. d
19. b
20. a
Chapter 4
21. c

22. a
23. a
24. d
25. b
26. b
27. c
28. b
29. a
30. c
Chapter 5
31. c
32. c
33. b
34. d
35. d
36. a
37. a
38. a
39. c
40. c
Chapter 6
41. b
42. a
43. c
44. b

45. a
46. c
47. a
48. c
49. a
50. a
Chapter 7
51. d
52. a
53. c
54. a
55. b
56. c
57. a
58. a
59. a
60. a
Chapter 8
61. a
62. c
63. c
64. b
65. b
66. d
67. a

68. c
69. c
70. a
Chapter 9
71. b
72. b
73. a
74. b
75. b
76. d
77. c
78. a
79. d
80. c
Chapter 10
81. c
82. c
83. b
84. b
85. d
86. c
87. b
88. c
89. d
90. d

Chapter 11
91. b
92. b
93. c
94. d
95. a
96. c
97. b
98. d
99. a
100. b

Chapter 12
101. a
102. a
103. a
104. a
105. d
106. a
107. a
108. a
109. d
110. a

Chapter 13
111. d
112. a
113. b
114. a
115. a
116. b
117. d
118. d
119. b
120. a

Chapter 14
121. c
122. b
123. d
124. d
125. b
126. b
127. d
128. a
129. b
130. b

II. Chapter 2
1. cardiologist
2. adenectomy
3. otoplasty
4. lithotripsy

5. geriatrics
6. cardiac
7. chirospasm
8. mucoid
9. neonatologist
10. phlebitis

Chapter 3
11. hypodermic or subcutaneous
12. microscopy
13. calculi
14. asymptomatic
15. lipoma
16. erythrocyte
17. mycology
18. polydipsia
19. anaerobic
20. bradycardia

Chapter 4
21. sign
22. chronic
23. auscultation
24. endoscope
25. radiopaque
26. thermotherapy
27. analgesic
28. prognosis
29. percussion
30. narcotic

Chapter 5
31. recumbent
32. blepharoplegia
33. acral
34. chiroplasty
35. hematuria
36. mucolytic
37. posterosuperior
38. viscera
39. abdominothoracic
40. cephalopelvic

Chapter 6
41. myasthenia
42. paraparesis
43. arthritis
44. decalcification
45. coccygeal
46. subchondral
47. scapular
48. osteomyelitis

49. arthroscope
50. iliopubic

Chapter 7
51. phlebectomy
52. antihypertensive
53. cardiomegaly (megalocardia)
54. lymphadenopathy
55. myocarditis
56. hypertension
57. arteriopathy
58. aortitis
59. tachycardia
60. lymphangioma

Chapter 8
61. rhinoplasty
62. tracheotomy
63. laryngeal
64. aphonia
65. bronchopneumonia or bronchopneumonitis
66. alveolar
67. sinusitis
68. antitussives
69. bronchiectasis or bronchiectasia
70. diaphragmatic or phrenic

Chapter 9
71. amylase
72. pancreatolithotomy or pancreatolithectomy
73. anorexia
74. cholecystography
75. hypoglycemia
76. duodenal
77. hyperemesis
78. choledochal
79. gastric
80. hepatomegaly

Chapter 10
81. pyelitis
82. urethral
83. nephromalacia
84. renal
85. ureteroplasty
86. anuria

87. lithotrite
88. nephrolithiasis
89. cystostomy
90. cystoscopy

Chapter 11
91. prostatectomy
92. hysteroptosis
93. cephalic
94. gonorrhea
95. prostatic
96. amenorrhea
97. neonate
98. oophorectomy
99. salpingitis
100. ovarian

Chapter 12
101. bacteriostatic
102. axillary
103. cyst
104. lipoma
105. aspiration
106. onychopathy
107. bullae
108. fissures
109. xerosis or xeroderma
110. hidradenitis

Chapter 13
111. craniotomy
112. aphagia
113. hemiplegia
114. phobia
115. neurorrhaphy
116. diplopia
117. tinnitus
118. encephalomalacia
119. anesthesia
120. hypnotics

Chapter 14
121. polydipsia
122. euthyroid
123. hypophysectomy
124. adenectomy
125. adenoma
126. acromegaly
127. gigantism
128. goiter
129. thyroidectomy
130. polyuria

Bibliography

Applegate EJ: *The anatomy and physiology learning system,* ed 3, Philadelphia, 2006, Saunders-Elsevier.

Bedolla M: *Essential Spanish for healthcare,* New York, 1997, Living Language.

Bonewit K: *Clinical procedures for medical assistants,* ed 7, Philadelphia, 2008, Saunders-Elsevier.

Dorland's illustrated medical dictionary, ed 31, Philadelphia, 2007, Saunders-Elsevier.

Dunmore CW, Fleischer RM: *Medical terminology: exercises in etymology,* ed 3, Philadelphia, 2004, Davis.

Ignatavicius DD, Workman ML, Mishler MA: *Medical-surgical nursing: critical thinking for collaborative care,* ed 6, Philadelphia, 2010, Saunders-Elsevier.

Joyce EV, Villanueva ME: *Say it in Spanish: a guide for health care professionals,* ed 3, Philadelphia, 2004, Saunders.

Leonard PC: *Building a medical vocabulary,* ed 7, Philadelphia, 2009, Saunders-Elsevier.

Lewis SM, Heitkemper MM, Dirksen SR: *Medical-surgical nursing: assessment and management of clinical problems,* ed 7, St Louis, 2008, Mosby-Elsevier.

Mosby's medical, nursing, and allied health dictionary, ed 8, St Louis, 2009, Mosby-Elsevier.

Seidel HM, Ball JW, Dains JE, et al: *Mosby's guide to physical examination,* ed 6, St Louis, 2006, Mosby-Elsevier.

Thomas CL, editor: *Taber's cyclopedic medical dictionary,* ed 20, Philadelphia, 2005, Davis.

Velásquez de la Cadena M, Gray E, Iribas JL: *The new revised Velásquez Spanish and English dictionary,* Clinton, NJ, 1985, New Win Publishing.

Illustration and Photo Credits

Chapter 1
Figure 1-1 from Polaski AL, Tatro SE: *Luckmann's core principles and practice of medical-surgical nursing*, Philadelphia, 1996, Saunders.

Chapter 2
Figure 2-2 from Seidel HM, Ball JW, Dains JE, Benedict GW: *Mosby's guide to physical examination,* ed 4, St Louis, 1999, Mosby.

Figure 2-3 from Callen JP et al: *Color atlas of dermatology,* ed 2, Philadelphia, 2000, Saunders.

Figure 2-4 from Lewis SM, Heitkemper MM, Dirksen SR, et al: *Medical-surgical nursing: assessment and management of clinical problems,* ed 7, St Louis, 2007, Mosby-Elsevier.

Figure 2-5 from Seidel HM, Ball JW, Dains JE, Benedict GW: *Mosby's guide to physical examination,* ed 5, St Louis, 2003, Mosby.

Figure 2-9 from Moore KL, Persaud TVN: *The developing human: clinically oriented embryology,* ed 6, Philadelphia, 1998, Saunders.

Figure 2-10 from Zitelli BJ, Davis HW: *Pediatric physical diagnosis,* ed 4, St Louis, 2002, Mosby.

Figure 2-11 courtesy Walter Tunnessen, MD, University of Pennsylvania, School of Medicine, Philadelphia.

Figure 2-12 from Weston WL, Lane AT: *Color textbook of pediatric dermatology,* St Louis, 1991, Mosby.

Chapter 3
Figure 3-2 courtesy Department of Dermatology, College of Medicine, Houston, Texas.

Figure 3-4 from Sanders MJ: *Mosby's paramedic textbook,* ed 3, St Louis, 2005, Mosby.

Figure 3-5 from Zitelli BJ, Davis HW: *Atlas of pediatric physical diagnosis,* ed 4, St Louis, 2002, Mosby.

Figure 3-6 from Kamal A, Brockelhurst JC: *Color atlas of geriatric medicine,* ed 2, St Louis, 1991, Mosby.

Figure 3-7 from Emond RT, Welsby PD, Rowland HA: *Colour atlas of infectious diseases,* ed 4, London, 2003, Mosby Ltd.

Figure 3-8 A from Bonewit K: *Clinical procedures for medical assistants,* ed 6, Philadelphia, 2004, Saunders.

Figure 3-9 from Chipps EM, Clanin NJ, Campbell VG: *Neurologic disorders,* St Louis, 1992, Mosby.

Chapter 4
Figures 4-1 and **4-2** from Seidel HM, Ball JW, Dains JE, Benedict GW: *Mosby's guide to physical examination,* ed 6, St Louis, 2006, Mosby-Elsevier.

Figure 4-3 D from Potter PA, Griffin A: *Fundamentals of nursing,* ed 7, St. Louis, 2009, Mosby-Elsevier.

Figures 4-4 A, B from Seidel HM, Ball JW, Dains JE, Benedict GW: *Mosby's guide to physical examination,* ed 5, St Louis, 2003, Mosby; **C** from Seidel HM, Ball JW, Dains JE, Benedict GW: *Mosby's guide to physical examination,* ed 6, St. Louis, 2006. Mosby.

Figure 4-5 from Ignatavicius MS, Workman ML: *Medical-surgical nursing: critical thinking for collaborative care,* ed 5, Philadelphia, 2006, Saunders-Elsevier.

Figure 4-6 from Phipps WJ, Monahan FD, Sands JK, et al: *Medical-surgical nursing,* ed 8, St Louis, 2007, Mosby-Elsevier.

Figure 4-8 from Ballinger PW, Frank ED: *Merrill's atlas of radiographic positions and radiologic procedures,* vol 1, ed 9, St Louis, 1999, Mosby.

Figure 4-9 A courtesy Siemens, Inc; **B** from Seeley RS, Stephens TD, Tate P: *Anatomy and physiology,* ed 3, St Louis, 1995, Mosby.

Figure 4-10 A from Mourad LA: *Orthopedic disorders,* St Louis, 1991, Mosby; **B** courtesy Professor A. Jackson, Department of Diagnostic Radiology, University of Manchester; **C** courtesy Siemens, Inc.

Figure 4-11 from Hagen-Ansert S: *Textbook of diagnostic ultrasonography,* ed 6, 2006, St Louis, Mosby-Elsevier.

Figures 4-12 and **4-13** from Ballinger PW, Frank ED: *Merrill's atlas of radiographic positions and radiologic procedures,* vol 2, ed 10, St Louis, 2003, Mosby.

Figure 4-14 from Frank ED, Long BW, Smith BJ: *Merrill's atlas of radiographic positioning and radiologic procedures,* ed 11, St Louis, 2007, Mosby-Elsevier.

Chapter 5

Figure 5-2 A and **D** from Herlihy B, Maebius, NK: *The human body in health and illness,* ed 2, Philadelphia, 2003, Saunders; **B** and **C** from Gartner LP, Hiatt JL: *Color textbook of histology,* ed 2, Philadelphia, 2001, Saunders.

Figure 5-3 from Ignatavicius MS, Workman ML, Mishler MA: *Medical-surgical nursing across the health care continuum,* ed 5, Philadelphia, 2006, Saunders-Elsevier.

Figure 5-5 from Ballinger PW, Frank ED: *Merrill's atlas of radiographic positions and radiologic procedures,* vol 1, ed 10, St Louis, 2003, Mosby.

Figure 5-8 from Thompson JM, Wilson SF: *Health assessment for nursing practice,* St Louis, 1996, Mosby.

Figure 5-10 from Lewis SM, Heitkemper MM, Dirksen SR, et al: *Medical-surgical nursing: assessment and management of clinical problems,* ed 7, St Louis, 2007, Mosby-Elsevier.

Figure 5-13 from *Dorland's illustrated medical dictionary,* ed 31, Philadelphia, 2007, Saunders-Elsevier.

Figure 5-14 from Hart CA, Broadhead RL: *Colour atlas of pediatric infectious diseases,* London, 1992, Mosby-Wolfe.

Figure 5-15 from Applegate E: *The anatomy and physiology learning system,* ed 2, Philadelphia, 2000, Saunders.

Figure 5-16 Copyright Dennis Kunkel Microscopy, Inc, 1994.

Figure 5-17 from Gartner LP, Hiatt JL: *Color textbook of histology,* ed 2, Philadelphia, 2001, Saunders.

Figure 5-18 from Applegate E: *The anatomy and physiology learning system,* ed 2, Philadelphia, 2000, Saunders.

Figure 5-19: **B** from Murray PR, Rosenthal KS, Kobayashi GS, Pfaller MA: *Medical microbiology,* ed 3, St Louis, 1994, Mosby; **D** from Forbes BA, Sahm DF, Weissfeld AS: *Bailey & Scott's diagnostic microbiology,* ed 11, St Louis, 2002, Mosby; **F** from Atlas RM: *Principles of microbiology,* St Louis, 1995, Mosby.

Chapter 6

Figure 6-6 from Frank ED, Long BW, Smith BJ: *Merrill's atlas of radiographic positioning and radiologic procedures,* vol 1, ed 11, St Louis, 2007, Mosby-Elsevier.

Figure 6-7 from Ballinger PW, Frank ED: *Merrill's atlas of radiographic positions and radiologic procedures,* vol 1, ed 10, St Louis, 2003, Mosby.

Figure 6-12 from Canale ST: *Operative orthopaedics,* ed 9, St Louis, 1998, Mosby.

Figure 6-14 from Black JM, Hawks JH: *Medical-surgical nursing: clinical management for positive outcomes,* ed 8, Philadelphia, 2005, Saunders.

Figure 6-15 from Herlihy B, Maebius NK: *The human body in health and illness,* ed 2, Philadelphia, 2003, Saunders.

Figure 6-17 from Zitelli BJ, Davis HW: *Atlas of pediatric physical diagnosis,* ed 5, St Louis, 2007, Mosby-Elsevier.

Figure 6-18 from Swartz MH: *Textbook of physical diagnosis: history and examination,* ed 2, Philadelphia, 1994, Saunders.

Figure 6-20 A from Ballinger PW, Frank ED: *Merrill's atlas of radiographic positions and radiologic procedures,* vol 1, ed 10, St Louis, 2003, Mosby; **B** courtesy Zimmer, Inc, Warsaw, Ind.

Chapter 7

Figure 7-7 from Ballinger PW, Frank ED: *Merrill's atlas of radiographic positions and radiologic procedures,* vol 3, ed 10, St Louis, 2003, Mosby.

Figure 7-9 from Braunwald E.: *Heart disease: a textbook of cardiovascular medicine,* ed 6, Philadelphia, 2001, Saunders.

Figure 7-12 from Lewis SM, Heitkemper MM, Dirksen SR, et al: *Medical-surgical nursing: assessment and management of clinical problems,* ed 7, St Louis, 2007, Mosby-Elsevier.

Figure 7-18 from Stone DR, Gorbach SL: *Atlas of infectious diseases,* Philadelphia, 2000, Saunders.

Figure 7-19 from Behrman R, Kliegman R, Jenson HB: *Nelson's textbook of pediatrics,* ed 17, Philadelphia, 2004, Saunders.

Chapter 8

Figure 8-3 from Wilson SF, Thompson JM: *Respiratory disorders,* St Louis, 1990, Mosby.

Figure 8-5 from Kumar V, Robbins SL, Cotran RS: *Pathologic basis of disease,* ed 7, Philadelphia, 2005, Saunders.

Figures 8-6 and **8-7** from Ignatavicius MS, Workman ML, Mishler MA: *Medical-surgical nursing across the health care continuum,* ed 5, Philadelphia, 2006, Saunders-Elsevier.

Chapter 9

Figure 9-2 modified from Liebgott B: *The anatomical basis of dentistry,* St Louis, 2001, Mosby.

Figure 9-6 from Damjanov I, Linder J: *Pathology: a color atlas,* St Louis, 2000, Mosby.

Figure 9-7 from Beare PG, Myers JL: *Adult health nursing,* ed 3, St Louis, 1998, Mosby.

Chapter 10

Figure 10-6 A from Zakus S: *Mosby's clinical skills for medical assistants,* St Louis, 2001, Mosby; **B** from Belchetz PE, Hammond P: *Mosby's colour atlas and text of diabetes and endocrinology,* London, 2003, Mosby, Ltd; **C** from Bonewit-West K: *Clinical procedures for medical assistants,* ed 6, St Louis, 2004, Saunders.

Figure 10-7 from Brunzel NA: *Fundmentals of urine and body fluid analysis,* ed 2, St Louis, 2004, Saunders-Elsevier.

Figure 10-8 from Price S, Wilson L: *Pathophysiology: clinical concepts of disease processes,* ed 6, St Louis, 2003, Mosby.

Figure 10-9 from Bontrager KL, Lampignano J: *Textbook of radiographic positioning and related anatomy,* ed 6, St Louis, 2005, Mosby.

Figure 10-10 from Kumar V, Abbas AK, Fausto N, Mitchell RN: *Robbins' basic pathology,* ed 8, Philadelphia, 2007, Saunders-Elsevier.

Figure 10-11 from Lewis S, Heitkemper MM, Dirksen SR: *Medical-surgical nursing: assessment and management of clinical problems,* ed 6, St Louis, 2004, Mosby.

Figure 10-14 courtesy Department of Pathology, Duke University School of Medicine, Durham, NC.

Figure 10-16 from Athanasoulis CA et al: *Interventional radiology,* Philadelphia, 1982, Saunders.

Chapter 11

Figure 11-6 from Black JM, Hawks JH: *Medical-surgical nursing,* ed 8, Philadelphia, 2009, Saunders-Elsevier.

Figure 11-7 from Greer I, Cameron I, Kitchner H, Prentice A: *Mosby's colour atlas and text of obstetrics and gynecology,* London, 2001, Mosby, Ltd.

Figure 11-11 A reproduced with the permission of the Royal College of Obstetricians and Gynaecologists; **B** from Symonds EM, MacPherson MBA: *Colour atlas of obstetrics and gynecology,* London, 1994, Mosby-Wolfe.

Figure 11-14 from Zitelli BJ, Davis HW: *Atlas of pediatric physical diagnosis*, ed 4, St Louis, 2002, Mosby.

Figure 11-16 from Svane G, Potchen EJ, Sierra A, Azavedo E: *Screening mammography: breast cancer diagnosis in asymptomatic women,* St Louis, 1993, Mosby.

Figure 11-20 from Polaski AL, Tatro SE: *Luckmann's core principles and practice of medical-surgical nursing*, Philadelphia, 1996, Saunders.

Figure 11-22 from Forbes BA, Sahm DF, Weissfeld AS: *Bailey & Scott's diagnostic microbiology,* ed 10, St Louis, 1998, Mosby.

Figure 11-23 courtesy Antoinette Hadd, MD, Indiana University School of Medicine, Indianapolis.

Figure 11-24 from Noble J, editor: *Textbook of primary care medicine,* ed 3, St Louis, 2001, Mosby.

Figures 11-25 and **11-26** courtesy Glaxo SmithKline, Research Triangle Park, NC.

Chapter 12

Figure 12-2 from Bork K, Brauninger W: *Skin diseases in clinical practice,* ed 2, Philadelphia, 1998, Saunders.

Figure 12-4 from Noble J, editor: *Textbook of primary care medicine,* St Louis, 2001, Mosby.

Figures 12-5 and **12-6** from Noble J, editor: *Textbook of primary care medicine,* St Louis, 1996, Mosby.

Figure 12-8 from *Dorland's illustrated medical dictionary,* ed 31, Philadelphia, 2007, Saunders-Elsevier.

Figure 12-9 from Behrman R, Kliegman R, Arvin A: *Nelson's textbook of pediatrics,* ed 17, Philadelphia, 2004, Saunders.

Figure 12-10 from Auerbach PS: *Wilderness medicine: management of wilderness and environmental emergencies,* ed 5, St Louis, 2007, Mosby-Elsevier.

Figure 12-11 A from Ignatavicius DD, Workman ML, Mischler MA: *Medical-surgical nursing across the health care continuum,* ed 5, Philadelphia, 2006, Saunders-Elsevier; **B** from Habif TP: *Clinical dermatology: a color atlas guide to diagnosis and therapy,* ed 4, St Louis, 2004, Mosby-Elsevier.

Figure 12-14 From Habif TP: *Clinical dermatology: a color atlas guide to diagnosis and therapy,* ed 3, St Louis, 1996, Mosby.

Chapter 13

Figure 13-5 B from Thibodeau GA, Patton KT: *Anatomy and physiology*, ed 5, St Louis, 2003, Mosby.

Figure 13-7 from Polaski AL, Tatro SE: *Luckmann's core principles and practice of medical-surgical nursing*, Philadelphia, 1996, Saunders.

Figure 13-9 from Zitelli BJ, Davis HW: *Atlas of pediatric physical diagnosis*, ed 3, St Louis, 1997, Mosby.

Figure 13-11 from Monahan FD, Sands JK, Neighbors M, et al: *Phipps' medical-surgical nursing: health and illness perspectives*, ed 8, St Louis, 2007, Mosby-Elsevier.

Figure 13-12 A courtesy Department of Neurological Surgery, Vanderbilt University Medical Center, Nashville.

Figures 13-12 B and **13-13** from Ignatavicius DD, Workman ML: *Medical-surgical nursing: critical thinking for collaborative care*, ed 5, Philadelphia, 2006, Saunders-Elsevier.

Chapter 14

Figure 14-2: **A** from Thompson JM, Wilson SF: *Health assessment for nursing practice*, St Louis, 1996, Mosby; **B** from *Dorland's illustrated medical dictionary*, ed 30, Philadelphia, 2003, Saunders.

Figure 14-3 from Mendeloff AI, Smith DE, editors: Acromegaly, diabetes, hypermetabolism, proteinuria and heart failure, *Clin Pathol Conf Am J Med* 20:133, 1956.

Figure 14-4 from Ignatavicius DD, Workman ML, Mishler MA: *Medical-surgical nursing across the health care continuum*, ed 3, Philadelphia, 1999, Saunders.

Figure 14-5 from Zitelli BJ, Davis HW: *Atlas of pediatric physical diagnosis*, ed 4, St Louis, 2002, Mosby.

Figure 14-6 courtesy Ewing Galloway.

Figure 14-7 from Black JM, Hawks JH: *Medical-surgical nursing*, ed 7, Philadelphia, 2005, Saunders.

Figure 14-8 from Monahan FD, Neighbors M: *Medical-surgical nursing: foundations for clinical practice*, ed 2, Philadelphia, 1998, Saunders.

Index

A

abbreviations
  dangers of, 7
  finding, 367-368
  list of, 365-366
  overview of, 6-7
abdomen, 108
abdominal adhesions, 106
abdominal hernias, 110, 110f
abdominal paracentesis, 108, 109f
abdominal quadrants, 108, 108f
abdominocentesis, 108
abdominopelvic cavity, 106
abdominothoracic, 108
abrasions
  dermabrasion, 311
  overview of, 306
abruptio placentae, 278
abscess
  defined, 307
  pyogenic membranes and, 115
  skin injuries and, 307f
absorption, of drugs, 369
absorption function, of digestive system, 212
accessory organs of digestion, 220f
  overview of, 219-220
  structures of digestive system, 214
  word parts, 220t
accessory skin structures
  disorders of, 309
  overview of, 302
acne vulgaris
  defined, 307
  disorders of accessory skin structures, 309
  treating, 310
acquired immunodeficiency syndrome (AIDS), 122-123
acral, pertaining to extremities, 110
acrocyanosis, 110
acrodermatitis, 110
acrohypothermy, 110

acromegaly
  defined, 344
  enlargement of the extremities, 110
  progression of, 344f
acronyms, in abbreviations, 7
active immunity, 121
acute disease, 78
acute respiratory failure, 194
ADD (attention deficit disorder), 330
adenectomy, 347
adenoidectomy, 184
adenoids, 182
adenoma, 344
ADH (antidiuretic hormone), 244, 343
ADHD (attention deficit hyperactivity disorder), 330
adhesions, abdominal, 106
adipose tissue
  of female breast, 280
  layers of skin, 300
  liposuction and, 310
adjectives, combining suffixes with, 13
adrenal glands, 339
adult respiratory distress syndrome (ARDS), 201
adverse drug reactions, 370
afferent (sensory) nerves, 317-318
agoraphobia, 330
AIDS (acquired immunodeficiency syndrome), 122-123
akinesia, 326
albinism, 61f, 307
albuminuria, 244
alimentary canal (or tract), 214-219
alimentation, 212
allergies, 123
Alzheimer disease, 330
amenorrhea
  menstrual irregularities, 270
  treating, 275
amniocentesis, 26f, 279
amnion, 276, 278
amniotic sac, 278
amniotomy, 279
amylase, 213
analgesics, 332
anaphylaxis, 123

Page numbers followed by f indicate figures; t, tables.

anaplasia, 99
anastomosis, 230
anatomic position, of body, 101, 101f
anemia, 118
anesthesia, 326
anesthesiologists, 23
anesthetics
    CNS and, 332
    local and general, 23
    spinal, 157
anesthetist, 23
angina pectoris, 172
angiocardiography, 174
angiography, 174
angiomas, 174
angioplasty, 180
ankylosed spine (poker spine), 154
ankylosis, 154
anorexia, 224
anorexia nervosa, 224, 330
anorexiant, 229
anoxia, 194
antepartum, 277
anteroposterior (AP) projection, 105f
antiarrhythmics, 179-180
antiarthritics, 158
antibiotics, 204
antibodies, 121
anticoagulants
    overview of, 117-118
    treating blood clots, 180
anticonvulsant drugs, 332
antidiarrheal drugs, 229
antidiuretic hormone (ADH), 244, 343
antiemetics, 229
antigens
    body defenses, 121
    hypersensitivity to, 123
antihistamines, 204
antihypertensive drugs, 180
antiinflammatory drugs, 157
antilipidemic drugs, 180
antimicrobial medicine, 311
anti-osteoporotics, 156
antiparkinsonian drugs, 332
antiperspirants, 311
antipyretics, 332
antithyroid drugs, 347
antitussives, 204
anxiety disorders, 330
aorta
    radiography of, 174
    structures of cardiovascular system, 166-170
aortic, 170
aortogram, 174
aortography, 174
aortoplasty, 180
AP (anteroposterior) projection, 105f

aphagia, 326
aphasia, 326
aplasia, 98
apnea, 194
appendectomy, 14, 230
appendicitis, 226
appetite suppression, 229
ARDS (adult respiratory distress syndrome), 201
areola, of female breast, 280
arrhythmia, 172
arterial, pertaining to arteries, 170
arteries
    arteriogram revealing blockage, 174f
    arteriography, 174
    blood leaving heart via, 167
    blood vessels of heart, 170
    coronary arteries, 169f
    stenosis of renal artery, 246
arteriogram, 174, 174f
arteriography, 174
arterioles, 167, 170
arthralgia, 154
arthritis
    hand deformity characteristic of rheumatoid arthritis,
        154f
    musculoskeletal system, 153-154
    rheumatoid arthritis (RA), 154
    treating, 157
    types of, 154
arthrocentesis, 158
arthrodynia, 154
arthropathy, 154
arthroplasty, 158
arthroscopy
    of knee joint, 155f
    overview of, 154
    removing torn cartilage, 158
arthrotomy, 154
articulation, 146
ascites, 108, 109f
asepsis, 310
aseptic wounds, 306
asphyxiation, 202-203
aspiration, 311
aspirin, treating arthritis with, 157
asthma, 201
astigmatism, 326
atelectasis, 201
atherectomy, 180
atrioventricular (AV) valves, of heart, 168, 169f
atrium, 168, 168f
atrophy
    of epidermis, 305f
    secondary skin lesions, 305
attention deficit disorder (ADD), 330
attention deficit hyperactivity disorder (ADHD),
        330
augmentation mammoplasty, 29, 30f

auscultation
  aspects of physical examination, 82f
  basic examination procedures, 82
autism, 330
autonomic nervous system, 318
AV (atrioventricular) valves, of heart, 168, 169f
axilla, 302
axon, 319

B
bacilli, 124
bacteria
  in body fluids, 123f
  types of pathogens, 124
  in urine, 245
bactericidal, 310
bacteriostatic, 310
balance (equilibrium), 324
balloon angioplasty, 180, 181f
barium enema, 221
barium meal, 221
barium swallow, 221
benign, 123
benign prostatic hyperplasia (BHP), 284, 285f
bicuspid (mitral) valve, of heart, 168, 169f
bile, 219-220
biliary, 219-220
biliary calculus. *See* gallstone (biliary calculus)
biliary lithotripsy, 230f
biliary tract, 221
biopsy
  defined, 311
  of lung, 205
  of lymph nodes, 184
  overview of, 29
  percutaneous bladder biopsy, 255
  percutaneous liver biopsy, 231
  percutaneous renal biopsy, 255
bioterrorism, 124
bipolar disorders, 330
birth canal, 264
bladder
  catheter inserted into, 84f
  cystoscope of, 249f
  normal bladder compared with cystocele,
    251f
  organs of urinary system, 240
  storing/expelling urine from, 243
blepharal, 110
blepharoplasty, 110
blepharoplegia, 110
blepharospasm, 110
blepharotomy, 110
blood
  as body fluids, 116-119
  bone function in formation of blood cells, 133
  bone marrow transplants for stimulating
    production of, 158

blood (*Continued*)
  changes in numbers of formed elements of, 119t
  coagulation of, 117f
  composition of, 117f
  overview of, 116-119
  stained, 118f
blood clots
  intravascular thrombolysis, 180
  treating, 180
blood pressure
  antihypertensive drugs, 180
  basic examination procedures, 80-81
  measuring, 81f
  overview of, 170
blood urea nitrogen (BUN), 245-246
blood vessels
  arteries and veins, 166f
  capillary bed showing relationship of, 167f
  diseases, disorders, and diagnostic terms, 174-178
  overview of, 170
  surgical and therapeutic interventions, 180-181
body
  bioterrorism, 124
  cavities, 106
  defenses and immunity, 120-124
  directional terms, 102t
  fluids, 111-120
  organization of, 97-111, 98f
  pathogens, 123-124
  reference planes, 101
body cavities
  abdominopelvic, 106
  catheterization of, 83, 84f
  cranial and spinal, 106
  dorsal and ventral, 106, 106f
  endoscopy of, 83
  overview of, 106
  thoracic, 106
body fluids
  bacteria in, 123f
  blood, 116-120
  collecting for diagnosis, 78-79
  compartments of, 112f
  overview of, 111-119
  water, 111
  word parts, 112t
body regions
  combining forms for, 107t
  overview of, 107-111
body systems
  in body organization, 100
  major, 100t
  overview of, 100t
  resisting disease or disorder, 120
body temperature, 79-80, 80f
bone marrow
  aspiration from posterior iliac crest, 151f
  function in formation of blood cells, 133

bone marrow *(Continued)*
    leukemia and, 151
    transplants, 158
bones
    anterior view of skeleton, 135f
    articulation, 146
    association with muscle, cartilage, and tendon, 134f
    dislocation of, 149
    excision of (ostectomy), 156
    fractures of, 149
    of hand, 142f
    of head, 138f
    infections, 150-151
    of lower extremity, 143f
    major bones of the body, 136t
    overview of, 135-145
    of pelvis, 141f
    of rib cage, 140f
    treating fractures, 155-156, 156f
    of vertebral column, 139f
    vertical axis of body, 135
Botox (clostridium botulinum toxin), 310, 311f
Bowman's capsule, 242
bradykinesia, 326
bradypnea, 194, 195f
brain
    assessing, 324
    electroencephalography, 324
    skull (cranium) encasing, 321
    structures of, 321f
brand names, of drugs, 370
breastbone, 135
breathing, 79, 191. *See also* respiratory system
breech presentation, of fetus, 278
bronchiectasis, 201
bronchodilators, 204
bronchogram, 201
bronchography, 201
bronchoscopy, 200f
bulbourethral glands, 282
bulimia, 224
bullae, 303, 304f
BUN (blood urea nitrogen), 245-246
bunionectomy, 157
burns
    skin injuries, 306
    tissues involved in, 307f
bursae, articulation and, 146
bursitis, 154

C
CABG (coronary artery bypass grafts), 180, 181f
CAD (coronary artery disease), 172
calcium, bones role in release of, 133
calcium channel blockers, 180
cancer. *See also* tumors
    biopsy of lymph nodes for detecting, 184
    of connective tissue, 151

cancer *(Continued)*
    of gastrointestinal system, 223
    of kidney, 247f
    of lung, 201
    lymphatic, 182
    mammogram, 281f
    myelosuppression for treating, 158
    of skin, 309
    treating breast cancer, 280
    of uterus, 273
canker sores, 226
cannula, 83
capillaries
    blood vessels of heart, 170
    structures of cardiovascular system, 167
    surrounding nephrons, 242f
carbohydrates, 213
carcinoma
    of gastrointestinal system, 223
    of lung, 201
cardiac (heart) muscles, 146, 147f
cardiac catheterization, 171, 171f
cardiomegaly, 172
cardiomyopathy, 170-171
cardiopulmonary bypass, 178, 179f
cardiopulmonary resuscitation (CPR), 179
cardiovascular system
    blood vessels, 166f, 170
    diseases, disorders, and diagnostic terms of blood vessels, 174-178
    diseases, disorders, and diagnostic terms of heart, 170-173
    function of, 165-166
    heart, 166f, 168-169
    structures of, 166-170
    surgical and therapeutic interventions for blood vessels, 180-181
    surgical and therapeutic interventions for heart, 178-179
cardioversion, 179
cartilage
    association with bone, muscle, and tendon, 134f
    excision of (chondrectomy), 156
    overview of, 145
    removing torn, 158
casts, for treating fractures, 155
cathartics, 229
catheter
    bladder, 84f
    cardiac, 171, 171f
    urinary, 84f, 245, 252
catheterization, 83
catheterize, 83
cavities, body. *See* body cavities
CBC (complete blood count), 118
CDC (Centers for Disease Control and Prevention), 124
cells
    anaplastic changes, 99
    in body organization, 98
    erythrocytes (red blood cells), 116

cells *(Continued)*
  formation of blood cells, 133
  intracellular and extracellular body fluids, 111
  leukocytes (white blood cells), 116
  nervous system, 319
  phagocytic/phagocytes, 119
  stem cells, 100
cellular pathology, 22
cellulitis, 150, 307
Centers for Disease Control and Prevention (CDC),
    124
central nervous system (CNS)
  divisions of nervous system, 318f
  organization of nervous system, 319
  overview of, 321
centrifuge, for spinning blood, 116
cephalalgia, 326
cephalgia, 110
cephalic presentation, of fetus, 278, 278f
cephalodynia, 110
cephalometry, 110
cephalopelvic, 109
cerebellum, 321
cerebral aneurysm, 325
cerebral concussion, 326
cerebral contusion, 326
cerebral hemorrhage, 326
cerebral palsy, 326
cerebrospinal fluid (CSF), 321
cerebrovascular accident (CVA), 324-325
cerebrum, 321
cervical, 265
cervical dilation, 278
cervical nerves, 322, 322f
cervical polyp, 271
cervicocolpitis, 271
cervix uteri
  cervical pap smear, 267f
  conization of the cervix, 275
  hysteroscopy of, 269f
  overview of, 265
cesarean section, 278-279
CHD (coronary heart disease), 172
cheilitis, 226
chemicals, in body organization, 97
chemoreceptors, 322
chemotherapy, 280
chest cavity
  abnormal conditions of, 197f
  lungs and organs in, 193
chest x-ray, 105f
CHF (congestive heart failure), 172
childbirth, 276-279
chiroplasty, 111
chiropodist, 111
chiropody, 111
chirospasm, 111
cholecystectomy, 230

cholecystic, 220
cholecystitis, 228
choledochal, 220
choledocholithiasis, 221
cholelithiasis, 221, 221f, 228
cholestasis, 228
cholesterol
  antilipidemic drugs, 180
  risk of hardening of arteries associated with, 174
chondral, pertaining to cartilage, 145
chondrectomy, 156
chondrosarcoma, 151
chorion, 276
chorionic villus sampling, 279
chronic disease, 78
chronic fatigue syndrome, 148
chronic obstructive pulmonary disease (COPD), 201, 204
circulatory system
  cardiovascular system. *See* cardiovascular system
  function of, 165-166
  lymphatic system. *See* lymphatic system
circumcision, 285
circumduction, of joints, 146
cirrhosis, 228
classes, of drugs, 370
clean-catch midstream technique, for urine collection, 245
climacteric, 266
clinical depression, 330
clinical pathology, 22
clinical psychology, 24
clinical studies, 78-79
clitoris, 263
closed reduction, of fracture, 156
clostridium botulinum toxin (Botox), 310, 311f
coagulation (clotting), of blood, 117-118, 117f
cocci, 124
coccygeal nerves, 322, 322f
cochlea, 324
colitis, 226
collagen injections, 310
colonoscopy, 222, 222f
colopexy, 29
color, combining forms related to, 61-63, 61t-62t
colostomy, 29, 230
colpitis, 271
colpoplasty, 275
colporrhaphy, 275
colposcopy, 268f
coma, 326
combining forms
  blood vessels, 170t
  body fluids, 112t
  body regions, 107t
  body structures, 14f, 27, 27t-28t
  color related, 61-63, 61t-62t
  combining word parts to write terms, 6f
  for medical specialties, 16t
  miscellaneous, 66t-67t

combining forms *(Continued)*
  radiology, 85t
  respiratory structures, 193t
  suffixes related to, 63, 63t-64t
  term building and, 5t
  treatment related, 91t
  for word roots, 3
combining vowels
  inserting between word roots, 3
  rules regulating use of vowel at end, 5
complement, in body defense, 120-121
complete blood count (CBC), 118
compound fracture, 149, 149f
compression, of spinal cord, 327f
computed radiography, 85
computed tomography (CTs)
  assessing brain and spinal cord, 324
  cardiac diagnosis with, 172
  types of diagnostic imaging, 86, 87f
concussion, cerebral, 326
congenital defects
  heart, 172
  musculoskeletal system, 153
congestive heart failure (CHF), 172
conization of the cervix, 275
connective tissue
  cancers arising from, 151
  cartilage, 145
  diseases, 153-154
  ligaments, 146
  overview of, 98, 99f
contact dermatitis, 307
contraception
  effectiveness of methods, 274t
  options for, 273-274
  overview of, 270
contrast imaging, in radiography, 88, 89f
controlled substances, 369-370
contusions (bruises), 306
COPD (chronic obstructive pulmonary disease), 201,
  204
cornea, 323
coronary arteries
  heart tissues and, 169f
  overview of, 169
coronary artery bypass grafts (CABG), 180, 181f
coronary artery disease (CAD), 172
coronary heart disease (CHD), 172
cortisone, 342
costectomy, 156
cough, antitussives for, 204
Coumadin (warfarin), 180
COX-2 (cyclooxygenase-2) inhibitors, 158
CPR (cardiopulmonary resuscitation), 179
cranial cavity, 106
craniectomy, 156
craniocele, 153

cranioplasty, 156, 331
craniotomy, 156, 331
cranium. *See* skull (cranium)
cretinism, 344, 345f
cryosurgery, 311
cryptorchidism, 284
CSF (cerebrospinal fluid), 321
CTs. *See* computed tomography (CTs)
curettage, 275, 311, 311f
cutaneous, 300
CVA (cerebrovascular accident), 324-325
cyanosis, 307
cyclooxygenase-2 (COX-2) inhibitors, 158
cyst
  differentiation of types of skin lesion, 303f
  overview of, 303
cystectomy, 252
cystic, 241
cystocele
  defined, 250, 271
  normal bladder compared with cystocele, 251f
cystoscope, of bladder, 249f
cystostomy, 254
cytoplasmic projections, 319

D
dactylitis, 111
dactylography, 111
dactylospasm, 111
dandruff (plaque), 303, 304f
debridement, 311
decongestants, 204
defecation, 212
defenses, body, 120-124
defibrillators, 172
degenerative joint disease (DJD), 153-154
degenerative joint disease (osteoarthritis), 153-154
dehydration, 224
dendrites, 319
depression, clinical, 330
dermabrasion, 311
dermatitis, 37f, 307
dermis layer, of skin, 300
description, prefixes related to, 58t
diabetes, 228
diabetes insipidus
  diabetes mellitus (DM) compared with, 344t
  overview of, 343
diabetes mellitus (DM), 223
  diabetes insipidus compared with, 343, 344t
  insulin deficiency causing, 245
  treating, 229, 347-348
diagnosis
  basic examination procedures, 79-82
  common tests and procedures, 83
  defined, 78
  radiology for, 85-90

diagnosis *(Continued)*
  signs and symptoms, 78-79
  suffixes related to, 33, 33t-34t
diagnostic imaging. *See* radiograph/radiography
diagnostic terms
  cardiovascular system, 170-174
  digestive system, 221-228
  integumentary system, 303-305
  musculoskeletal system, 148
  reproductive system of female, 266-273
  reproductive system of male, 284-285
  respiratory system, 194-202
  urinary system, 244-252
dialysis, 253
diaphragm
  dividing thoracic and abdominopelvic cavities, 106
  hiatal hernia causing structural abnormality, 227f
  respiratory function of, 193
diarrhea, 223
diastolic blood pressure, 80-81, 81f
diencephalon, 321
digestive system, 214
  accessory organs of digestion, 219-220
  alimentary tract, 214-219
  causes of bleeding, 227f
  diseases and disorders of esophagus, 226
  diseases and disorders of gallbladder, 228
  diseases and disorders of intestines, 226-228
  diseases and disorders of liver, 228
  diseases and disorders of mouth, 226
  diseases and disorders of pancreas, 228
  diseases and disorders of stomach, 226
  function of, 212-213
  structures of, 214, 215f
  surgical and therapeutic interventions, 229-231
digoxin, 179-180
dilation and curettage (D&C), 275
diplegia, 326
diplopia, 326
direct inguinal hernia, 110f
direction
  body terms related to, 102t
  prefixes related to, 54-56, 54t-56t
discoid lupus erythematosus (DLE), 307-308, 308f
disease-modifying antirheumatic drugs (DMARDs),
    158
diseases
  acute and chronic, 78
  pathology of, 22
diseases and disorders
  of cardiovascular system, 170-174
  of connective tissue, 153-154
  of digestive system, 221-228
  of esophagus, 226
  of gallbladder, 228
  of integumentary system, 303-305, 307-309
  of intestines, 226-228

diseases and disorders *(Continued)*
  of liver, 228
  of mouth, 226
  of musculoskeletal system, 148
  of nervous system, 324-329
  of pancreas, 228
  psychologic, 329-330
  of reproductive system of female, 266-273
  of reproductive system of male, 284-285
  of respiratory system, 194-202
  of stomach, 226
  of urinary system, 244-246
diskectomy, 157
disks
  herniated, 149
  surgical and therapeutic interventions, 157
dislocation
  of bones from joint, 149
  radiograph of dislocated finger, 149f
disorders. *See* diseases and disorders
distribution, of drugs, 369
diuretic, 254
diverticulitis, 226-227
diverticulum, 226-227
DJD (degenerative joint disease), 153-154
DLE (discoid lupus erythematosus), 307-308, 308f
DM (diabetes mellitus). *See* diabetes mellitus (DM)
DMARDs (disease-modifying antirheumatic drugs),
    158
dorsal cavity, 106, 106f
dose, drug, 369
Down syndrome, 279
  facial characteristics of, 279f
drug abuse, 369-370
drug addiction, 369-370
drug administration, 369
drugs
  overview of, 369-373
  pharmacology of, 7
  transdermal delivery, 56f
ductus deferens (vas deferens), 282
duodenal ulcer, 227
duodenitis, 227
dwarfism, 345, 345f
dyslexia, 326
dysmenorrhea, 270
dysphagia, 226, 326
dysphasia, 326
dysplasia, 98
dyspnea, 194
dysrhythmia, of heart, 172

E
ears
  equilibrium, 324
  as sense organ, 322
  structure of, 323, 323f

echocardiogram, 172, 172f
echocardiography, 172
echograms, 88
ectopic pregnancy, 277
ED (emergency department), 23-24
EDD (expected date of delivery), 278
edema, 111
efferent (motor) nerves, 318
electrocardiogram, 171
electrocardiograph, 171
electrocardiography, 66f, 171
electroencephalogram, 324
electroencephalography, 69f, 324
electrolysis, 311
electromyography, 326
electrosurgery, 311
elimination
    of body waste, 212
    of drugs, 369
emaciation, 224
embryo, 276f
emergency department (ED), 23-24
emergency medicine, 23-24
emergency room (ER), 23-24
emesis, 223
emetics, 229
emphysema, 202
encephalitis, 326
encephalocele, 326
encephalomalacia, 328
encephalomeningitis, 328
encephalopathy, 328
endocarditis, 170-171
endocardium, 169, 169f
endocrine glands, 339, 339f
endocrine system
    diseases, disorders, and diagnostic terms,
        342-346
    function of, 338
    hormones, 341, 342t
    major glands of, 339f
    structures of, 339-342
    surgical and therapeutic interventions, 347-348
endometrial ablation, 275
endometriosis, 271
endometritis, 271
endometrium, 265, 276
endoscopic retrograde cholangiopancreatography
        (ERCP), 221
endoscopy
    cardiac catheterization used with, 171
    fiberoptic, 154
    flexible endoscope, 84
    overview of, 83
    of upper gastrointestinal tract (UGI), 222f
endotracheal intubation, 203, 203f
English, translating medical terms into Spanish,
        378-380

enteral feeding tubes
    overview of, 229
    placement of, 229f
enterostasis, 228
enzymes, role in digestion, 213
epicardium, 168, 169f
epidemiology/epidemiologists, 24
epidermis
    atrophy of, 305f
    layers of skin, 300
epididymis, 282
epidural hematoma, 324
epilepsy, 328
episiotomy, 279
epithelial tissue, 98, 99f
eponyms, 6
equilibrium (balance), 324
ER (emergency room), 23-24
ERCP (endoscopic retrograde cholangiopancreatography),
        221
erythema, 307-308
erythroblastosis fetalis, 279
erythrocytes (red blood cells)
    diseases and disorders, 118
    overview of, 118
    RBC (red blood count), 118
    types of cells, 116
erythropoiesis, 119
erythropoietin, 119, 238
esophageal varices, 226
esophagitis, 226
esophagoscopy, 222
esophagostomy, 229
esophagram, 221
esophagus, 226
estrogen, 266
ESWL (extracorporeal shock wave lithotripsy), 26f,
        254-255
eupnea, 194, 195f
euthyroid, 343
examination procedures, basic, 79-82
excretion, 238
exocrine glands, 339
exophthalmos, 342-343, 343f
expected date of delivery (EDD), 278
expiration (exhalation), 191
extension, of joints, 146
external fixation, treating fractures, 156
extracellular fluids, 111
extracorporeal shock wave lithotripsy (ESWL), 26f,
        254-255
extraembryonic membranes, 276
extrauterine
    overview of, 264
    pregnancy, 277
extremities
    acral, 110
    as body region, 107

extremities (*Continued*)
  bones of lower extremity, 143f
  paralysis of, 149
eyes
  as sense organ, 322
  structure of, 323, 323f

F

fallopian tubes, 264, 265f
family practice, 15
fascia, 146
fats (lipids)
  nutrient classes, 213
  testing levels of, 174
FDA (Food and Drug Administration), 369
Federal Emergency Management Agency (FEMA),
    124
feet, treating, 111
FEMA (Federal Emergency Management Agency),
    124
female breasts
  in female reproductive system, 280-281
  milk production, 262
  structure of, 281f
  surgical and therapeutic interventions,
    280
females
  external reproductive structures, 263
  internal reproductive structures, 264-266
  sexually transmitted diseases (STDs), 286
  sterilization, 273
  structures of reproductive system, 262-266
femoral hernias, 110, 110f
fertilization, 276, 276f
fetus, 264
  development of, 276-277
  fetal monitoring, 279
  fetal presentation, 278, 278f
  pertaining to (fetal), 276-277
  sonography of, 88f
fibrillation, 172
fibromyalgia, 148
fibrosarcoma, 151
fingernails, 111, 302
fingers/toes, 111, 149f
fissures, skin, 305, 305f
fistula
  overview of, 271
  sites of vaginal, 271f
flatulence, 224
flexible endoscope, 84
flexion, of joints, 146
fluids, body. *See* body fluids
fluoroscope/fluoroscopy, 88
follicles, 302
folliculitis, 309
Food and Drug Administration (FDA), 369
forensic medicine, 24

fractures
  of bones, 149
  classification of, 149f
  treating, 155-156
  vertebral column, 327f
freckles (macules), 303, 304f
frontal plane, of body, 101, 101f
frostbite, 308
fungi, 124
furuncle, 308

G

gallbladder
  accessory organs of digestion, 219
  diseases and disorders of, 228
gallstone (biliary calculus)
  common locations of, 221f
  overview of, 221
  treating, 230f
gamma cameras, 88
gamma knife, 331f
gastrectomy, 230, 231f
gastric bypass, 229
gastritis, 226
gastrocele, 226
gastroduodenostomy, 230
gastroenteritis, 226
gastroesophageal reflux disease (GERD), 226
gastrointestinal tract
  pharmaceuticals for, 229
  upper and lower, 214
gastroplasty, 229
gastroscopy, 222
gastrostomy, 229-230
general anesthetics, 23
generic names, of drugs, 370
genital herpes, 288f
genital warts, 289f
genitalia
  external female, 263, 263f
  internal female, 264-266
  male, 282-284, 282f
  midsagittal and anterior views of female, 264f-265f
  overview of, 261-262
genitourinary (GU) organs, 286
GERD (gastroesophageal reflux disease), 226
gestation, 277-278. *See also* pregnancy
gestational diabetes mellitus, 223
gigantism, 345, 346f
gingivitis, 226
glands
  endocrine, 339, 339f
  exocrine, 339
  removing, 347
glans penis, 282
glaucoma, 328
glia, 319
glial cells, 319

glomerular filtration, 242, 243f
glomerulus, 242, 242f
glossitis, 226
glucose, 213
glucose strips, for urine testing, 244f
glycosuria, 223, 244, 343
goiters, 342-343
gonads
    function of, 261-262
    in male reproductive system, 282
gonorrhea, 287f
gout, 154
gram-negative intracellular diplococci, 287f
gravida (primigravida), 277
Greek
    source of medical terms, 1, 2t
    word roots used for diseases, conditions, diagnosis, and
        treatment, 3
growth hormone
    deficiency of, 345f
    as performance enhancing drug, 342
GU (genitourinary) organs, 286
gynecologist, 262
gynecology
    overview of, 262
    reasons for seeking gynecologic care, 270

H
hair
    accessory skin structures, 302
    in integumentary system, 299
hands
    radiograph/radiography of, 142f
    treating, 111
HCG (human chorionic gonadotropin), 276-277
head
    as body region, 107
    cephalometry, 110
heart
    cardiac (heart) muscles, 134, 146, 147f
    cardiac catheterization, 171, 171f
    in cardiovascular system, 166f
    circulation of blood through, 168f
    congenital defects, 172
    diseases, disorders, and diagnostic terms, 170-173
    overview of, 168-169
    surgical and therapeutic interventions, 178-179
heart attack, 173, 173f
heart failure, 172
heart murmur, 173
heart rate, basic examination procedures, 79
Heimlich maneuver, 202, 203f
hemangioma, 174
hematology, 116
hematomas
    head injuries, 324, 325f
    overview of, 117

hematopoiesis, 119, 133
hematuria, 244
hemiplegia, 328
hemodialysis, 117, 253
hemoglobin, 118
hemolysis, 117
hemorrhoidectomy, 180, 230
hemorrhoids, 228
hemothorax, 197f
heparin, as anticoagulant, 180
hepatitis, 228
hepatomegaly, 228
hernias
    abdominal, 110f
    hiatal, 226, 227f
    overview of, 110
herniated disks, 149
hiatal hernia, 226, 227f
hidradenitis, 309
history, medical, 82
HIV (human immunodeficiency virus), 122-123
homeostasis, 100, 165
hormonal system. See endocrine system
hormone replacement therapy (HRT), 275
hormones
    female, 266
    hyposecretion and hypersecretion, 338
    male, 283
    overview of, 341-342
    releasing, 339
    treating deficiencies, 347
    treating excesses, 347
hospitalists, 24
HRT (hormone replacement therapy), 275
human body. See body
human chorionic gonadotropin (HCG), 276-277
human immunodeficiency virus (HIV), 122-123
humpback (kyphosis)
    compared with scoliosis, 153f
    as congenital defect, 153
hydrocele, 284, 285f
hydrocephalus, 115, 325
hyperacidity, 226
hyperemesis, 223
hyperextension, of spinal cord, 327f
hyperflexion, of spinal cord, 327f
hyperglycemia, 223, 343
hyperinsulinism, 345
hyperkinesia, 328
hyperlipemia, 223
hyperlipidemia, 173, 223
hyperopia, 328
hyperparathyroidism, 345
hyperplasia, 98, 99f
hyperpnea, 194, 195f
hypersecretion, of endocrine hormones, 338
hypersensitivity, to antigens, 123

hypertension, 173
hyperthyroidism
    overview of, 342-343
    treating, 347
hypertrophy
    compared with hyperplasia, 99f
    of organs, 99
hyperuricemia, 154
hyperventilation, 194
hypoglycemia, 223, 228, 345
hypoparathyroidism, 345
hypophysectomy, 347, 347f
hypophysis, 339
hypopigmentation, 308
hypopituitarism, 346-347
hyposecretion, of endocrine hormones, 338
hypotension, 173
hypothalamus, 321
hypothyroidism, 343
hypoxia, 194
hysterectomy, 275
hysteroptosis, 272, 272f
hysterosalpingogram, 269f
hysteroscopy, 269f

I

ibuprofen, for treating arthritis, 157
ichthyosis, 308
ICU (intensive care unit), 24
ileostomy, 230-231
immunity
    active and passive, 121
    types of specific, 122f
immunization, 121
immunocompromised persons, 122
immunodeficiency diseases, 122-123
immunosuppressants, 122
immunosuppressive agents, 122
immunosuppressive therapy, 252
implantation
    extrauterine, 277
    fertilization, 276
    overview of, 276f
in utero, 264
in vitro fertilization (IVF), 274-275
incision
    as invasive procedure, 85
    of joint, 154
    skin injuries, 306
incisional hernia, 110f
indirect inguinal hernia, 110f
infarction, 173
infections
    musculoskeletal, 150-151
    opportunistic, 122-123
    pathogens and, 124
    urinary tract, 245, 251

infertility
    overview of, 270
    treating, 274-275
inflammation
    abdominal adhesions caused by, 106
    antiinflammatory drugs, 157
    arthritic disorders, 153
    body defenses, 120-121
influenza, 202
    vaccinations for, 204
ingestion function, of digestive system, 212
inguinal hernias, 110f
    overview of, 110
inhalation (inspiration), 191
injections
    collagen injections, 310
    intradermal injections, 55t
    intramuscular injections, 55t
    intravenous injections, 55t
    subcutaneous injections, 55t
    using prefixes in naming types of, 55f
inspection, basic examination procedures, 82
inspiration (inhalation), 191
insulin
    diabetes mellitus (DM) and, 223, 245
    external insulin pump, 348f
    pancreas producing, 220
    role of hormones in diabetes mellitus, 341
    treating diabetes mellitus, 347-348
integumentary system
    accessory skin structures, 302
    diseases, disorders, and diagnostic terms, 303-305
    disorders of accessory skin structures, 309
    disorders of skin, 307-309
    function of, 299
    skin injuries, 306
    skin layers, 300-301, 300f
    skin lesions, 303-305
    structures of, 300-302
    surgical and therapeutic interventions, 310-311
intensive care unit (ICU), 24
intensivists, 24
interferon, 120-121
internal fixation, treating fractures, 156
internal medicine, 15
internist, 15
interns, 15-16
interstitial fluids, 111
interventions, therapeutic. *See* therapeutic interventions
intestines
    diseases and disorders of, 226-228
    divisions of large intestine, 219f
    divisions of small intestine, 218f
intracellular fluids, 111
intracerebral hematoma, 324
intradermal injections, 55t
intramuscular injections, 55t

intrauterine, 264
intrauterine devices (IUDs), 273, 274t
intravascular thrombolysis, 180
intravenous injections, 55t
intravenous urogram, 249f
intubation
    endotracheal, 203f
    types of, 203
invasive procedures, 85
involuntary (smooth) muscles, 134, 146, 147f
irritable bowel syndrome, 228
islets of Langerhans, in pancreas, 339, 339f
IUDs (intrauterine devices), 273, 274t
IVF (in vitro fertilization), 274-275

J

jaundice, 63f, 221
jejunostomy, 229
joints
    arthritic disorders of, 154
    arthroscopy, 154
    articulation of, 146
    dislocation of, 149
    incision of, 154
    removing fluid (arthrocentesis) from synovial joints, 158
    replacement (arthroplasty) of, 158
    sprains, 150

K

Kaposi sarcoma, 288f
keloid, 306
keratin, 301
ketone bodies, 245
ketonuria, 245
kidney dialysis, 253
kidney stones, 254, 254f
kidneys
    anatomical features of, 241
    blood urea nitrogen reflecting kidney function, 245-246
    cancer of, 247f
    functions of, 238
    normal kidney compared with polycystic kidney, 251f
    organs of urinary system, 240
    radiograph/radiography of, 246
    sectional view, 241f
knee joint, arthroscopy of, 155f
kyphosis (humpback)
    compared with scoliosis, 153f
    as congenital defect, 153

L

labia, 263
labor, in pregnancy, 278
laboratory tests, 78-79
laceration, of skin, 306
lacrimal, 323
lacrimation, 323

lactase, 213
lactation, 280
lactiferous duct, 280
lactose, 213
laminectomy, 157
laparoscope/laparoscopy
    defined, 275
    of female reproductive system, 268f
    laparoscopic cholecystectomy, 231
    laparoscopic nephrectomy, 252
    overview of, 109
laparotomy, 109, 275
laryngeal polyp, 199f
laser lithotripsy, 230f
last menstrual date (LMD), 278
Latin
    source of medical terms, 1, 2t
    word roots used for body structures, 3
laxatives, 229
LE (lupus erythematosus), 154, 308f
letters, in abbreviations, 7
leukemia, 119, 151
leukocytes (white blood cells), 116, 119
leukocytopenia, 119
leukocytosis, 119
leukopenia, 119
LGI (lower gastrointestinal tract), 214, 228
ligaments
    connective tissue, 146
    sprains and, 150
lipase, 213
lipids (fats)
    nutrient classes, 213
    testing levels of, 174
lipoma, 308
liposuction, 310, 310f
lithotripsy, 26f, 254-255
lithotrite, 254-255
liver
    accessory organs of digestion, 219
    biopsy, 231
    diseases and disorders of, 228
    functions of, 219-220
LMD (last menstrual date), 278
lobectomy, 205
lobules, of female breast, 280
local anesthetics, 23
local effects, of drugs, 369
lower gastrointestinal tract (LGI), 214, 228
lower respiratory tract (LRT), 193
lumbar nerves, 322, 322f
lumbar puncture, 157, 157f
lumpectomy, 29, 280
lungs
    biopsy, 205
    carcinoma of the lung, 201
    organs of respiration, 193
    vital capacity (VC), 194

lupus erythematosus (LE), 154, 308f
lymph, 182
lymph nodes
    biopsy for detection of cancer, 184
    structures of lymphatic system, 182
lymph vessels, 182
lymphadenectomy, 184
lymphadenitis, 184, 184f
lymphadenoma, 184
lymphadenopathy, 184
lymphangiograms, 184
lymphangiography, 182-184
lymphangioma, 174
lymphangitis
    overview of, 182-183
    streptococcal, 183f
lymphatic carcinoma, 182
lymphatic system
    diseases, disorders, and diagnostic terms,
        182-184
    function of, 165-166
    overview of, 183f
    structures of, 182
    surgical and therapeutic interventions, 184
lymphedema, 33f, 184
lymphoma, 182

M

macules (freckles), 303, 304f
magnetic resonance imaging (MRI)
    assessing brain and spinal cord, 324
    cardiac diagnosis with, 172
    lab tests for endocrine disorders, 343
    types of diagnostic imaging, 86, 87f
malabsorption syndrome, 224
males
    hormones, 283
    sexually transmitted diseases (STDs), 286
    sterilization, 273
    structures of reproductive system, 282-284, 282f
malignancies
    musculoskeletal system, 151
    pathogens and, 123
malignant melanoma, 308
malnutrition, 224
mammalgia, 280
mammary glands, 280
mammogram, 280, 281f
mammography, 280-281
mammoplasty, 29
mandibular arch, 217f
mastalgia, 280
mastectomy, 29, 280
mastitis, 280
mastodynia, 280
mastopexy, 280
mastoptosis, 280
medical abbreviations. *See* abbreviations

medical terms. *See* word terms/word building
medicine, 15
medulla oblongata, 321
melanocytes, 308
memorization techniques, 25
Meniere disease, 328
meninges, 321
meningitis, 328
meningocele, 328
menopause
    hormone replacement therapy (HRT), 275
    overview of, 266
menorrhagia, 270
menses, 266
menstruation
    irregularities of, 270
    overview of, 266
mercury manometer, 81f
metabolic disturbances, of musculoskeletal system,
        151-152
metabolism
    digestive system and, 212
    of drugs, 369
metastasis/metastasize, 123
metrorrhagia, 270
MI (myocardial infarction), 173, 173f
microtia, 30f
midsagittal plane, of body, 101, 101f
mitral (bicuspid) valve, of heart, 168, 169f
moles (papules), 303, 304f
mons pubis, 263
motor (efferent) nerves, 318
mouth
    diseases and disorders of, 226
    as sense organ, 322
MRIs. *See* magnetic resonance imaging (MRI)
mucolytics, 204
multiple myeloma, 151
multiple sclerosis, 328
Multistix, for urine testing, 244f
muscles
    association with bone, cartilage, and tendon, 134f
    fascia, 146
    infections, 150-151
    injuries to, 150
    major skeletal muscles, 148f
    overview of, 146-147
    relaxants, 157
    straining, 150
    surgical procedures, 157
    types of, 134, 146, 147f
muscular dystrophy, 153
muscular tissue, 98, 99f
musculoskeletal system
    arthritis and connective tissue diseases, 153-154
    articulation and structures associated with, 146
    cartilage, 145
    congenital defects, 153

musculoskeletal system *(Continued)*
  diseases, disorders, and diagnostic terms, 148-155
  function of, 133
  infections, 150-151
  major bones of the body, 135-145
  metabolic disturbances, 151-152
  muscles and structures associated with, 146-147
  stress and trauma injuries, 149-150
  structure of, 134-148
  surgical and therapeutic interventions, 155-158
  tumors and malignancies, 151
myasthenia gravis, 148, 328
mycodermatitis, 308
myelin sheath, 319
myelitis, 328
myelography, 328
myelosuppression, 158
myocardial infarction (MI), 173, 173f
myocardial ischemia, 173
myocarditis, 170
myocardium, 169, 169f
myocele, 150
myocellulitis, 150
myofibrosis, 148
myoma, 272
myometrium, 265
myopia, 328
myoplasty, 157
myxedema, 346

N
nails
  accessory skin structures, 302
  finger and toe, 111
  in integumentary system, 299
narcolepsy, 328
nasal cannula, administering oxygen via, 204
nasoduodenal tubes, 229
nasogastric tubes, 229
nasojejunal tubes, 229
nasolacrimal, 323
nasotracheal intubation, 203
neck, as body region, 107
necrosis
  overview of, 308
  tissues, 308f
negation, prefixes related to, 58t
neonatal period, 277
neonate, 277
neonatology, 19b
nephrectomy, 252
nephrolithotomy, 255
nephrons
  capillaries surrounding, 242f
  functions of, 243f
  glomerulus and tubules of, 242
  overview of, 240

nephropexy, 255
nephroscope, 255
nephroscopy, 255
nephrosis, 250
nephrostomy, 255
nephrotomograms, 246, 246f
nephrotomography, 246
nephrotomy, 255
nephrotoxic, 250
nerve blockade, for pain, 332
nervous system
  central nervous system, 321
  diseases, disorders, and diagnostic terms, 324-329
  divisions of, 318f
  function of, 317-318
  nerves of spinal cord, 322f
  organization of, 319
  peripheral nervous system and sense organs, 322-324
  psychologic disorders, 329-330
  surgical and therapeutic interventions, 331-332
nervous tissue, 98, 99f
neuralgia, 328
neurasthenia, 330
neurilemma, 319
neuritis, 328
neuroglia, 319
neuroglial cells, 319
neurolysis, 331
neurons
  overview of, 319
  structure of, 319f
neuropathy, 328
neuroplasty, 331
neurorrhaphy, 331
neuroses, 330
neurosurgeon, 23
newborns, 19b
nitroglycerin, as vasodilator, 180
nodules, 303
  differentiation of types of skin lesion, 303f
noninvasive procedures
  for diagnosis of heart disease, 171
  vs. invasive procedures, 85
nonspecific resistance, of body to disease or disorder, 120
nonsteroidal antiinflammatory drugs (NSAIDs), 157
normal range, for bodily substances, 79
nose, 322
nouns, combining suffixes with, 13
NSAIDs (nonsteroidal antiinflammatory drugs), 157
nuclear medicine, 89f
nuclear scans, 88
nullipara, 277
numbers, prefixes related to, 51, 52t
nutrition, 212

O

obesity, 223, 229
obstetricians, 277
obstetrics
    overview of, 277
    word parts, 277t
occlusion, of arteries, 173
OCs (oral contraceptives), 273-274, 342
omphalic, 109-110
omphalitis, 110
omphalocele, 110
omphalorrhagia, 110
omphalorrhexis, 110
onychectomy, 111
onychomycosis, 111, 308
onychopathy, 111, 309
oophorectomy, 275
oophoritis, 272
oophorosalpingitis, 272
open heart surgery, 178
open reduction, treating fractures, 156
ophthalmoscopy, 83
opportunistic infections, 122-123
oral contraceptives (OCs), 273-274, 342
orchidectomy, 285
orchiditis, 284
orchidoplasty, 285
orchiopexy, 285
orchiotomy, 285
organisms, in body organization, 100
organs
    accessory organs of digestion, 214, 219-220, 220f
    in body organization, 98
    in chest cavity, 193
    endoscopy of, 83
    hypertrophy of, 99
    of respiration, 192f, 193
    of urinary system, 240f
orotracheal intubation, 203
orthopedic surgeons
    overview of, 23
    treatment of fractures, 155-156
orthopedics, 134
orthopedist, 134
orthopnea, 194
ostectomy, 156
osteitis, 150
osteitis deformans (Paget disease), 152
osteoarthritis (degenerative joint disease), 153-154
osteochondritis, 150-151
osteomalacia, 152
osteoporosis
    changing curvature of spine, 152
    hormone replacement therapy (HRT) and, 275
    metabolic disturbances, 151-152
    treatment of, 156
anti-osteoporotics, 156

OTC (over the counter) drugs, 369
otoscopy, 31f
ova (eggs)
    fertilization, 276
    production of, 261
ovarian carcinoma, 272, 272f
ovarian cyst, 272, 272f
ovaries
    function of, 261
    glands of endocrine system, 339
    location of, 266
    overview of, 264
ovulation, 266
oxygen, administering, 204f

P

PA (posteroanterior) projection, 105f
pacemakers
    artificial, 179f
    cardioversion, 179
    sinoatrial (SA) node as, 178
Paget disease (osteitis deformans), 152
pain, nerve blockade for, 332
palatine tonsils, 182
pallor, signs of anemia, 118
palpation, basic examination procedures, 82, 82f
pancreas
    accessory organs of digestion, 219
    diseases and disorders of, 228
    insulin produced by, 220
    islets of Langerhans in, 339
pancreatitis, 228
pancreatolithectomy, 231
pancreatolithiasis, 221
panic attacks, 330
pap smear, 267f
papules (moles), 303, 304f
paracentesis, 205
paracentesis, abdominal, 108, 109f
paranasal sinuses, 198f
paraparesis, 149
paraplegia, 149, 328
parathyroid, 339
parenteral administration, of drugs, 369
paresis, 149
Parkinson disease, 328
paroxysmal, 201
parturition, 277. See also childbirth
passive immunity, 121
pathogens, 123-124
pathologic/pathological, 22
pathology, of disease, 22
pediculosis, 308
pelvic inflammatory disease (PID), 273
pelvis
    bones of, 141f
    region of trunk, 109

penis, 282
percussion, basic examination procedures, 82, 82f
percutaneous bladder biopsy, 255
percutaneous liver biopsy, 231
percutaneous nephrostomy, 252
percutaneous renal biopsy, 255
pericarditis, 171
pericardium, 168
perimetrium, 265
peripheral nervous system (PNS)
    divisions of nervous system, 318f
    organization of nervous system, 319
    overview of, 322-324
peritoneal dialysis, 253
peritoneum, 106
peritonitis, 108
perspiration, 302
PET (positron emission tomography)
    cardiac diagnosis with, 172
    combining tomography and radioactive substances, 88-90
petechiae, 308
phagocytic/phagocytes, 119
phagocytosis, 120-121
pharmaceuticals, 7, 88, 369
pharmacokinetics, 369
pharmacology
    of drugs, 7
    overview of, 369-373
pharyngeal tonsils, 182
phlebectomy, 180
phobias, 330
photoreceptors, 322
phrenic, pertaining to diaphragm, 193
physical examination
    aspects of, 82f
    basic procedures, 82
physical therapy, for treating arthritis, 157
PID (pelvic inflammatory disease), 273
pilomotor muscles, 302
pineal gland, 339
pituitary gland
    as master gland, 339
    surgical removal, 347f
pituitary tumors, 347
placebo, 369
placenta, 276
placenta previa, 279
plaque (dandruff), 303, 304f
plasma, 116
platelets (thrombocytes), 116, 118
pleura, 193
pleural cavity, 193
pleurisy, 202
pleuritis, 202
plurals, rules for plural form of medical terms, 8, 9t
PMS (premenstrual syndrome), 273
pneumectomy, 205

pneumonectomy, 205
pneumonoconiosis, 202
pneumothorax, 197f
PNS. See peripheral nervous system (PNS)
poker spine (ankylosed spine), 154
polyarthritis, 154
polycystic kidney disease, 250, 251f
polydipsia, 223, 343
polyp, 250
polyphagia, 223
polyuria, 223, 343
pons, 321
position, prefixes related to, 54-56, 54t-56t
positron emission tomography (PET)
    cardiac diagnosis with, 172
    combining tomography and radioactive substances, 88-90
posterior plane, of body, 101f
posteroanterior (PA) projection, 105f
postnatal, 277
postpartum, 277
prefixes
    combining word parts to write terms, 6f
    miscellaneous, 57-58, 57t-58t
    overview of, 3-4
    radiologic, 85t
    recognizing in terms, 58-60
    related to numbers or quantities, 51, 52t
    related to position or direction, 54-56, 54t-56t
    term building and, 5
    using to form words, 51
    using to write terms, 60-61
pregnancy
    ectopic or extrauterine, 277
    gestation period, 278
    labor, 278
    overview of, 276-279
    trimesters of, 278
premenstrual syndrome (PMS), 273
prenatal, 277
prepuce, 282
prescriptions, 369
primary skin lesions, 303, 304f
primigravida, 277
proctoscope, 222
proctoscopy, 222
progesterone, 266
prognosis, 78
programmed learning, as learning method, 17
pronation, 105f
prone position, 105f
pronunciation, of medical terms, 8b
prostate gland, 254, 283-284
prostatectomy, 286
prostatic carcinoma, 284
prostatitis, 284
protease (proteinase), 213
proteins, 213

proteinuria, 244
protozoa, 124
psoriasis, 308
psychiatry/psychiatrists, 24
psychologic disorders, 329-330
psychology, 317
psychosis, 329
psychosomatic, 329
pulmonary (semilunar) valves, of heart, 168, 169f
pulmonary embolism, 197f, 202
pulmonary ventilation, 191
pulmonologist, 194
pulse, basic examination procedures, 79, 80f
purgatives, 229
pustules, 303, 304f
pyelolithotomy, 255
pyelostomy, 255
pyogenic membranes, 115
pyromania, 330
pyuria, 244

Q

quadriparesis, 149
quadriplegia
    overview of, 328
    spinal chord injuries, 149
quantities, prefixes related to, 51, 52t

R

RA (rheumatoid arthritis). *See* rheumatoid arthritis (RA)
radial pulse, 80f
radiation therapy. *See* radiotherapy
radiograph/radiography. *See also* x-rays
    of aorta, 174
    comparing male and female pelvis, 141f
    diagnostic, 85-86
    of dislocated finger, 149f
    of hand, 142f
    of intestinal tract, 221
    of kidneys, 246
    lymphangiography, 182-184
radiologic studies, 78-79
radiology, 85-90
radiolucent substances, 86
radiopaque substances, 86
radiopharmaceuticals
    defined, 369
    nuclear medicine and, 89f
    overview of, 88
radiotherapy
    nuclear medicine and, 90f
    radiation oncology, 90
    treating tumors, 90
    treatment of breast cancer, 280
red blood cells. *See* erythrocytes (red blood cells)
red blood count (RBC), 118
reduction, for treating fractures, 155-156

reduction mammoplasty, 29
reference planes, of body, 101
regions, of body. *See* body regions
renal, 241
renal angiography, 246
renal arteriogram, 246, 246f
renal failure, 250
renal function, 245-246
renal insufficiency, 250
reproductive system
    diseases, disorders, and diagnostic terms of female,
        266-273
    diseases, disorders, and diagnostic terms of male,
        284-285
    external structures of female, 263
    female breasts, 280-281
    function of, 261-262
    internal structures of female, 264-266
    pregnancy and childbirth, 276-279
    sexually transmitted diseases, 286-288
    structures of female system, 262-266
    structures of male system, 282-284, 282f
    surgical and therapeutic interventions for females,
        273-275
    surgical and therapeutic interventions for males,
        285-286
resistance, of body to disease or disorder, 120
respiration, 191
respiratory rate, 79
respiratory system
    diseases, disorders, and diagnostic terms, 194-202
    function of, 191-211
    organs of respiration, 192f
    structures of, 192-194
    surgical and therapeutic interventions, 202-205
retina, 323
retinal detachment, 328, 329f
retinopathy, 328
retrograde urography, 251
rheumatoid arthritis (RA)
    hand deformity characteristic of, 154f
    overview of, 154
    treating, 158
rheumatoid spondylarthritis, 154
rhinoplasty, 205
rib cage
    bone structures in vertical axis of body, 135
    bones, 140f
    excision of (costectomy), 156
rotation, of joints, 146
routes of administration, drugs, 369

S

SA (sinoatrial) node, of heart, 178
sacral nerves, 322, 322f
sagittal plane, of body, 101
saliva, 220

salivary glands
    accessory organs of digestion, 219
    overview of, 220
    sialography, 221
salpingectomy, 275
salpingitis, 273
salpingocele, 273
salpingo-oophorectomy, 275
salpingorrhaphy, 275
sarcomas, 151
SARS (severe acute respiratory syndrome), 202
scabies, 308
schizophrenia, 329
scleroderma, 309
scleroprotein, 301
scoliosis
    compared with kyphosis, 153f
    as congenital defect, 153
scrotum, 282
sebaceous glands
    accessory skin structures, 302
    in integumentary system, 299
    overview of, 302
seborrhea, 309
seborrheic dermatitis, 309
seborrheic keratosis, 303, 303f
sebum, 302
secondary skin lesions, 305, 305f
secundipara, 277
semen, 283
semicircular canals, 324
semilunar (pulmonary) valves, of heart, 168, 169f
seminal vesicles, 283-284
semipermeable membranes, 53f
sense organs, 322-324
sensory (afferent) nerves, 317-318
sepsis, 310
septal defects, 173
septic wounds, 310
severe acute respiratory syndrome (SARS), 202
sexually transmitted diseases (STDs), 286-288, 287t-289t
shingles, 328
shock, 173
shock wave lithotripsy, 230f
shortened words, in abbreviations, 7
shortness of breath (SOB), signs of anemia, 118
shoulder presentation, of fetus, 278
shunts
    overview of, 331
    ventriculoperitoneal shunt, 330
sialography, 221
side effects, of drugs, 370
SIDS (sudden infant death syndrome), 202
sigmoidoscopy, 222
signs, in diagnosis, 78-79
silicosis, 202
simple fracture, 149, 149f

sinoatrial (SA) node, of heart, 178
sinuses, paranasal, 198f
size, prefixes related to, 57t
skeletal muscles
    major skeletal muscles of body, 148f
    as muscle type, 146, 147f
skin
    accessory structures, 302
    injuries, 306
    layers, 300-301, 300f
    lesions, 303-305, 303f
    as sense organ, 322
skin cancer, 309
skin grafts, 306
skin injuries
    overview of, 306
    treating, 310-311
skin lesions
    differentiation of types of, 303f
    overview of, 303-305
skull (cranium)
    bone structures in vertical axis of body, 135
    bony structures of head, 138f
    brain and spinal cord encased by, 321
    surgical interventions, 156
sleep apnea, 194
smooth (visceral or involuntary) muscles, 134, 146, 147f
SOB (shortness of breath), signs of anemia, 118
somatic cells, 98
somatic nervous system, 318
sonograms, 88
sonography
    of fetus, 88f
    types of diagnostic imaging, 86-88
Spanish
    pronunciation of medical terms, 374-377
    translation of medical terms, 378-380
specialties/specialists of medicine
    combining forms for, 16t
    suffixes related to, 14-17, 15t
specific/selective immunity
    of body to disease or disorder, 121
    types of, 122f
specimens, in diagnosis, 78-79
spelling, of medical terms, 2
sperm (spermatozoa)
    fertilization, 276
    in male reproductive system, 282
    overview of, 284
    production of, 261-262
spermatocidal, 284
spermatogenesis, 283
spermicides, 273-274
spina bifida, 153
spinal anesthesia, 157
spinal cavity, 106

spinal column
    bone structures in vertical axis of body, 135
    fractures, 327f
    lumbar puncture, 157, 157f
    osteoporosis changing curvature of spine, 152
    spinal anesthesia, 157
    types of vertebrae, 139f
spinal cord
    closed spinal cord injuries, 327f
    injuries, 149
    nerves of, 322f
spinal tap. See lumbar puncture
spirilla, 124
spirometry, 194, 195f
spleen, 182
splenectomy, 184
splenomegaly, 184
spondylarthritis, 154
spondylomalacia, 152
sprain, 150
stained blood, 118f
STDs (sexually transmitted diseases), 286-288, 287t-289t
stem cells, 100
stenosis
    of arteries, 173
    of renal artery, 246, 246f
stereotactic radiosurgery, 331
stereotaxis, 331f
sterilization, male and female, 273
stethoscope
    function of, 82
    measuring blood pressure, 81f
stomach
    diseases and disorders of, 226
    divisions of small intestine, 218f
    surgical interventions reducing capacity of, 229
stomatitis, 226
stones
    of gallbladder. See gallstone (biliary calculus)
    of kidneys. See kidney stones
strain, muscle, 150
streptococcal lymphangitis, 183f
stress injuries, 149-150
stress tests, of heart, 171
striated muscles, 147f
subcutaneous adipose tissue, 300
subcutaneous injections, 55
subdural hematoma, 324
sudden infant death syndrome (SIDS), 202
sudoriferous glands, 302
suffixes
    combining forms related to, 63-64, 63t-64t
    combining word parts to write terms, 6f
    common or important, 38, 38t-39t
    medical specialties and, 14-17, 15t
    overview of, 3-4
    surgical procedures, 25-26, 25t-26t

suffixes (Continued)
    in symptoms or diagnosis, 33, 33t-34t
    term building and, 5t
    treatment related, 91t
    using to write terms, 13-14
supination, 105f
supine position, 105f
suprapubic catheter, 252
surgery
    defined, 22-23
    suffixes related to, 25-26, 25t-26t
surgical and therapeutic interventions
    blood vessels, of cardiovascular system, 180-181
    digestive system, 229-231
    heart, 178-179
    integumentary system, 310-311
    musculoskeletal system, 155-158
    nervous system, 331-332
    reproductive system of female, 273-275
    reproductive system of male, 285-286
    respiratory system, 202-205
    urinary system, 252-255
susceptibility, of body to disease or disorder, 120
sweat glands
    as accessory skin structure, 302
    in integumentary system, 299
symptoms
    diagnosis and, 78-79
    suffixes related to, 33, 33t-34t
synovial joints
    articulation and, 146
    removing fluid from (arthrocentesis), 158
syphilitic chancre, 287f
systemic effects, of drugs, 369
systems, body. See body systems
systolic blood pressure, 80-81, 81f

T
tachypnea, 194, 195f
target organ, of hormones, 339
tarsoptosis, 153
taste buds, 322
TB (tuberculosis), 202
teeth, designation of permanent teeth of lower jaw, 217f
temperature, measuring body temperature, 79-80, 80f
tendinitis, 150
tendons
    association with bone, muscle, and cartilage, 134f
    inflammation of (tendinitis), 150
    role in attaching muscles to bones, 146
    sprains, 150
    surgical procedures, 157
tendoplasty, 157
tenomyoplasty, 157
TENS (transcutaneous electrical nerve stimulation), 332f
terms. See word terms/word building

testes
  function of, 261-262
  glands of endocrine system, 339
  in male reproductive system, 282
testicular torsion, 284, 285f
testosterone, 283
tests, diagnostic, 78-79, 83
tetraparesis, 149
tetraplegia, 149
thalamus, 321
therapeutic, 91
therapeutic interventions. *See also* surgical and therapeutic
    interventions
  overview of, 90-96
  word parts related to treatment, 91t
therapeutics, 369
therapists, 24
thermometers, for measuring body temperature, 79-80
thermoreceptors, 322
thoracentesis, 205, 205f
thoracic cavity, 106
thoracic nerves, 322, 322f
thoracocentesis (thoracentesis), 109
thorax, 108
thrombocytes (platelets), 116, 118
thrombocytopenia, 118
thrombolytic agents, 180
thrombosis, 118
thymus, 182
thyroid, 339, 343f
thyroidectomy, 347
thyrotoxicosis, 346
TIA (transient ischemic attack), 325
time, prefixes related to, 57t
tinnitus, 328
tissues
  abnormalities in development, 98-99
  in body organization, 98
  involved in burns, 307f
  major types of, 99f
  necrosis of, 308f
toenails, 111
toes, 157
tonsillectomy, 184
tonsillitis, 184
tonsils, 182
topical medication, for skin injuries, 310
torso (trunk)
  as body region, 107
  pelvis region of, 109
tracheostomy
  removing airway obstruction, 202-203
  tube for, 203f
tracheotomy, 202-203
traction, for treating fractures, 155-156
trade names, of drugs, 370
transabdominal, 279

transcutaneous electrical nerve stimulation (TENS), 332f
transdermal drug delivery, 56f, 310
transient ischemic attack (TIA), 325
transtracheal oxygen, 204
transurethral microwave thermotherapy (TUMT), 286
transurethral needle ablation (TUNA), 286
transurethral prostatectomy, 286
transurethral resection of prostate (TURP), 286
transurethral resection (TUR), 254
transverse plane, of body, 101f
trauma injuries
  musculoskeletal system, 149-150
  skin injuries, 306
treatment, word parts related to, 91t
triage, 23-24
trichosis, 309
tricuspid valve, of heart, 168, 169f
triglycerides, 174
trimesters, of pregnancy, 278
tripara, 277
tubal ligation, 275
tubercles, 202
tuberculosis (TB), 202
tubular reabsorption, 242, 243f
tubular secretion, 242, 243f
tubules, 242f
  of nephrons, 242
tumors. *See also* cancer
  benign vs. malignant, 21f
  of blood vessels, 174
  musculoskeletal system, 151
  pituitary, 347
  radiotherapy for, 90
TUMT (transurethral microwave thermotherapy), 286
TUNA (transurethral needle ablation), 286
TUR (transurethral resection), 254
TURP (transurethral resection of prostate), 286
tympanic thermometer, 80
Type 1 diabetes, 223, 347-348. *See also* diabetes mellitus
    (DM)
Type 2 diabetes, 223, 347-348. *See also* diabetes mellitus
    (DM)

U
UGI (upper gastrointestinal tract). *See* upper gastrointestinal
    tract (UGI)
ulcers, gastrointestinal, 226
ulcers, secondary skin lesions, 305, 305f
ultrasonography/ultrasound
  echocardiogram, 172
  of fetus, 88f
  obstetric uses of, 277
  types of diagnostic imaging, 86-88
ultraviolet therapy, 53f
umbilical hernias, 110, 110f
umbilicus/umbilical, 109-110
ungual, 302

unipara, 277
upper gastrointestinal tract (UGI)
   bleeding, 226, 227f
   endoscopy of, 222f
   overview of, 214
upper respiratory tract (URT), 193
urea, 239
ureteral, 241
ureteral catheterization, 252
ureteroplasty, 255
ureters, for kidneys, 240
urethra, 240
urethral, 241
urethral catheterization, 252
urethritis, 286
urinalysis (UA), 244
urinary, 240
urinary catheterization, 245, 252
urinary diversion, 253f
urinary incontinence, 251
urinary retention, 251
urinary system
   diseases, disorders, and diagnostic terms, 244-246
   function of, 238-239
   organs of, 240f
   structures of, 240-244
   surgical and therapeutic interventions, 252-255
urinary tract infection (UTI), 245, 251
urination, 238
urine
   clean-catch midstream technique for collecting,
      245
   process of forming/expelling, 242, 243f
   tests, 244, 244f
urinometer, 244f
urogram, intravenous, 249f
urologist, 239
urology, 239
URT (upper respiratory tract), 193
urticaria, 309
uterine cancer, 273
uterine cavity, 269f
uterus
   cancer of, 273
   internal reproductive structures of female, 264-266
   location of ovaries relative to, 266
   overview of, 264
UTI (urinary tract infection), 245, 251

V

vaccinations, 122, 204
vagina
   colposcopy of, 268f
   overview of, 264
vaginal, 264
vaginal speculum, 267f
vagotomy, 231

valves, of heart, 168, 169f
varicose veins, 178f
vasectomy, 286, 286f
vasoconstriction, of blood vessels, 174
vasodilation, of blood vessels, 174
vasodilators, 180
vasovasostomy, 286
VC (vital capacity), 194
veins
   blood vessels of heart, 170
   structures of cardiovascular system, 167
   surgical excision of, 180
   varicose, 178f
venae cavae
   inferior and superior, 168b
   structures of cardiovascular system, 167
venereal disease, 286
venous, 170
ventilation, 191
ventilators, 202-203
ventral cavity, 106, 106f
ventricle chamber, of heart, 168, 168f
ventricular heart defects, 172
ventriculoperitoneal shunt, 330
venules
   blood vessels of heart, 170
   structures of cardiovascular system, 167
verbs, combining suffixes with, 13
vertebral column. *See* spinal column
vertebroplasty, 156
vesicles, 303, 304f
viruses, 124
visceral or involuntary (smooth) muscles, 134, 146,
      147f
visceral pericardium, 168
vision, photoreceptors in, 322
vital capacity (VC), 194
vital signs, basic examination procedures, 79
voided specimens, 245
voiding, 238
voiding cystourethrogram, 251
vowels, combining, 3, 5
vulva, 263, 263f
vulvitis, 273

W

warfarin (Coumadin), 180
water component, body fluid, 111
WBC (white blood count), 118
weapons of mass destruction (WMD), 124
weight loss, treatments for, 229
wheals, 303, 305f
wheezing, 201
white blood cells (leukocytes), 116, 119
white blood count (WBC), 118
within normal limits (WNL), 79
WMD (weapons of mass destruction), 124

WNL (within normal limits), 79
word association, memorization techniques, 25
word parts
    accessory organs of digestion, 220t
    blood related, 116t
    body fluid related, 112t
    combining forms, 3
    combining to write terms, 5-6, 6f
    common or important, 40-41, 41t
    digestive system, 213t-215t
    endocrine system, 340t-341t
    female reproductive system, 262t
    integumentary system, 301t
    list of, 381-385
    list of word parts in English terms, 386-390
    male reproductive system, 283t
    in medical terminology, 1
    nervous system and psychologic, 320t
    obstetric terms, 277t
    prefixes. *See* prefixes
    radiology, 85t
    suffixes. *See* suffixes
    treatment related, 91t
    urinary system, 239t-240t
    word roots, 2-3
word roots, 2-3

word terms/word building
    abbreviations. *See* abbreviations
    combining word parts, 5-6, 6f
    list of word parts in English terms, 386-390
    plurals, 8, 9t
    prefixes. *See* prefixes
    proper names, 6
    rules for, 7t
    Spanish pronunciation of medical terms, 374-377
    suffixes. *See* suffixes
    using prefixes to write terms, 60-61
    word roots, 2-3
wounds. *See* skin injuries
writing medical terms, 2

X

xerosis, 309
x-rays. *See also* radiograph/radiography
    diagnostic use, 85-86, 86f
    of intestinal tract, 221
    positioning patient for chest x-ray, 105f
    radiopaque quality of bones and, 134
    therapeutic, 90

Z

zygote, 276